# Where to from Here?

## Keeping Medicare Sustainable

Stephen Duckett

Queen's Policy Studies Series
School of Policy Studies, Queen's University
McGill-Queen's University Press
Montreal & Kingston • London • Ithaca

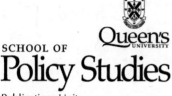

SCHOOL OF

# Policy Studies

Publications Unit
Robert Sutherland Hall
138 Union Street
Kingston, ON, Canada
K7L 3N6
www.queensu.ca/sps/

**Library and Archives Canada Cataloguing in Publication**

Duckett, S. J.
        Where to from here? : keeping medicare sustainable / Stephen Duckett.

(Queen's policy studies series)
Includes bibliographical references.
ISBN 978-1-55339-318-4

        1. Health care reform—Canada. 2. Medical care—Canada. 3. National health insurance—Canada. I. Queen's University (Kingston, Ont.). School of Policy Studies II. Title. III. Series: Queen's policy studies series

RA395.C3D83 2012          362.10971          C2012-900029-9

# Word cloud of proposals made in this book

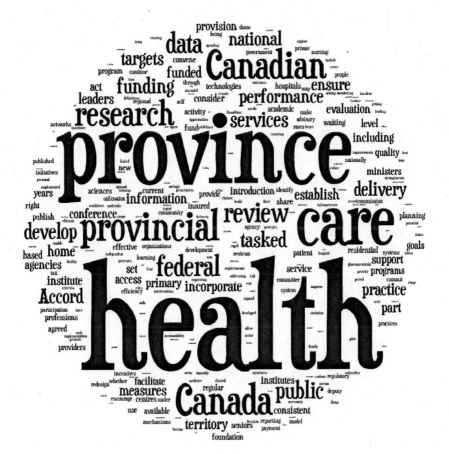

A word cloud provides a visual summary of a text: the size of the font reflects the different frequency of the words used in the chapter. The word clouds in this volume were generated using Tagul (www.tagul.com, retrieved 14 September 2011) and are used with permission.

# CONTENTS

# ACKNOWLEDGEMENTS

Although this is a single-authored book, that implies only that I take sole responsibility for its contents. I was helped in writing this book by both institutions and people. Having access to the online resources of the University of Alberta Library made it possible for me to hunt down references in an incredibly convenient way. Colleagues in my previous workplaces have helped to shape my thinking on many of the issues in this book over the years: former colleagues in Alberta Health Services, especially, have helped me translate Antipodean ideas into this colder climate.

A number of people commented on drafts: Irfan Dhalla, Annalise Kempton, Terri Jackson, Richard Lewanczuk, Steven Lewis, Joan McGregor, Anita Molzahn, Tom Noseworthy, Adrian Peetoom, Andrea Robertson, Heather Toporowski, Bill Trafford, Sharon Willcox, and an anonymous PhD student at Queen's University. The book has been immeasurably improved by their willingness to give of their time and advice, for which I thank them. They may not agree with how I incorporated their advice, of course. I still retain responsibility for errors of fact and ideology. The word clouds in this volume were generated using Tagul (www.tagul.com, retrieved 14 September 2011).

Finally, my family has been incredibly supportive. Thank you, Terri and Sarah, for everything.

# INTRODUCTION

Medicare's principles of universal, publicly funded access to health care are under challenge. Every few weeks commentators question the sustainability of Medicare, continuing what a *CMAJ* (2002) editorial referred to as "the national pastime." But why? What are the challenges to sustainability? And what changes to Medicare might be desirable while still consistent with the underlying principles of Medicare that have made it a Canadian icon and "a defining aspect of ... [Canadian] citizenship" (Commission on the Future of Health Care, 2002). The 2014 discussion on the refinancing of Medicare, the negotiation of how funds flow from the federal government to the provinces and territories (hereafter, provinces), represents another watershed moment for health care in Canada when these issues will come to the forefront of the policy agenda. But those negotiations, important as they are, should be seen as part of a continuous process of ensuring that health care in Canada is sustainable, equitable, and responsive to changing needs.

These are the issues tackled in this book.

It's a book about directions: *Where to from Here?* The subtitle, *Keeping Medicare Sustainable*, captures the thesis of this book that Medicare *is* sustainable, now and into the future. But historically, health care costs have risen faster than gross domestic product: health care is consuming a larger share of national income. This inevitably means that health costs come under careful scrutiny, and each incremental expenditure, especially expenditure from the public purse, is questioned. So sustainability is not a one-time decision—as if we could take some action and it's fixed. Sustainability is an ongoing quest. It requires an emphasis on value for money. Processes need to be established that evaluate changes in policy and new spending proposals fairly and in a way consistent with the values of Canadians.

Medicare's sustainability should, of course, be part of the policy agenda. There are other legitimate calls on public and private spending, and responding to every proposal for additional health spending is not in the best interest of anyone—and certainly not those of us who support universal, equitable access to health care. *Uncontrolled* spending is a challenge to Medicare. The more that health spending can be portrayed as a voracious monster, eating up public budgets or causing unpopular tax increases, the more Medicare's fundamental design principles of universal, publicly financed health care will be under challenge.

So this book takes as its premise that the sustainability agenda is critical to the future of Medicare. The issue then becomes, How do we ensure sustainability?

If Canada is to continue with a sustainable health system, actions need to be taken now. These are not actions that impinge on the core elements of Medicare. No need to introduce substantial private funding. No need to change the five *Canada Health Act* criteria for provincial compliance with Medicare arrangements in any major way. No need to undermine the trust that Canadians exhibit in their health system (Abelson, Miller, & Giacomini, 2009). No need to revisit the values shared by Canadians. There need be no access/quality/sustainability trade-off; all three are achievable. But the money currently spent on health care—and the inevitable increase in spending that will occur as the population and economy grow—must be invested wisely to achieve "social efficiency" (Bohm, 1987). Essentially, social efficiency occurs when the next dollar spent on any program yields the same level of additional benefit for the public as the next dollar spent on any other program. This also requires that each service funded under any program is operating efficiently, with no waste. Big asks, but critical to the sustainability agenda.

Efficiency should not be about mindless service cuts, penny pinching and cost-cutting. It's about managing better, to ensure services are run efficiently with no waste. It's about making wise investments in public health and primary care to reduce future demand elsewhere in the system. And this can be done.

This book draws on my experience in both Australia and Canada. In Australia I had a long history working in the public sector dealing with access, efficiency, and quality issues. As an academic and as a senior manager, I was a staunch defender of Australia's Medicare. In Canada, I was the inaugural president and chief executive officer of Alberta Health Services, now the largest health care provider in Canada, managing the merger of the predecessor entities and setting the policy framework for how the new organization would work.

This book draws heavily on that experience. Much of what is in this book is based on the directions we (my former colleagues and I) charted in Alberta Health Services and began implementing prior to my abrupt resignation. Where I propose in subsequent chapters that *Provinces should ...*, we had often already started that process in Alberta. This is a reality-based book, written with an eye to the achievable, what is politically feasible today. It does not propose a single policy "big bang" but rather makes a range of suggestions, adopting the path of multiple "opportunities for cumulative incremental change that could enhance the effectiveness, efficiency, and responsiveness" of health care in Canada (Hutchison, Abelson, & Lavis, 2001, p. 123) as the more productive way to achieve change. I write out of concern that if we do not address the continuing sustainability challenges, Medicare's fundamentals will be undermined.

## The politics of implementation

Designing an equitable, efficient, and high-quality health system is what Rittel and Webber (1973) would classify as a "wicked problem" as opposed to a tame one: there is no clear right answer, just solutions that are better or worse. There will be no time when the policy maker can sit back and say the problem has been solved and we have reached nirvana. There will be competing frames about how to describe the current issues, and framing will affect the viable solution-set. What's more, health system problems may be the result of issues created in the wider environment, and that environment is a contested, highly political terrain.

As Rudolf Virchow famously pointed out in 1848,

> Medicine is a social science, and politics is nothing else but medicine on a large scale. Medicine as a social science, as the science of human beings, has the obligation to point out problems and to attempt their theoretical solution: the politician, the practical anthropologist, must find the means and their actual solution. (cited in Sigerist, 1941, p. 93)

In this book I am trying to balance both sciences: pointing out problems but also attempting to find actual solutions. The health sector is rife with internal and external politics that shape and constrain our ability to find solutions. Policies are about resource allocation: what will be spent, on whom, by whom, and through whom. Distributional decisions will involve winners and losers, not only in monetary terms but also in terms of other aspects of utility. In health care this might include changes in autonomy or status.

The health sector in Canada consumes about 10 percent of gross domestic product; that is, ten cents of every dollar spent in Canada is spent on people who work in the health sector or on goods and services used in the health sector. The health sector is one of the country's largest industries, and employees in the health sector represent a significant proportion of the total workforce[1] and of voters. This in turn means that political aspects of health sector decision making must take into account the impact of the decision not only on health sector goals (access, quality, sustainability) but also on employment and stakeholder interests. The health sector creates employment and opportunities for businesses, and confers status and prestige on medical and other leaders—all of which may impinge on decision making.

However, stakeholders' interests are not necessarily coincident with health sector goals, no matter how they might masquerade. Health care politics in Canada has been characterized as reflecting a historical accommodation between the medical profession and the state (Tuohy, 1999). This accommodation is made most visible in the negotiated agreements in each province between the medical profession and the provincial government about setting physician fees.[2] These agreements are not neutral in their effect: they incorporate implicit and explicit policies about fee relativities and hence what total income a physician working in a particular specialty can expect. This inevitably involves decisions about which specialties—including family practice—are to be privileged and which not. By recognizing and putting a price on new procedures, the agreements encourage or discourage their adoption.

To move toward health system reform in Canada, it will be necessary to recognize the power and position of these agreements. Yet we must also open up these agreements to greater scrutiny, and ensure that the incentives, culture, and values enshrined in the agreements are consistent with the policy directions required to meet changing health system needs.

For better or for worse, implementation has to recognize the reality of the position of stakeholders in the Canadian health care system, and change will sometimes require political courage. The history of Medicare in Canada is not one without conflict: the introduction of Medicare in Saskatchewan was preceded by a doctors' strike (Taylor, 1978), and strikes and strife accompanied Medicare's implementation in Quebec and the abolition of extra-billing in the 1980s (Boychuk, 2008a; Heiber & Deber, 1987; Taylor, 1978). So tough decisions have been made in the past and potentially might be made in the future.

## Pursuing all three goals: Access, quality, and sustainability

I write this book as an economist: one who sees economics as being about the *equitable* distribution of resources. This orientation means I place a high value on value for money: eliminating waste, prioritizing services that prevent illness or involve early intervention, and prioritizing low-technology interventions. The more we emphasize value for money, the more we can eke out publicly allocated funds to ensure services are available for all when they are needed, without having to (re)introduce financial barriers to access.

Too often I hear that the three goals of access, quality, and sustainability are not simultaneously achievable: "pick any two" is proposed as the only reality. But the "pick any two" compromise is a failure of leadership and management. As I will demonstrate in this book, there are a host of reforms that can and should be made in the health system that enhance sustainability, while simultaneously improving access and quality.[3]

Service change in the health sector is not easy: it often involves disruption of the existing order, new tasks to undertake, changes to roles, changes to established routines, changes to employment locations. Although it is possible to win stakeholder support for that change, it is always a challenge to embed change with no backsliding.

Health sector change does not simply involve one decision to implement policy X. Policy X almost inevitably involves a myriad of implementation steps, each engaging different decision makers, until the real experience of front-line workers and health consumers/patients changes. American political scientist Aaron Wildavsky hypothesized that the multiple steps involved in large-scale implementation processes almost guaranteed that the final policy as implemented would look little like the original conception. He summarized the disconnect (between the original decision and the working out on the ground) in the lengthy subtitle to his book on implementation: "How great expectations in Washington are dashed in Oakland or, why it's amazing that federal programs work at all, this being a saga of the Economic Development Administration as told by two sympathetic observers who seek to build morals on a foundation of ruined hopes" (Pressman & Wildavsky, 1973).

So is the quest for value for money in the health sector a vain one? Will stakeholder interests, long decision paths, organizational inertia, and poor leadership conspire to maintain a status quo that is comfortable for the insiders but shifts costs of addressing future challenges unnecessarily onto taxpayers or those who will miss out on care? I'm an optimist and think not. It is possible to build coalitions inside and outside the health sector to argue for necessary change.

Change is more likely if a clear case for change can be made, and here information helps. United States' Supreme Court Justice Louis Brandeis (1914, p. 92) argued, "Publicity is justly commended as a remedy for social and industrial diseases. Sunlight is said to be the best of disinfectants; electric light the most efficient policeman."

Data about disparities, inefficiencies, variation in practice patterns, and different processes, outputs, and outcomes by province will help arm those seeking change (whether they be inside or outside the health sector) and highlight areas where action is necessary. The Health Council of Canada's (2009b) *Value for Money* report is a good start in this regard.

In addition to good information, new structures and expectations need to be put in place or strengthened. Identifying the need for change, arguing for it, and implementing it is the clear responsibility of health service leaders, leaders of the health professions and health academics, together with political leaders. I have found in my career that being part of making the health system better can be very exciting and is a great motivator.

Canada's health system has not adapted well to changing needs. As I will show later in this book, much needs to be done to better position the health system to respond to the increase in chronic diseases, for example. To some extent this need for improvement reflects poorly on all of us who have exercised leadership roles in the health sector, and presents a challenge for those who still do so.

The prescriptions in this book have a rationalist orientation. As I said earlier, I'm an economist and an emphasis on rational decision making is part of that territory. In my view a key role for health service leaders is to argue the case for a (more) rational allocation of resources and the right priorities, with value for money as an important criterion. Placating political interests, while creating short-term comfort and often personal financial and career advancement, should not be the *sine qua non* of those leadership roles, much as it might appear that this is the current practice.

The media has a role to play, too. Even the quality broadsheet media too often falls into the tabloid trap of chasing scandals (assuming that all management decisions are wrong and all managers are venal), trumpeting (unevaluated) new technologies, or dwelling on the self-serving in the interest of conflict and a good story. Part of the role of health academics should be to support journalists to be more evaluative in their stories.[4]

So my thesis is that it is possible to strengthen rational decision-making in the health sector: information, new structures, and good leadership will help with stakeholder engagement to make progress on all three goals of access, quality, and sustainability. I agree with Sullivan and Baranek (2002, p. 92) that "what is required is action to create informed public discussion and propel political leadership."

## Organization of this book

The first chapters of the book set the scene: Chapter 1 discusses the *Canada Health Act*, the 2004 Accord, and current provincial funding of health care. Chapter 2 addresses the sustainability discourse and makes the case that Medicare is sustainable. The next chapters outline some of the needed actions in public health and health promotion (Chapter 3), in health care delivery including primary care (Chapter 4), with new drugs and technologies (Chapter 5), for seniors and long-term care (Chapter 6), and in hospitals and acute care (Chapter 7). The final three chapters address the workforce reform agenda (Chapter 8), alternative paths (Chapter 9), and the steps necessary to move forward (Chapter 10).

Specific recommendations for reform are proposed throughout the book and listed in the Appendix. Many of these are proposed for consideration in the context of the negotiation of the 2014 Accord. But given the decentralized nature of health care in Canada, not all of these recommendations are directed at the federal government, and many are independent of the Accord itself. Many are directed at provinces and regions, and implementation of these recommendations need not wait until 2014.

# Word cloud: Medicare and its context

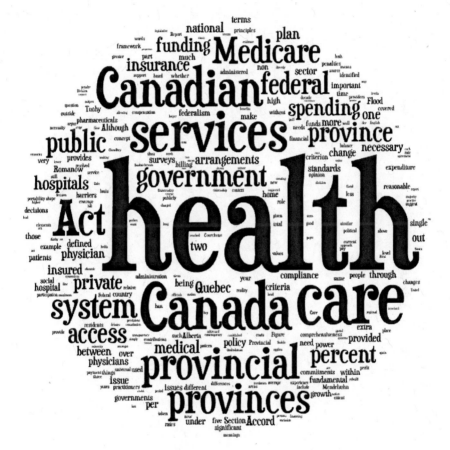

# CHAPTER 1

# MEDICARE AND ITS CONTEXT

The Medicare we know is underpinned by three governmental regulatory and financial factors: the *Canada Health Act* that defines what Medicare is, the 2004 Accord that defines expectations and the flow of taxpayers' funds from the federal government to provinces, and decisions of the provincial governments about the funding and shape of services. These government decisions are constrained by the constitutional division of powers and take place within the larger value framework and professional collegiality that characterize Canadian health policy (Courchene, 2003; Tuohy, 1999).

Medicare has come to mean more to Canadians than a financing system for health care; it is no longer simply about how government funding assures them access to care. Rather, as the Romanow Report of 2002 highlighted, it's about values, and about how Canadians relate to and care about each other (Commission on the Future of Health Care, 2002). Glouberman and Zimmerman (2002, 2004) suggest that "Medicare is a symbolic replacement for railroads as that which holds the country together ... and an indication of Canadian social generosity" (2004, p. 24).[5]

Medicare signals in a very real sense a different approach to health care and community from that adopted by the larger neighbour to the south. Medicare thus has a very special place in Canadian politics, to be preserved.

## The *Canada Health Act*

The *Canada Health Act* is the current legislative description of Canada's national health financing system, Medicare. Health insurance in Canada traces its antecedents to Saskatchewan's innovations in the 1940s for hospital insurance and the 1950s for medical insurance (Taylor, 1978), which led to the national commitments in the 1950s for hospitals (*Hospital Insurance and Diagnostic Services Act, 1957*) and in the 1960s for medical care *(Medical Care Act, 1966)*. In turn, the framework set by these original pieces of legislation continues today. The *Medical Care Act, 1966* for example, provides that provincial insurance arrangements must be comprehensive (s. 2(e)), publicly administered, portable to cover those "temporarily absent" from the province, and universal. Universal benefits are defined as covering, after a phasing-in period, at least 95 percent of residents of the province (s. 4(1)).[6]

The original funding arrangements involved cost-sharing between the federal government and the provinces. These arrangements were replaced in the 1970s by defined grants and "tax room"; the federal government reduced its tax rates to allow provinces to increase theirs with no additional impact on consumers, and the provinces gained more control of funding (*Federal-Provincial Fiscal Arrangements and Established Programs Financing Act, 1977*).

The latest iteration for the legislative framework is the *Canada Health Act, 1984*, which among other things addressed issues relating to "extra-billing," where medical practitioners charged above the provincial fee schedule, thus creating access barriers to medical care (Stevenson, Williams, & Vayda, 1988; Tuohy, 1988).

For something so important to Canadians, the legislative framework is surprisingly short (the English version has around 4,000 words), articulating broad principles of scope and governance, and how funds will flow. The relative brevity is in part a reflection of Canadian federalism. The Canadian Constitution vests the provinces with exclusive power over hospitals, with the place of "health" somewhat vague: provinces have power within a province but the national Parliament can make laws about health when the issue is national (Braën, 2002, 2004; Gibson, 1996; Leeson, 2002, 2004). The language of a Supreme Court decision of the late 1930s about unemployment insurance suggests that the federal Parliament does not have power to make laws about health insurance (Choudhry, 2000). The *Canada Health Act* is not made under any assumed "health" power, but under the spending power. It is an Act about principles that apply across the whole country: the details and implementation are left to the provinces to flesh out.

The *Canada Health Act* articulates the broad "primary objective of Canadian health care policy" as being

> to protect, promote and restore the physical and mental well-being of residents of Canada and to facilitate *reasonable access* to health services without financial or other barriers. (s. 3, emphasis added)

Consistent with its place as a "spending" Act, the provisions of the Act itself are more mundane. Essentially the Act provides for two things:

1. The federal government will make available a "Canada Health and Social Transfer" to the provinces (the health part of which was worth $27 billion nationally in 2011/12).
2. If provinces want their share, they must establish a complying program for "insured health services and extended health care services" (*Canada Health Act*, s. 4).

"Insured health services" are defined to include hospital and physician services, the former defined broadly to include both inpatient (accommodation, medical and nursing services, and pharmaceuticals) and outpatient services. "Extended health care services" are defined in the Act to include nursing home, home care, and adult residential and ambulatory health care services "as more particularly defined in the regulations," but no such regulations have been promulgated.

Medicare, in common with other welfare state provisions, has a redistributive ("Robin Hood") function, combating social exclusion so people who are less well-off can get access to necessary care, but it also has benefits for everyone by allowing equalization of payments over the life cycle (a "piggy bank" function). The latter function recognizes that contributions (via tax or mandated premiums) are equalized over a person's life, but health needs are typically greatest after the person retires and has less income to pay for any care needs (Arrow, 1963; Barr, 2001).

For Canadians, what Medicare means is access to hospitals and physicians, for services they need, without any upfront payment. Although there are no financial barriers to access, Canadians wait for care: for elective procedures and in emergency departments. Many Canadians do not have a regular family physician. And, as Chief Justice Beverley McLachlin noted, "access to a waiting list is not access to health care" (*Chaoulli v. Quebec*, 2005).

## *The five* Canada Health Act *criteria*

As well as defining access to what kinds of services, the *Canada Health Act* (s. 7) specifies five key criteria[7] for "complying" provincial health insurance arrangements:

- public administration
- comprehensiveness
- universality
- portability
- accessibility

Although simply stated, each of the criteria is somewhat contentious.

### Public administration

The public administration criterion relates solely to the administration of the health insurance plan, the two critical elements being that:

1. the health care insurance plan of a province must be administered and operated on a non-profit basis by a public authority appointed or designated by the government of the province; and

2.  the public authority must be responsible to the provincial government for that administration and operation (s. 8).

Nothing is currently included in the *Canada Health Act* about hospitals or other services being publicly administered—the Act only specifies that the insurer is to be public—and it is important to recognize that most physician services in Canada are provided by physicians working privately.[8]

Privatization of services in Canada is hotly debated. Opponents argue that privatization is inconsistent with both the principles of Medicare and the *Canada Health Act* (Church & Smith, 2006; Whiteside, 2009). The issue was considered by two recent reports on the Canadian health care system: the Kirby Report (Senate, 2002a) and the Romanow Report (Commission on the Future of Health Care, 2002). The two reports reached different conclusions and identified different value bases for Medicare and its evolution (Courchene, 2003).

Romanow consulted extensively with the public before framing his report and commissioned a synthesis of previous published opinion polls on health care (Mendelsohn, 2002). Romanow's starting value proposition, informed by the consultation process, was that "Canadians view Medicare as a moral enterprise, not a business venture," and he went on to argue for a limit on private provision:

> One of the most difficult issues with which I have had to struggle is how much private participation within our universal, single-payer, publicly administered system is warranted or defensible. On the one hand, I am confronted by the fact that the private sector is already an important part of our "public" system. The notion of rolling back its participation is fraught with difficulty. On the other hand, I am acutely aware of the potential risks to the integrity and viability of our health care system that might result from an expanded role for private providers. At a minimum, I believe governments must draw a clear line between direct health services (such as hospital and medical care) and ancillary ones (such as food preparation or maintenance services). The former should be delivered primarily through our public, not-for-profit system, while the latter could be the domain of private providers. (Commission on the Future of Health Care, 2002, p. xxi)

In contrast, Kirby was "agnostic about whether health service providers are government-owned, not-for-profit or for-profit enterprises" (Courchene, 2003, p. 4). This issue is discussed further in Chapter 9.

### Comprehensiveness

To meet the comprehensiveness criterion, "the health care insurance plan of a province must insure all insured health services provided by hospitals, medical practitioners or dentists" (s. 9).[9] Forget (2002) labels this criterion as "historically narrow, non-existent today and foolish for tomorrow" and argues that it should be deleted:

> The importance of renouncing "comprehensiveness" as a principle derives from the realization that to do otherwise is to deny a fundamental reality: the Canadian health care system is not now, never has been and should not even attempt to be all-encompassing. To retain the pretence of "comprehensiveness" is to irresponsibly refuse to adjust citizens' expectations to the reality of government commitments. (p. 19)

The comprehensiveness of Medicare is already constrained in two important ways. First, Medicare privileges hospital and physician services (to use Hutchison, Abelson, and Lavis's [2001] terms) in that it applies only to those services, leaving other important aspects of health care (such as access to pharmaceuticals outside hospitals) uncovered, subject to significant provincial variation, and weakening needs-based resource allocation (Birch & Gafni, 2005). The Organisation for Economic Co-operation and Development (OECD), in its 2010 survey of the Canadian economy, also highlighted this issue:

> All non-hospital and non-physician services–including pharmaceuticals, long-term/home care and therapeutic services–are outside Medicare. Despite provincial public safety nets and employer-provided private insurance for such services, gaps in coverage are frequent and out-of-pocket costs can be high. With sector-segmented finance, non-congruent incentives along the continuum of care may impede an optimal division of labour for a given patient and prevent efficient service integration for any given episode of illness. (2010a, p. 107)

A second constraint is that only "necessary services"[10] are encompassed within the ambit of insured services. "Necessary" is not defined but implies a dichotomy: services are either necessary or not. This is easier to determine for some services than others, cosmetic surgery being the classic example, but provincial exclusions also include reproductive health services and some counselling services (Tuohy, 2009). The dichotomous decision is not the reality of every day clinical practice (Glassman, Model, Kahan, Jacobson, & Peabody, 1997). Different players in the health system will have different perspectives on what is necessary and what is not (Rosenbaum, Frankford, & Moore, 1999), and as discussed in Chapter 7, the evidence about indications for interventions is sometimes uncertain (Wennberg, 2010). Little wonder that Griener (2002) referred to the "beguiling simplicity" of the term, and Glassman et al. (1997) labelled it "ambiguous." Caulfield (1996, p. 84) suggested that the term will "consistently defy a single concrete definition" and questioned the utility of trying to define it.

But decisions still need to be taken every day about what is in and what is out; what is deemed necessary and what is not. These decisions are taken at a range of levels in the system (federal, provincial, regional health authorities, delivery agencies—hospitals, home health care agencies, etc.—municipalities, individual practitioners, and individual patients) with varying degrees of transparency (Nauenberg, Flood, & Coyte, 2005). Decision makers' values are often not explicit and may or may not coincide with those of the broader population (Flood & Erdman, 2004; Flood, Tuohy, & Stabile, 2006).

Charles, Lomas, and Giacomini (1997) have argued,

> The concept of medical necessity has taken on different meanings over time, depending on the perceived policy needs of the day. During the decade following the introduction of universal medical care, the concept slept quietly, like Rip Van Winkle, embedded comfortably in legislation and attracting little policy attention. In the mid-1980s, policy makers "discovered" medical necessity, woke it from a long sleep, and capitalized on its malleability to attach different meanings to the concept in pursuit of their own policy agendas. The result is confusion over the array of meanings and how these are used in current health policy debates. The meaning of medical necessity is not intrinsic to it but, rather, depends on how people interpret and use the concept. (pp. 385-386)

In their very comprehensive review, Charles et al. suggest that the initial meaning (what physicians and hospitals do), provided a "federal floor" in terms of what was to be covered, and this narrowed over time to become "the maximum we can afford," a provincial ceiling. More contemporary meanings move into whether only cost-effective services are in scope (Flood, Stabile, & Tuohy, 2008a), an issue addressed in Chapter 10. Today the concept of "medical necessity" is used to justify restricting access to some services through "delisting" processes, which have ambiguous impacts on equitable access (Stabile & Ward, 2005).

### Universality

Universality is the heart of Medicare: a single payer covers everyone in a single system. In the words of the Act: "The health care insurance plan of a province must entitle one hundred per cent of the insured persons of the province to the insured health services provided for by the plan on uniform terms and conditions" (s. 10).

Universality is the defining difference between Canada's health system and that of the United States. Even post the Obama reforms, not all people in the United States will be covered for health care. Although Cacace and Schmid (2008) have identified a number of variables where the health systems of the two countries are converging, "single-payer" remains one of the "boo words" of American health care politics.

Although universality, per se, is not under challenge, there are many proposals to augment public funding with private health insurance for services covered under Medicare, effectively creating a dual track system of access, an anathema to both Kirby and Romanow.

Portability

The portability criterion of the *Canada Health Act* has two main elements:

1. The waiting period for new residents is limited to a maximum of three months.
2. The province's plan covers care received outside the province (s. 11).

Where care is received in Canada, the service is covered at the rate determined by the province for intraprovincial services. This becomes contentious when payment rates of one province diverge substantially from others, or when a province wants to restrict outflow of services in border regions for fiscal reasons (Cohen, 1993). Quebec imposes a maximum daily rate for reimbursement of non-urgent services.

Similar arrangements apply for physician services. In most cases, the physician simply bills the provincial plan and is reimbursed by it. Quebec again provides an exception. Apart from special arrangements applying in border areas, care for Quebec residents is paid at the lower of what is actually charged and what would have been paid in Quebec. In many cases Quebec residents need to pay for care directly and are subsequently reimbursed in line with these rules.

The portability criterion also applies to care received outside Canada, on the same basis as care in other provinces. In countries with health care systems similar to Canada's, this effectively means that Canadians can get care in emergencies in hospitals without any payment (e.g., the case for Canadians taken in an emergency to public hospitals in Australia). But the obligation under the *Canada Health Act* is to pay only at the same rate as applies within the province. This potentially leaves Canadians obtaining care in other countries, for instance the United States, with very significant out-of-pocket costs. Each province has established arrangements to pre-authorize care that receives a higher level of reimbursement, but these arrangements vary across the country, are often slow, and have little transparency in terms of decision making (Alberta Ombudsman, 2009; Ombudsman Ontario, 2007; Ombudsman Saskatchewan, 2010).

Accessibility

Finally, the accessibility criterion has two critical elements. The province must provide for

1. insured health services ... on a basis that does not impede or preclude, either directly or indirectly whether by charges made to insured persons or otherwise, reasonable access to those services by insured persons (s. 12 (1)(a)); and

2. reasonable compensation for all insured health services rendered by medical practitioners or dentists (s. 12 (1)(c)).

Both elements incorporate a test of "reasonableness": reasonable access for patients and reasonable compensation for providers. The *Canada Health Act* provides that federal funds to the province will be reduced to the extent that extra-billing occurs, effecting a "ban" on extra-billing. The provision of reasonable compensation to medical practitioners means that compensation above the negotiated tariff or fee schedule[11] can be labelled unreasonable, providing a justification for the ban. The ban on extra-billing was controversial from the start (Heiber & Deber, 1987; Stevenson, Williams, & Vayda, 1988; Tuohy, 1988) and initially subject to imperfect oversight (Choudhry, 2000), but is now part of what Canadians expect of Medicare (Mendelsohn, 2002). This expectation was expressed forcefully by then federal Health Minister Marleau: "Canadians do not want cash-register medicine—with or without an express line" (cited in Jackman, 1994, p. 54).

The provinces have set differing provincial rules about physician participation in their insurance plans (Flood & Archibald, 2001). This provides an opportunity for de facto circumvention of the "ban." The ban on extra-billing means that a physician (or dental surgeon) cannot charge an extra moiety to patients over and above what is paid by the provincial plan. But, physicians have a choice about their participation in the plan. In most provinces physicians have to elect to be all-in or all-out: If they accept any patients under the province's plan, then they cannot separately bill any patients for insured services; if they want to bill any patients directly, they have to bill all their patients. This works for physicians who practice solely in cosmetic surgery, for example.[12] In a few provinces, however, physicians can opt to participate in both modes: for some of their work they are in, and for some out (Sullivan & Baranek, 2002). But under this option, when the physician is working outside the plan, the patient must pay the full cost and there is no subsidy from the plan (Boychuk, 2008b; Flood & Archibald, 2001). Importantly, hidden subsidies exist under these arrangements in that complications of private care that lead to a subsequent hospital admission or treatment are publicly funded.

In addition to the mandatory penalty to be applied in provinces where extra-billing occurs, the *Canada Health Act* provides for discretionary penalties (effected through reduced transfer payments) where any of the other criteria are breached. Imposition of any penalty is a political act, which mitigates the effectiveness of the penalty provisions. Between March 2008 and March 2010, for example, a total of $140,120 was deducted from grants to the provinces as penalties (Health Canada, 2008a, 2010). Health Canada (2010) describes its compliance strategy as one where penalties are a last resort:

> Health Canada's approach to resolving possible compliance issues emphasizes transparency, consultation and dialogue with provincial and territorial health ministry officials. In most instances, issues are successfully resolved through

consultation and discussion based on a thorough examination of the facts. To date, most disputes and issues related to administering and interpreting the *Canada Health Act* have been addressed and resolved without resorting to deductions. Deductions have only been applied when all options to resolve an issue have been exhausted.... In instances where a *Canada Health Act* issue has been identified and remains after initial enquiries, Division officials ask the jurisdiction in question to investigate the matter and report back. Division staff discuss the issue and its possible resolution with provincial/territorial officials. Only if the issue is not resolved to the satisfaction of the Division after following the aforementioned steps, is it brought to the attention of the federal Minister of Health.

Choudhry (2000, p. 48) provides a much less sanguine assessment, referring to "a yawning gap" between the rhetoric and the reality of federal government enforcement of the *Canada Health Act*:

> The truth is that the federal government is largely unaware of the degree of provincial compliance with the *Canada Health Act* and, in suspected cases of provincial non-compliance, has followed the traditional norms of intergovernmental relations in Canada, shrouding its interactions with provincial governments in secrecy.

The Auditor General of Canada has also criticized Health Canada's compliance-monitoring approach, noting the time it takes for compliance issues to be resolved and the very low level of penalties imposed (Office of the Auditor General of Canada, 2002).

Financial penalties are, of course, not the only way to enforce compliance: given the very high levels of public commitment to the principles of the *Canada Health Act*, there are high local political costs for breaches. This public vigilance is clearly an important compliance-monitoring mechanism, which increases reputational costs of a province planning or condoning breaches.

Taken together, the five *Canada Health Act* criteria lead to policies that eliminate financial barriers at point of service for insured services (physicians, hospitals). But Medicare does not ensure equity of access. After standardizing for "need" (as measured by self-reported health status), compared with people living in the poorest 20 percent of households, people living in the wealthiest 20 percent of households have 40 percent more family physician visits, 65 percent more specialist visits, but 26 percent fewer hospital admissions (Allin, 2006); Curtis and MacMinn (2008) have also shown lower utilization of specialty services by poorer people. There are also significant differences in utilization rates between the provinces, driven primarily by differences in income and education (Allin, 2008).

The five *Canada Health Act* criteria are writ large in any discussion of health policy in Canada. Marmor, Okma, and Latham (2002, 2010) argue that these criteria have now attained the status of "values," albeit instrumental values, noting parenthetically that "it is no coincidence that nearly every contemporary report that calls for Medicare reform feels compelled to do so by alleging the consistency of their proposed reforms with the five criteria" (Marmor et al., 2002, p. 19).

## The 2004 Accord

The federal-provincial Medicare arrangements are subject to periodic re-negotiation, most recently in 2004, leading to a First Ministers' Accord on Health Care Renewal and the associated *10-Year Plan to Strengthen Health Care* (Health Canada, 2004). As political documents, they are of course full of high-sounding rhetoric, fine phrases, and commitments to good intentions (Edelman, 1988; Watson, 2003, 2004). Although Kent (2004) argues the commitments are more definite than previous agreements, they are still circumscribed, with adjectives carefully chosen to limit obligations, and words used to create ambiguity and the "veil of vagueness" often necessary to reach superficial agreement in public negotiations (Gibson & Goodin, 1999). This vagueness is exemplified in home care where the commitments do not specify "which services will be covered, by what time and for whom" (Motiwala, Flood, Coyte, & Laporte, 2005, p. 8).

The Accord was fashioned within the context of the contemporary realities of Canadian power-separating (rather than power-sharing) federalism (Jordan, 2009). Although as Banting (2005, p. 37) notes, "for the vast majority of Canadians, debates about federal-provincial fiscal arrangements have a highly soporific quality," the outcomes of federal-provincial negotiations shape Canadians' access to key health care services.

Federalism discussions raise the key question: Is the Canadian health system, well, "Canadian"? Or is it, as Detsky and Naylor (2003, p. 804) describe, "a collection of plans administered by the ten provinces and three territories" or Di Matteo's (2009, p. 32) "set of centralized provincial systems"? Boychuk (2008a) has highlighted the importance of provincial experimentation and provincial politics and the place of Quebec in the Canadian federation in shaping the evolution of Medicare.

As Banting (2005) puts the alternatives,

> The promise of social citizenship is the equal treatment of all citizens of the country. The promise of federalism is regional diversity in public policies, reflecting the preferences of regional communities and cultures. Stripped to its core, the logic of social citizenship holds that a sick baby should be entitled to public health care on the same terms and conditions wherever he or she lives in the country. Stripped to its core, the logic of federalism holds that the public health benefits to which a sick baby is entitled also depend significantly on the region in which he or she resides. Establishing a balance between these two logics is a central task in federal welfare states. (p. 39)

There are advocates for the polar extremes of social citizenship and federalism, and so policy debates are often aimed at shifting the balance in one or other direction. At present the way federalism plays out in the health care system leads to a middle position, with some Canadian standards (e.g., the *Canada Health Act* criteria) while allowing considerable provincial autonomy. Attitudes toward a greater federal government role versus greater provincial autonomy partly reflect views of the role of government (those who see a smaller role for government generally argue for a smaller role for the federal government). Generally, Liberals argue for a broader federal scope, and Conservatives for a narrower one (Bickerton, 2010; Mahon, 2008). Also influencing views about stronger versus weaker federal roles are views about the nature of the Canadian federation and whether "the division of powers represents a pact between the majority and minority nations comprising Canada" (Graefe & Bourns, 2009, p. 190). This is particularly relevant to Quebec:

> The notion of a national consensus and national standards, furthermore, implies the presence of only one nation. This has been disconcerting to the government of Quebec, which finds the notion of national standards doubly offensive. First, in political practice, *national* standards mean *federal* standards in areas of *provincial jurisdiction.* This, of course, is contrary to the federal principle, at least as understood by the government of Quebec. Second, national standards are interpreted in Quebec as the standards of the *English Canadian nation.* They are viewed as an imposition by the majority upon a minority nation. (Telford, 2003, p. 36)

Because the provinces are not equally wealthy (so-called horizontal fiscal imbalance[13]), interprovincial funds transfers, effected by the federal government, are used to support achievement of these minimum national standards everywhere in Canada. Transfers are increasingly contentious (Courchene, 2010), with Sears (2010, p. 26) colourfully describing the process as "Ottawa *merely laundering* the billions as they pass through (from the richest provinces) to Quebec and the Atlantic provinces" (emphasis added).

Federal governments have an array of instruments to influence policy including increasing funding (either generally to the field or in a targeted way), providing expertise, and holding to account (Boismenu & Graefe, 2004). All were used in the 2004 Accord, with new money predominating. Kent (2004) describes the outcome as "sugar daddy federalism." While the Accord is mostly rhetoric, it reflected important progress on funding. An identified pool of funds, specific to health care (the Canada Health Transfer), was established to flow from the federal government to the provinces for the period 2004–2014 (McIntosh, 2004). A new quantum of funding was determined with a new basis for escalation (currently 6 percent per annum). In terms of accountability, national wait-time goals were established, with agreement from provinces to identify priority areas for improvement and publish progress. Funds flowed to assist provinces to achieve the waiting-time commitments. Expertise was provided through a "Federal Adviser on Wait Times."

The duration of the funding agreement has given stability for a decade, allowing provinces to plan with relative certainty on a revenue source that accounts for about 20–25 percent of average provincial health spending.

### Provincial government funding

The *Canada Health Act* and the 2004 Accord provide a context, but only a context, for provincial decisions about how much to spend on health care, and relative priorities for that spending in terms of sector (hospitals, aged care) and location (rural, urban). It is those provincial priority choices (now and in the past) that shape Canadians' experience of the health care system. The Canadian Institute for Health Information (2010b) projected that almost two thirds (65.3 percent) of all health spending in Canada in 2010 would be through provincial governments, 29.5 percent from private sources (whether out-of-pocket or through insurance arrangements), and the balance (5.3 percent) from other government sources. Of the total private sector funding, 34 percent is spent on medications, 23 percent on dental services, and 18 percent on hospitals and other institutions (e.g., single room supplements).

The provinces vary significantly in how much they spend on health care, and in their public-private balance and rates of growth. Figure 1.1 shows comparisons in levels of spending across the provinces and territories. Territorial spending stands out as distinct from the pattern among the provinces. But there is significant variation in spending per capita among the provinces, after adjusting for the age and sex composition of the provincial population, from a high in Alberta, at $6,864 per head in 2010, to a low of $4,966 in Quebec, less than three quarters of the Alberta spend (Canadian average $5,614 per head). Provincial government expenditure follows a similar pattern (Alberta the highest at $4,704 per head, Quebec the lowest at $3,255).

The contribution of the private sector also varies across the provinces. Private sector contributions in Ontario make up one third of total health spending, compared with less than one quarter of total health spending in Newfoundland and Labrador, Saskatchewan, and Manitoba (22 percent, 23 percent, and 24 percent respectively; CIHIb, 2010). As would be expected because of the distinct roles for public and private sector funding in Canada, there is no evidence here to suggest that lower spending by provincial governments is offset by higher private sector contributions.

Depending on relative efficiency across the provinces, and the nature of provincial investments, prima facie one would expect that the variation in levels of spending would lead to differences in access or quality. However, a recent analysis of Alberta's comparatively high spending found no commensurate benefit in terms of outcomes (Duckett, Kramer, & Sarnecki, 2012).

## FIGURE 1.1
## Per capita health expenditure (age-sex adjusted) by province/territory, by source of funds, 2010

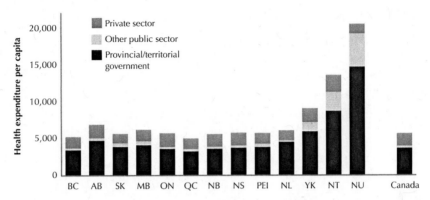

Source: Author's analysis based on the Canadian Institute for Health Information (2010b), *National Health Expenditure Trends*. Age-sex adjustment calculated by applying 2008 provincial government health spending adjustment (CIHI, 2010b, Table 6) to total 2010 expenditure.

Provincial governments make annual decisions as part of their budget processes about their health spending. Figure 1.2 shows the pattern of spending growth by province over the last three decades.

The pattern was for extremely high rates of spending growth in the 1970s (Canadian average above 10 percent in each year 1976–1983), with single-digit growth in most years thereafter. In both 1984 and 1986 provincial government health expenditure declined. However, differences are again seen between provinces. Alberta, for example, shows higher spending growth than other provinces in almost every year. Even larger provinces evidence significant volatility in growth patterns, almost "boom and bust" cycles (e.g., British Columbia went from 10.4 percent growth in 2002 to 2.2 percent in 2004), presumably creating management difficulties within hospitals and other funded units.

### Public perspectives on need for change

Although Medicare has been described as "iconic" and "the country's most cherished social program" (Epps & Flood, 2002, p. 749), this does not mean that Canadians are uncritical of their health system. Medicare is a financing arrangement for hospitals and physicians, and does not cover all aspects of health care. Financial barriers to access exist in parts of the system not covered, the most notable being pharmaceuticals.

**FIGURE 1.2**

**Percentage changes in provincial government health expenditure, current dollars, 1976–2010**

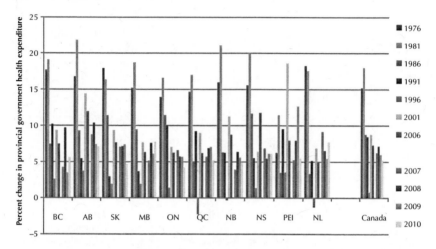

Note: Data from 1976 to 2006 are reported at five-year intervals. Annual percentage changes are shown from 2007 to 2010. The territories are excluded as, probably because of their small size, they experience much greater volatility in spending patterns.

Source: Canadian Institute for Health Information, NHEX database. Retrieved 11 August 2011 from http://apps.cihi.ca/MicroStrategy/asp/Main.aspx?&EVT=4001&REPORTid=5315E422488 4AB25EC396A863BC6F29B

The New York–based Commonwealth Fund has conducted international health surveys for more than a decade, with Canada being part of their coverage from the start.[14] One question in those surveys asks Canadians about the extent of health-system change thought necessary. Three standard choices are given:

- On the whole the system works pretty well, and only minor changes are necessary to make it work better ("minor change").
- There are some good things in our health care system, but fundamental changes are needed to make it work better ("fundamental change").
- Our health care system has so much wrong with it that we need to completely rebuild it ("complete rebuild").

As shown in Figure 1.3, about a fifth to a third of Canadians, a significant minority, think only minor change is necessary to the system, a proportion that appears to be increasing, with a corresponding decrease in the proportion who think the system needs a complete rebuild. However, since 2000, on average 50–60 percent of Canadians see much merit in the health system but still look to "fundamental change."

## FIGURE 1.3
## Canadians' perception of extent of change necessary to health system, 1998–2010 (percent distribution)

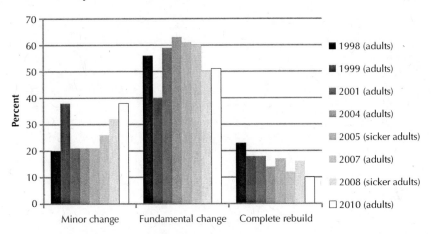

Source: Created with data from Duckett and Kempton (2012).

A response that "fundamental changes are needed" gives little guidance about the direction of change. Are respondents suggesting, as some commentators have proposed, that there should be a greater level of private funding in the Canadian health system (Skinner & Rovere, 2009)? Or are other fundamental changes envisaged? Unfortunately the data source used here does not allow us to tease out the whys. However, some things are clear from the surveys: Canadians experience long waits at almost every point of the care journey and face financial barriers in access to pharmaceuticals. A commitment to improve access, with some funding to support that, was a feature of the 2004 Accord, although clearly problems still exist. Respondents thus might be looking for big (fundamental) changes on access, but not a demolition of Medicare to achieve that. This interpretation is supported with the preamble to the question that "there are some good things in our health care system."

The results from the Commonwealth Fund surveys are consistent with other surveys of public opinion about the health system in Canada. Mendelsohn (2002), who reviewed findings from public opinion surveys for the Romanow Commission on the Future of Health Care in Canada, concluded that "Canadians have reached a mature, settled public judgment, based on decades of experience, that the Canadian health care model is a good one that should be preserved" (p. vii).

Incremental improvements identified in public opinion surveys reviewed by Mendelsohn related to primary care, home care and, to a lesser extent, access to pharmaceuticals. Soroka (2007) provided a more recent review of public opinion surveys and reached similar conclusions to Mendelsohn's earlier findings: strong support for the Medicare framework with recognition of the need for expansion of universal coverage into some specific areas. Coverage of home care was again supported, with weaker support for pharmaceutical coverage.

The *Canada Health Act,* in all its ambiguity, would seem not to be up for debate: its underlying principles have been consistently supported by Canadians for the last 50 years (Davidson, 2004). The second factor underpinning Medicare, the Federal-Provincial Accord, is due for renegotiation prior to the current Accord's expiry in 2014. Provincial funding for health care varies between provinces, and from year to year. How these factors combine in years to come will determine health care funding, and thus the shape of Canada's Medicare system.

# Word cloud: The sustainability discourse

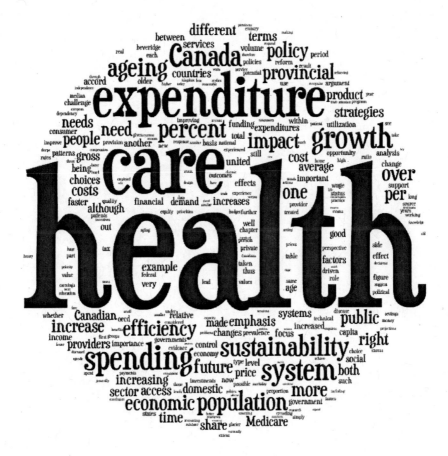

# CHAPTER 2

# THE SUSTAINABILITY DISCOURSE

Questions about the "sustainability" of Medicare arise in the media on a regular basis, possibly creating anxiety and concern in the public (Contandriopoulos & Bilodeau, 2009) that then contributes to further questioning of Medicare's sustainability. On the face of it, sustainability is simply about whether the health system of the future will be affordable and able to be staffed. Achieving sustainability means that the health system needs to be adept at preparing itself for the future. This involves changing delivery arrangements or policies to respond to emerging needs (what economists call achieving dynamic efficiency). Sustainability also requires that this response to emerging needs not be at the expense of mortgaging the future, spending now by borrowing from future generations; we must achieve what economists refer to as intergenerational equity (Stavins, Wagner, & Wagner, 2003).

Many commentators challenge the sustainability of Medicare, generally referring to the aging of the population which is feared will lead to increased demand for health care—health care that in Canada is predominantly funded from the public purse. Following this line of reasoning, aging is predicted to impact adversely on one or more economic indicators, including total health expenditure per capita or as a share of gross domestic product (GDP), and government spending in total or as a share of provincial government budgets. These indicators are understood to reflect the "affordability" of health care for any country, given its economic resources.

## The aging effect on health care: Glacier or avalanche/tsunami?

Older people use health care more than younger people. It is this visible reality that is most often the basis for apocalyptic projections of the future demand for health care. And there clearly will be more older people in Canada in the future (The boomers are coming! The boomers are coming!), even though the increase in the proportion of older people in the population is driven primarily by low fertility rates rather than aging per se (Simmons, 2011).

Paradoxically, Canada may be more exposed to fear mongering about the impact of aging, not because it is an older society (it is not), but because it is younger and so, too, is its self-image (McDaniel, 2002). The demographic transition (where population over 60 exceeds population under 15) has already occurred in many other developed countries, but is not projected to occur in Canada until 2016 (Trovato, 2011).

The simplistic "more older people, more problems" analysis is often all there is behind the forewarnings of an aging avalanche/tsunami[15] that will overwhelm the health system. Schulz (1998, p. 82) disparagingly refers to the basis of this argument as "voodoo demographics," a term picked up by Gee (2000). Reputable demographers now see a major part of their job as to "remove the preconceptions and inaccuracies" that surround debates about the impact of aging (Leone, 2010, p. 4). Distressingly, the apocalyptic argument implicitly conveys the impression that older people are simply a burden, belying any contributions of the past or their contemporary roles (which McDaniel, 2002, nicely refers to as "intergenerational interlinkages"). The apocalyptic scenario also ignores the reality that, over the long term, increased life expectancy leads to increased gross domestic product and GDP per capita[16] (Swift, 2011), which in turn will make increased health costs affordable.[17]

The logic behind the doomsayers' argument is flawed. One of the reasons there are more older people is that people are now healthier in old age than previously (Schoeni, Freedman, & Martin, 2008; Tomblin Murphy, Kephart, Lethbridge, O'Brien-Pallas, & Birch, 2009). A 75-year-old in the future will not have the same health care utilization patterns as a 75-year-old today; onset of illness will be delayed leading to a "compression of morbidity" (Fries, 1983, 2005).[18] Even modest reductions in the age-specific prevalence of chronic illness yield substantial reductions in utilization and savings (Denton & Spencer, 2010).

A number of studies have found that health expenditures are concentrated in the last years of life,[19] suggesting that health expenditure is therefore better predicted by years until death rather than years from birth (Felder, Werblow, & Zweifel, 2010; Moïse & Jacobzone, 2003; Riley & Lubitz, 2010; Scitovsky, 2005). Propper (2003) concludes that the impact of aging will thus be to push the high levels of health care expenditure to a later time in individuals' lives rather than to increase per capita expenditure. Palangkaraya and Yong (2009) go further, demonstrating that after proximity to death is taken into account, there is a (weak) negative relationship between aging and health expenditure.

Studies of health expenditure in Canada have found very moderate aging effects, if any. A research synthesis for the Canadian Health Services

Research Foundation (Constant, Petersen, Mallory, & Major, 2011) estimated that population aging contributed about 0.4 percent to 0.8 percent per annum to growth in health expenditure, and forecasting through to 2030 would only increase the estimate to between 0.95 percent and 1.3 percent per annum. Di Matteo (2010), echoing Palangkaraya and Yong (2010), showed that an increasing proportion of older people was associated with a decrease in health costs in four provinces. Tomblin Murphy et al. (2009) demonstrated that more recent cohorts have lower likelihood of reporting mobility issues at a given age, for example, and concluded that "planning based on past patterns of utilization or current age distributions of needs could therefore lead to over-provision of the capacity to meet the needs of what are no longer 'close to death' age groups" (p. 231).

A host of other studies have taken sophisticated approaches to disentangle the potential impacts of aging (well reviewed by Breyer, Costa-Font, & Felder, 2011; Dormont, Grignon, & Huber, 2006; Payne, Laporte, Deber, & Coyte, 2007). The overall conclusion points to a relatively small impact of aging on costs. Smith, Newhouse, and Freeland (2009, Technical Appendix), using data from OECD countries, concluded that aging effects accounted for between 3.5 percent and 8.8 percent of the increase in per capita health spending over the 40-year-period 1960 to 2000, providing little support to the doomsayers. In a recent study of British Columbia data over the period 1996 to 2006, Morgan and Cunningham (2011, p. 78) estimated the aging effect as leading to about a 1 percent increase in health expenditure per annum, describing this effect as "steady, predictable and modest."

Barer, Evans, and Hertzman's (1995) summary is still pertinent:

> The reality, as reflected in a steadily accumulating collection of research studies, is that to date the effects of aging per se on health care costs have been quite limited, accounting for only a small proportion of the observed escalation. Projections suggest that future effects, while not inconsequential, will appear gradually, and will be within the capacity of historical rates of economic growth. Yet these consistent research findings, like a lighthouse lost in the fog, have remained obscured by the persistent claims that the aging of the population will bankrupt our health care systems. (p. 195)

Expenditure growth is driven by two key factors—a rise in the prevalence of treated disease and an increase in the cost of each treated case—but the relative importance of the two factors is a subject of academic contention.[20] Change in treated prevalence is driven only in part by population factors that include aging but also other causes of increased prevalence of disease, such as stress and increased obesity.[21] It is also affected by changed treatment thresholds (sometimes driven by innovation, such as new drugs, sometimes by professional advice to consumers or consumer expectations). In other words, the increased prevalence of treated disease is due to both external and internal factors: population factors external to the health system, and policy and practice changes internal to the system. Even the exogenous factor of population effects could be impacted by policy choices, inside or outside the health system, for example, the prevalence of obesity.

The small and gradual impact of aging, referred to as a glacier in the title of a paper by Barer, Evans, and Hertzman (1995), leads to the conclusion that any impact of aging can be absorbed as part of the normal evolution and innovation in the health system (Hogan & Hogan, 2004; Sinha, 2011), a conclusion echoed by Reinhardt (2003) in his study of the impact of aging on health costs in the United States. If a glacier is the right analogy, then the appropriate policy response to this gradual impact of aging is incremental change over time, rather than a single tectonic shift in the 2014 Accord.

Nonetheless, some policy response is needed. Statistics Canada's (2010) medium projections for population growth suggest the population over 65 will double between 2011 and 2036, with the population over 85 increasing by 150 percent (from 675,000 to 1,700,000). Even assuming that compression of morbidity will occur, generating lower health-care utilization than currently, these increased numbers of people over 85 could potentially lead to overall increases in health service utilization. The extent of the utilization increase will depend on the extent to which the current over-60 cohort improves its relative health status in 2036, compared to people currently over 85. Assuming the current over-60 cohort has one-third lower utilization in 2036, still leads to the possibility of a two-thirds increase in demand in 2036. Another way of presenting this same effect is "a 2 percent impact per annum," not sounding nearly so dramatic, and within the bounds of reasonable incremental policy response.

As Carrière (2000) concluded,

> Instead of looking at population aging as another reason to dismantle what remains of our welfare state, it should be envisioned as an opportunity to transform those social programs that are ill-equipped to respond to the challenge.... The policy changes that will have to be made to respond to the challenge of population aging should not respond to false assumptions about its consequences on the health care system (or other social programs). Population aging is a slow process and we have time to adjust. The sooner we tackle the real problems, the smoother the transition will be. (pp. 41-42)

Just as a 75-year-old in 20 years' time will not have the same life expectancy and morbidity profile as a 75-year-old today, so too a 75-year-old in 20 years' time will have different political expectations and expectations of what the health system can do for him or her than does a 75-year-old today. It is not possible to fully incorporate these behavioural and possible political impacts into expenditure projections, but certainly different political and personal expectations may place upward pressure on health spending, in addition to a demographic effect (Breyer, Costa-Font, & Felder, 2011; Zweifel,

Steinmann, & Eugster, 2005). Nevertheless, this does not alter the overall tenor of the above discussion: the aging effect is likely to be moderate and can be absorbed by reasonably incremental policy adjustments.

## Sustainability of the tax base

The aging population effect is often presented in terms of the ratio of the over-65 population to the total population. This, combined with the proportion of people under 15, yields the "dependency ratio," so called because on average people under 15 are being supported by parents and through education, and people over 65 potentially receive income support and access to publicly funded health care. Both ends of the age spectrum are, in that sense, "dependent" on the taxpaying population of working age.[22] This language quickly morphs into the more value-laden "dependency burden" (Trovato, 2011, p. 48). Statistics Canada (2010) projections show the dependency ratio increasing from around 45 percent in 2011 to 65 percent in 2036, with most of that attributable to the growth in the percentage of people over 65 (20.4 percent to 39.1 percent).

But just as previous morbidity patterns do not reflect morbidity patterns of the future, the dependency ratio may not provide a reliable predictor of the extent of any tax base or workforce issues in the future. The size of the population between the ages of 15 and 65 is in fact not a reliable predictor of the size of the taxpaying or working population because of increasing average working years for males and increasing female participation in the labour market. Wolfson (2007) addresses this by calculating an "economic dependency ratio" (paid hours of work per capita), which has a more moderate impact into the future and, more importantly, is clearly amenable to policy intervention, for example in terms of policies to encourage people to remain in the workforce.

## What is happening to health expenditure in Canada and elsewhere?

As the economy grows, so too can expenditure on health care with no threat to sustainability (Dhalla, 2007). There is more of a debate, though, if health expenditure grows faster than the economy. Again, a moderately faster health-spending growth may be reasonable as some non-health expenditures are relatively fixed and do not increase with income, and so extra spending on health care can be reasonably absorbed out of the extra income.

Although aging may not be the principal cause of expenditure growth (and to some extent serves as a diversion), the cumulative impact of aging, practice change, and excess inflation in the health sector may well give rise for concern.

Health expenditure is growing as a share of gross domestic product in wealthy nations, with Canada no exception to this rule. Although "demand growth faster than income growth" meets the economist's classic definition of a luxury good (Newhouse, 1977), there is considerable controversy about applying that label to health care. For a start, there may be an aggregation or level-of-analysis problem, with what might be true at one level of analysis being false at another. Regardless of whether health care at the national or aggregate level is technically a luxury good, health care at the individual level might still be a necessity (Costa-Font, Gemmill, & Rubert, 2011; Di Matteo, 2003; Getzen, 2000; Parkin, McGuire, & Yule, 1987). Further, the definition of a luxury good refers to the link between demand and income, but the analysis is typically expenditure against income. Expenditure is the product of price and volume, with only the latter variable appropriately considered in analysis of whether the conditions pertinent to luxury good status exist.

In the health sector, excess price growth over productivity growth is endemic (the so-called Baumol [1967] hypothesis), and this may better explain the growth in GDP share (Hartwig, 2008; Smith, Newhouse, & Freeland, 2009). This suggests that policy options for the future should focus on improving efficiency and productivity, and on prices paid to providers rather than expenditure constraint per se (Oberlander & White, 2009; Vladeck & Rice, 2009).

Canada's health expenditure patterns are similar to other comparable countries. Figure 2.1 shows trends in health expenditure as a proportion of gross domestic product for Canada, the United Kingdom, the United States, and the average experience of western European countries.

The United States is an outlier in almost all comparative analyses of health expenditure (Aaron & Ginsberg, 2009; Anderson, Reinhardt, Hussey, & Petrosyan, 2003), consistently reporting higher spending than other countries. The United Kingdom and western European countries report very similar levels of health expenditure as a share of gross domestic product. Health expenditure consumed a larger share of gross domestic product in Canada than in other similar countries at the start of this period, but although still relatively high, spending levels in Canada now appear to be converging to those of other countries.

In terms of public expenditure, the United States (with public expenditure at 46.5 percent of total health expenditure in 2007) is again an outlier. Canada's public share (70.6 percent) is at the low end of the experience of other developed nations (e.g., United Kingdom stands at 82.6 percent, and the western European average is 76.7 percent).

Canada's trend in growth in public health expenditure is similar to growth patterns in other countries (see Figure 2.2). This convergence of spending patterns is not surprising, as policy ideas migrate from one country to another through both official channels and the work of individuals and interest groups (Clavier, 2010; Kimberly & de Pouvourville, 1993; Kimberly, de Pouvourville, & D'Aunno, 2008; Marmor, Freeman, & Okma, 2005; Steffen, 2005).

**FIGURE 2.1**
**Trends in health expenditure as share of gross domestic product, selected countries, 1988–2008**

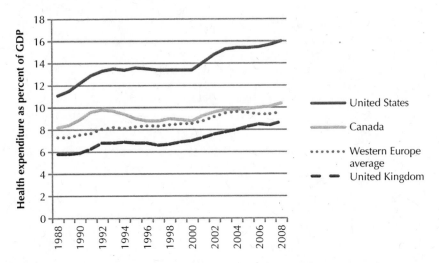

Note: The average for western Europe is the unweighted average of Austria, Denmark, France, Germany, Ireland, Italy, Luxembourg, Norway, Spain, Sweden, and Switzerland. Countries selected have continuous data series.

Source: Author's analysis of OECD (2010b) Health Data.

**FIGURE 2.2**
**Average annual growth rate in public health expenditure, selected countries, 2000–2008**

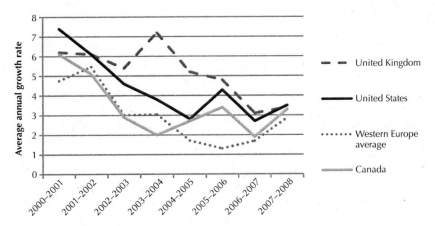

Source: Author's analysis of OECD (2010b) Health Data.

Although labelling different types of systems is a precarious enterprise (Freeman & Frisina, 2010), European systems have been classified according to their origins: the social insurance systems, first introduced into Germany by Bismarck, and the tax-financed, national health services, first introduced in the United Kingdom following a report by Lord Beveridge. Canada's health system shares many of the attributes of a Beveridge-type national health service, with the associated strengths and weaknesses. In general Beveridge systems are able to (and do) exercise tight fiscal discipline, whereas the more decentralized Bismarckian systems tend to face higher prices from the more independent providers (van der Zee & Kroneman, 2007; Wendt & Kohl, 2010). Or et al. (2010) conclude that "in terms of cost containment and affordability, Bismarck-type systems appear to be less successful than the Beveridge type. In contrast, Beveridge-type systems appear to be less successful in terms of access, defined as availability of services when required" (p. 290).

Canada's health system shares the access weakness with other Beveridge-type systems (Duckett & Kempton, 2012). In terms of reform directions, Or et al. (2010, p. 269) observe, "Most reforms in Beveridge-type systems have sought to increase choice and reduce waiting times while those in major Bismarck-type systems have focused on cost control by constraining the choice of providers."

## Crowding out

If sustainability of Medicare is not challenged by population aging, either through direct effects on health care or via the tax base, and if comparative trends in health expenditure do not suggest that Canada has a health-spending problem, either in total expenditure or in public expenditure on health (Mackenzie & Rachlis, 2010), why do we continue to hear forecasts of troubled times ahead?

Another sustainability argument relates to the concept of "financial sustainability" in contrast to "economic sustainability" (Thomson et al., 2009). Economic sustainability focuses on whether a good return is being made on investments in health care, specifically whether the return on health investments exceeds their opportunity costs. Financial sustainability does not explicitly consider the (economic) value proposition, but looks at the level of health spending and so represents a political rather than an economic judgment. Commentators who focus on financial sustainability emphasize the level of health spending that can be "afforded" at prevailing or desired levels of taxation. The health share of spending is driven by both the numerator and the denominator of that index, and so increasing health share may be the result of policies about provincial revenues (e.g., a desire to be a "low tax" province) rather than excess health spending. As Thomson et al. (2009) have pointed out, there are a number of problems with adopting financial sustainability as the principal goal of health policy. Strategies to achieve financial sustainability may impact adversely on other social and economic objectives (financial protection, health gain) and even efficiency (if cost-effective interventions are not introduced).

The variant of the financial sustainability argument seen in the Canadian discourse is that increases in spending on health care will be beyond the "capacity" of provincial governments to fund. Ontario premier Dalton McGuinty articulated this position, ludicrously suggesting that "at these rates [of increase], there will come a time when the Ministry of Health is the only Ministry we can afford to have and we still won't be able to afford the Ministry of Health" (cited in MacKinnon, 2004, p. 603).

Of course this argument assumes that governments either have no understanding of how to influence growth in health spending, or no power to act; neither reflects well on their skills and acumen. Whether projected growth in expenditure actually occurs depends, of course, on policy responses, including policies to improve efficiency and control costs (to be discussed below).

Premier McGuinty has not been the only one to bemoan provincial health-spending increases; a number of authors have suggested that increases in health spending are crowding out other important areas of expenditure such as higher education. MacKinnon (2004, p. 603), for example, claimed that "the scramble by governments to find more money for health care is resulting in the neglect or severe underfunding of other critical priorities." Simpson (2005) discusses the impact of the health sector's iconic status on provincial spending flexibility in entertaining journalistic language:

> Icons are hard to change, by the very fact that they are icons. Icons are supposed to have an everlasting quality, like the ones hanging in an Orthodox church. They are certainly difficult to attack, since they are viewed so reverentially that any aspersion cast upon them risks furious denunciations. (p. 48)

Although different expenditure data sources may yield different results (Béland, 2007), real per capita provincial spending on health care is certainly increasing faster than provincial government income, and health care is taking up an increasing share of provincial budgets (Di Matteo, 2010). Depending on the basis for the forecast, if unconstrained, health spending will take up a larger proportion of provincial gross domestic product in the future: from an average of 7.7 percent in 2008 to between 8.0 percent and 13.1 percent in 2035 (Di Matteo, 2010), leading to the argument that spending on other provincial priorities will be crowded out.

But the need to address relative priorities, which is at the heart of the "crowding out" case, is not new: the very basis of the discipline of economics is that resources are scarce and priority decisions need to be made, in households, provinces, and nations. As Simpson (2005, p. 48) points out, "We have been making tradeoffs, whether we know it or not, in favour of health care in every Canadian province for 30 years. We are still making them, and we will apparently continue to do so."

It is no surprise that trade-offs are being made by provincial govern-ments; that is the stuff of politics and economics. Priority choices are made at each budget time, influenced by a host of factors. Education costs might legitimately decline in the face of the impact of lower birth rates on school populations, and this independent of any health care effect. But what is the evidence to support "crowding out"? Can changes in eligible school populations, for example, account for any decline in education expenditure? Landon, McMillan, Muralidharan, and Parsons (2006) have undertaken just such a study. They concluded,

> There is either no relationship between health spending and other expenditures (as in the case of social services and education) or a positive relationship (as in the all other or residual expenditures categories) in which case health and other expenditures move in the same direction. Hence, the statistical evidence … provides no support for the hypothesis that, during the sample period, health expenditures crowded out either non-health provincial program spending in aggregate or any major category of provincial government spending. Indeed, the results imply the opposite—that health and non-health expenditures tend to move in tandem. (p. 131)

Importantly, total provincial program expenditures increased during the period studied (1988–2004), driven in part by reduction in debt-servicing costs. This highlights the importance of looking at the whole picture when examining health shares of provincial government expenditures. In addi-tion to variation in other program expenditure categories, there is both a numerator and a denominator that vary: a decline in the tax base can also cause an increase in health share (Dhalla, 2007).

The size of government (and the tax structure to support the desired range and level of public services) is the result of political choices. Political parties (and political commentators) have different predispositions to sup-port public provision, public subsidies to private provision, or personal/ private responsibility for aspects of health care. Their positions reflect, in part, different emphases on the values of welfare, equality, and liberty (Yeo, Emery, & Kary, 2009) and their place on the left/right spectrum of Canadian politics (Cochrane, 2010). It should come as no surprise that questioning of the sustainability of Medicare is often accompanied by calls for a greater role for private funding (Skinner & Rovere, 2009).

The sustainability of provincial governments (not just their health port-folios) requires long-run alignment of spending and revenue. Therefore, in addition to pursuing efficiency strategies, governments could consider rev-enue-side strategies, including increases in general taxation or hypothecated ("earmarked") health taxes, to meet future increases in health expenditure requirements (Dhalla, Guyatt, Stabile, & Bayoumi, 2011). Different types of taxes impact differently on equity, and have different political impacts, with less visible taxes (natural resource revenues, corporate taxes) eliciting smaller negative voter impact at elections (Landon & Ryan, 1997).

The lack of evidence for the crowding-out hypothesis leaves an important question unanswered: Is it reasonable that health and other expenditures move in tandem? From a social efficiency perspective, efficiency is maximized if the next dollar of expenditure on one function (such as health) generates the same benefits as the next dollar spent on any other function. This requires assessment of costs and benefits on a common basis across portfolios. This does not happen and, in any event, does not recognize the political factors in budgeting (Braybrooke & Lindblom, 1970; Self, 1975; Wildavsky, 1988).

Health advocates have an advantage in the politics of budgets: health spending is seen as "deserving" and as supporting a good cause. Health charities benefit from this perception as well. But there is little evidence that spending more on health is worthwhile: indeed, on average across OECD countries, a 1 percent increase in total health spending would yield an increase in average life expectancy of only approximately 10 days (Joumard, Hoeller, André, & Nicq, 2010).

Given the importance of broader socioeconomic factors in determining health status (discussed further in Chapter 3), there is a real opportunity cost in health care expenditure being privileged in the budget process over expenditure in other portfolios that might provide a greater impact on longevity or its equitable distribution. A challenge for health sector leadership is to drive system reform so that better outcomes can be achieved from existing health expenditure: spending smarter to meet emerging needs.

## The other factor in expenditure increases: Prices

Total expenditure is the result of the multiplication of prices and volumes—both factors can impact on sustainability. The aging effect focuses attention on volumes, argued above to be manageable over the long term. The price effect also needs to be considered.

Health costs are increasing faster than gross domestic product, resulting in an increase in the share of gross domestic product spent on health over time (see Figure 2.1). Although some of this increase is driven by volume changes (some due to aging, most due to other factors), some is also driven by health prices rising faster than the rest of the economy. The OECD (2010a, p. 127) summarized the relative contributions:

> According to a decomposition of public health spending growth per capita over the period 1981–2002 into the effects of age, income and a residual capturing both relative price and age-adjusted per capita utilisation, the residual explains 23% of the total in Canada, *versus* an OECD average of 28%. With long-run price growth presumably above the OECD average, this could suggest somewhat below average per capita volume growth in Canada.

The OECD is thus reinforcing the importance of price growth, and with wages accounting for the majority of health spending, wage growth is a particularly important factor in accounting for changes in health spending. Galarneau (2003) examined wage growth over the period 1990 to 2000 (see Figure 2.3). She found that median earnings for all employed Canadians increased by 3.3 percent in real terms; those employed in the health sector experienced an increase in median earnings more than twice that experienced by those employed in other sectors (6.4 percent vs. 3.1 percent). Within the health sector, health professionals experienced increases in median earnings of 15.1 percent, with some groups exhibiting faster increases. Support workers in the health sector also experienced faster rates of growth than the average employed person. Other groups, such as technical personnel, experienced median earnings growth in line with inflation, that is, no real growth in median incomes.

**FIGURE 2.3**
**Percent increase in real median annual earnings, various sectors and professions, Canada, 1990–2000**

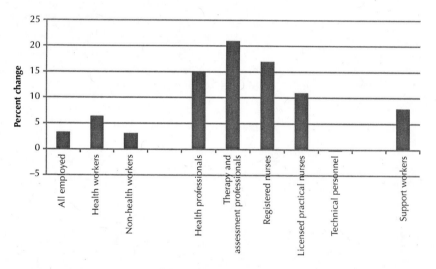

Note: These data are for all employed persons, including full time and part time. The growth in median incomes is thus affected by both wage rates per hour and hours worked. Average hours worked for support staff increased faster than the Canadian average over the reporting period (7.6 percent vs. 5.5 percent); hours worked for technical professionals grew slower (3.5 percent). Health professional hours grew at approximately the same rate as other employees.
Source: Galarneau (2003).

Wage growth significantly faster than inflation (and faster than other groups in the economy) is thus one of reasons for an increasing share of gross domestic product being devoted health. Given Canada's proximity to the United States, remuneration of Canadian health workers, who have portable skills, is influenced by wage trends in that country. The very high wage rates paid in the United States (and other price effects) is one of the reasons for the high health-care costs in that country, a pattern that needs to be avoided in Canada (Anderson, Reinhardt, et al., 2003).

Obviously people working in the health sector, as with all employees, should be remunerated fairly, but excess wage growth has the potential to challenge sustainability of the sector. One response to excess wage growth is to change the skill mix, discussed further in Chapter 8.

## Responding to the glacier

Canada needs to ensure it is positioned well to address the emerging health issues of the future. Children born this year will be alive for practically all of the rest of this century. We know the importance of experiences in utero and early childhood development on health (Anderson, Shinn, et al., 2003; Felitti et al., 1998; Shonkoff, 2010; Shonkoff & Phillips, 2000) and the positive economic return of investments in the early years of life (Currie, 2009; Killburn & Karoly, 2008). So the actions being taken today will have long-reaching consequences—for individuals, for the health care system, and for the whole of Canadian society. Similarly, in terms of inaction: decisions we do not make today might mean we need to take different decisions in the future.

If Canada is to continue with a sustainable health system, actions need to be taken now. These need not be actions that impinge on the core elements of Medicare. In my view, there is no need to introduce substantial private funding; no need to change the five criteria for complying with Medicare arrangements in any major way; no need to revisit the values shared by Canadians. There need be no access/quality/sustainability trade-off, as all three are achievable. But the money currently spent on health care (and the inevitable increase in spending to occur as the population and economy grow) needs to be invested wisely, to achieve social efficiency (Bohm, 1987). "Spending smarter" (to use Flood, Stabile, and Tuohy's [2008c] terminology) will be a consistent theme of the chapters of this book.

### Improving efficiency

Although improving efficiency would be widely endorsed as an objective of health policy, improving efficiency is not synonymous with budget cuts. Expenditure increases may improve efficiency, if the marginal benefits exceed the marginal costs (e.g., some investments in early childhood). And all this is an ongoing process, not just something that happens in 2014. The health care system is dynamic, with new pressures requiring new responses. Partly for this reason, Altman,Tompkins, Eilat, and Glavin (2003) suggest that cost-control successes are inevitably time limited. Expenditure and cost controls need to focus on multiple strategies and be renewed on a continuous basis.

One could argue that the quest to improve health care in Canada has a moral dimension: Is it legitimate to take actions that impinge on equity, for example, if there is still waste in the health system or if we could improve outcomes by shifting resources from program A to program B? Brook and Lohr (1986, 1991) asked rhetorically, "Will we need to ration *effective* care?" In essence they argue that if we spend smarter and eliminate ineffective services, enough resources will be available to provide beneficial care to all who need it.

Sustainability demands that expenditure be actively managed, and this is not simple. Health care is a labour-intensive industry: what a payer sees as health care expenditure is seen as health care income by providers. Although payers have an interest in constraining health expenditure, providers have an interest in increasing health expenditure (or at the very least, changing the distribution of health expenditure from other providers to themselves). As Evans (1990a) has pointed out, these opposing forces in health care financing debates lead to opposing strategies, termed tension and compression. These forces of tension and compression can also lead to "shear"—strategies to transfer costs from one group to another, the most common Canadian suggestion here being to shift costs onto consumers, with consequential adverse equity impacts.

A number of authors have reviewed the instruments, strategies, or targets of health cost control (White, 1999). In broad general terms, cost-control strategies can attempt to influence the behaviour of suppliers or providers (such as hospitals and medical practitioners—the economists' "supply side"), or consumers' behaviour on the demand side (Carrin & Hanvoravongchai, 2003; Rice, 2002). Given that total health care expenditure is determined by multiplying price of services by the volume provided, strategies can also be categorized into those two broad targets: control of price or control of volume (Hepburn, 2006). Table 2.1 portrays these choices and provides an example of policy instruments in each cell.

**TABLE 2.1**
**Targets of health care cost control**

|  | *Demand side* | *Supply side* |
|---|---|---|
| Price | Consumer copayments | • Design/structure of payment schedule (e.g., activity-based funding)<br>• Private sector provision to "improve efficiency" |
| Volume | Assessment processes for eligibility | • Regulating capacity<br>• Cost-effectiveness and utilization review |

Use of any strategy might evoke a reaction (and a need for strategies) in other cells; for example, squeezing providers on price may result in providers' increasing their volume to achieve a target income. Also, instruments and policies focusing on one area need to take account of the interaction with, and consequences for, potential substitutes. For example, very high copayments for prescription medication in community settings may result in consumers increasing their use of hospital emergency services.

In aggregate, health expenditure, health revenues, and health incomes are identical, but the benefits are distributed differentially. Interests in the health sector are thus differentially affected by the policies shown in Table 2.1. For example, providers are generally opposed to supply-side strategies focused on price, which are designed to reduce provider income. Providers thus can typically be expected to attempt to focus on strategies in the other cells in Table 2.1, in particular, cost shifting or attempting to focus policy attention on the demand side (Evans, 1997), with an emphasis on consumer copayments. But the evidence for the effectiveness of consumer copayments in reducing demand is very slight indeed (Carrin & Hanvoravongchai, 2003), so slight that this focus of policy attention has been described as a walking zombie that refuses to die (Barer, Bhatla, Evans, & Stoddard, 1993; Evans, Barer, & Stoddart, 1995).

There is now an extensive literature (recently reviewed in Joumard, André, and Nicq, 2010) demonstrating the weak link between levels of expenditure (and inputs generally) and health outcomes. This underlines the importance of ensuring that health expenditure management also focuses on social efficiency, to ensure that the right investments are made (see discussion in next chapter and Chapter 5).

## A proposed direction

So returning to the glacier problem. Assuming incremental changes to policy are required, what should they be? Although not every preventive strategy is a sensible economic investment (Russell, 1986), there *are* a few public health interventions that should be made to reduce the prevalence of treated disease. But most of the change that is necessary will be in terms of the health system, particularly how chronic care is managed, and in terms of improving efficiency.

The object of a reformed Canadian health system can be articulated simply:

*The right person enables the right care in the right setting, on time, every time.*

Each of these words is important.

*Right person*: This presages a workforce reform agenda to ensure that the full potential of all health workers is used, that all work to their full scope of practice, with physicians doing what physicians should do, registered nurses likewise, and aides used to their full potential. This makes sense from a job-satisfaction perspective, as well as an economic perspective.

*Enables*: The health problems of today are not the same as yesterday when Medicare was designed. Although acute/episodic disease and trauma are still important, health utilization is increasingly about managing chronic diseases. In that context, health system discourse needs to recognize the importance of "co-production": that the person with the disease is an important partner in the care (Hunter & Ritchie, 2007; Le Grand, 2003), and that a key health system reform strategy is about ensuring *informed* demand (Flood, Stabile, & Tuohy, 2008c). So the language here is about changing the role of the health provider to "enabling" care, supporting the person with chronic disease to manage his or her care, and supporting the family or caregivers in that endeavour.

*Right care:* Knowledge about what is best care is increasing rapidly, but that new knowledge is often not implemented in clinical practice for a decade or so after it is first established (Carroll et al., 1997; Glasziou & Haynes, 2005; Haynes & Haines, 1998). Purposive steps need to be taken to identify best care, develop protocols to facilitate use in practice, and benchmark outcomes as part of the knowledge development cycle. "Right care" also implies that the care is provided efficiently.

*Right setting:* Different care settings have different strengths and weaknesses from the perspective of the patient, the clinician, and the economist. Higher-volume settings tend to have better clinical outcomes, but concentration of care imposes travel and dislocation costs on patients and their families. For seniors, as an example, different types of settings allow more or less independence. An important concept here is the "least restrictive alternative" that arose from the disability and mental health deinstitutionalization movements, but unfortunately has acquired a plethora of meanings (Bachrach, 1980). Simply put, following this orientation, an emphasis is placed on maintaining independence as much as possible for the patient/resident in seniors' accommodation, with care at home if possible through services coming into the home, or via telephone consults, and in local, community settings. By extrapolation it includes an emphasis on primary care rather than secondary care, an emphasis on ambulatory care rather than inpatient care, and an emphasis on getting patients home as quickly as possible.

*On time:* The phrasing of the *Canada Health Act* criterion of "reasonable access" explicitly addresses financial barriers to access, but long waits also impede access. Since the 2004 Accord, policy attention has focused on waits for a small list of elective procedures and diagnostic services, but the access agenda needs to be broadened to include waits to see a specialist, and waits in an emergency. Timeliness of access across the whole continuum of care thus needs to be assured and demonstrated.

*Every time:* This emphasizes consistency, in terms of right care (in the right setting) and on time, thus linking to both timely access and good quality. Baker et al. (2004) estimated that one in every 15 patients admitted to Canadian hospitals experiences an adverse event. The safety and quality agenda is thus a critical one. Achieving that requires cultures that allow learning from mistakes. "Every time" also connotes "for everybody," emphasizing the importance of equity in access and provision.

## 2014 looms

The 2004 Accord expires in 2014, providing both an opportunity and a threat to the future of Canadians' experience of Medicare. First, the threat. Federal funding under the existing Accord is a significant funding source for the provinces. The 2004 Accord both boosted the base and enshrined 6 percent escalation. The environment for 2014 looks very different from 2004 on two fronts, politics and the economy. The 2004 Accord was negotiated by Liberal Prime Minister Paul Martin, from a party traditionally associated with a greater public sector role, and whose father (when Minister of National Health and Welfare) had played a key role in the introduction of national hospital insurance in Canada (Taylor, 1978). Current Prime Minister Harper's Conservatives, in contrast, favour smaller government, and a concomitant smaller federal role. Moreover, the economy is different too:

> The 2004 Martin health care deal and the tremendous growth in federal transfers it has fuelled were both made possible by the expansion of the national economy, which continued throughout most of the first decade of the 21st century until the fall of 2008. At that point the international recession hit with a vengeance, and the federal and provincial governments suddenly found themselves in deficits due to plunging revenues and the rising stimulus spending needed to support their economies. (Norquay, 2010, p. 17)

During the 2011 election campaign, Prime Minister Harper committed to continuation of the 6 percent escalation, at least for a period. However, a deficit environment puts at risk 6 percent escalation for the full length of the next Accord and makes the possibility of further increases in funding remote. Any changes to health care should therefore be formulated within that budget envelope.

The outcomes of negotiations between the provinces and the federal government are clearly affected by the skills of the participants. A cohesive group of strong provincial leaders, working as a team with articulate spokespeople, will likely achieve the best outcomes. The preconditions for unity, with leaders known to each other, may not now be present (Sears, 2010), not auguring well for a good outcome from a provincial perspective.

Another potential threat is that the renegotiation of the Accord is, by definition, a reopener of the existing Medicare convention. An open agenda provides as much scope for proposals to challenge and limit Medicare as to expand it. The challenge to Medicare is currently couched as questioning its "sustainability," especially in the face of demographic change, as discussed above.

The Accord also presents an opportunity to reaffirm or expand. The rhetoric of the 2004 Accord gave hope for a new basis for home care, a hope largely unfulfilled. This might be revisited. The contemporary challenge may also be to address coverage of pharmaceuticals (considered in Chapter 5) and public health (next chapter).

Reform of Medicare and the Canadian heath care system should not be cast as being simply about more money, from whatever source (federal transfers, private funding). So the 2014 Accord, which will be principally about money and its sources, is not the only opportunity for reform. Addressing the gaps in care in this country is as much if not more about system redesign (ensuring the right person enables the right care in the right setting, on time, every time) and improved efficiency (technical and social). It is about changes that can be made within every province, within every health service, and at every point of the care continuum.

## Values and principles

The changes that need to be made must be consistent with the enduring values of Canadian health care (Davidson, 2004) and build on the trust exhibited by Canadians in the health system (Abelson et al., 2009). It is important, therefore, to recognize how health care cost-control strategies, which focus on the efficiency attributes of the health system, interact with the other system values such as equity: the introduction of extensive consumer copayments will have a differential impact on the poor. Some strategies to affect volume, by restricting consumer choice, may also have an adverse impact on consumer and provider acceptability (Flynn & Smith, 2002).

The relative emphasis on, or choice of, different reform strategies, design choices, and investment priorities is and should be shaped by values and where you sit in the health care system—principally, consumer or provider. Ethical frameworks are now often incorporated in policy documents, although sometimes as window dressing rather than shaping the policy (Giacomini, Kenny, & DeJean, 2008), with consequential limited effects on policy (Sabik & Lie, 2008). Moving beyond rhetoric and vagueness (Gibson & Goodin, 1999) is difficult, and it may not be possible to reach agreement in the community on priority choices at any level of detail (Sabik & Lie, 2008).

Policy and value choices abound impacting access, management, and sustainability issues. Some examples of choices and orientations are as follows: [23]

1.  *Concern for disadvantaged populations and addressing unmet needs.* Health needs are unevenly distributed in the population and vary by age, aboriginality, location, employment status, and other factors. Where should the emphasis be in terms of improving the average level of health status in Canada? To what extent should the focus be on improvement in health status of the most disadvantaged versus policies targeted at the majority population? What is the right mix of interventions here, and how much weight in economic appraisal should be placed on distributional goals?

2.  *An emphasis on the least restrictive alternative.* System design should recognize the importance of facilitating independence for the patient/ resident in seniors' accommodation: the emphasis should be on primary care rather than secondary care, on ambulatory care rather than inpatient care, and on getting patients home as quickly as possible. The trade-off is between promoting independence consistent with safety and efficient provision.

3.  *Weighing the three perspectives on value: patient, clinician, and economic.* Patients want to be treated with dignity; they want speedy access, good facilities, and good care. But patients are not well placed to judge the technical quality of care: Was the right procedure performed? Was the procedure performed appropriately? This dimension of health-system value can be judged only by clinicians. Health systems need to be sustainable from a societal perspective, and so assessments need to be made from both efficiency and effectiveness perspectives. Economic choices are made every day: If money is spent for one purpose, it is not available for another (the concept of opportunity cost). What should be the criteria used in evaluating spending priorities? All three perspectives (patient, clinician, economic) on value are important. But what should be the relative emphasis on each? Where should an organization start in terms of its improvement effort?

4.  *The use of economic incentives.* Although the principal criterion for decision-making in the health sector should not be a one-dimensional focus on technical efficiency, economic incentives have a role in shaping system development. What is the place of financial incentives on providers (e.g., activity-based funding, "pay for performance") and staff (pay at risk)?

5.  *Different provider forms.* In what circumstances should care be in organizations directly administered by the public sector? What is the role of not-for-profit organizations? Is it appropriate to have for-profit providers (other than professional corporations) involved in care? Do we view larger versus smaller professional corporations differently?

None of these choices have been framed as simple alternatives, for example, to use economic incentives or not. Rather, the phrasing highlights the choice of the balance or emphasis of this dimension in system design or management. Nor have these policy choices been phrased as "slogans" (e.g., "managed care") where the antonym is absurd and the phrase itself can have a variety of meanings (Marmor, 2007). Instead, the continuous nature of the choice is emphasized.

Decisions are taken about each of these issues every day, both implicitly and explicitly. In making a budget announcement to expand services at a hospital, a provincial government has implicitly considered the form of delivery (this service will not be contracted to another provider), the relative priority of providing this need versus another, and so on. The alternative options considered (the "road not taken") are rarely announced at the same time as a service expansion.

Choices about the future of health care involve trade-offs and tensions across a range of dimensions (Glouberman & Zimmerman, 2002, 2004). Economic tensions are often the most visible and vocally expressed (e.g., public vs. private funding), but other dimensions of tensions include governance (centralized vs. decentralized), knowledge (evidence-based vs. experience-based medicine) and institutional (primary vs. acute care struggles). These tensions need to be acknowledged before they can be addressed.

I have already nailed my flag to the mast and indicated my concern for and focus on efficiency. It is my contention that improvements in efficiency (technical and social) are the way to protect access to and quality of health care in Canada. Subsequent chapters of this book outline proposals for desirable changes and what investments are necessary to improve the Canadian health care system.

# Word cloud: Improving the public's health

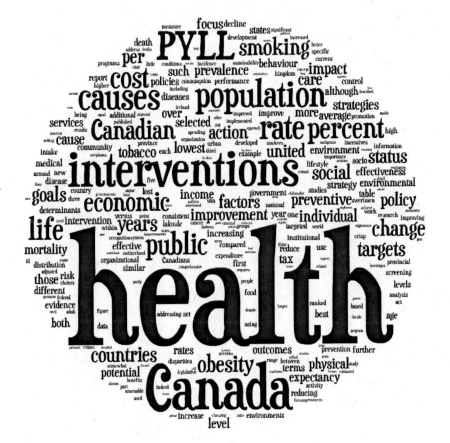

In this chapter I propose the following policy initiatives:

- Consistent with the language of the 2004 First Ministers' statement, a pan-Canadian set of goals and targets for improving the health status of *all* Canadians should be developed by governments to cover the period of the next Accord. Once developed, each province should publish its own goals and targets, consistent with the national goals and targets, and report progress against those targets. Regional health authorities and other organizations should also consider the development of goals and targets consistent with the national goals and targets.
- Provinces and regional health authorities should publish regular reports on disparities in health outcomes.
- The Canadian Health Services Research Foundation should be tasked to review the evidence on the use of tax incentives to promote public health objectives, including the case for a targeted tax on sugar-sweetened beverages.
- Federal, provincial, and territorial leaders should commission an evaluation of the existing Canadian Strategy for Cancer Control and recommend how it might be enhanced to reduce smoking prevalence further.
- The Public Health Agency of Canada should commission a comprehensive economic evaluation of potential policies to improve health status (and its distribution) in Canada and ensure that the evaluation is updated every five years.
- The *Canada Health Act* should be amended to include "cost-effective preventive interventions" as part of required insured services.

# CHAPTER 3

# IMPROVING THE PUBLIC'S HEALTH

Whichever way you measure it, the health of the average Canadian is improving and has been doing so for decades. Unfortunately though, health status improvement in Canada is not occurring at the same rate as in other comparable countries (Fang & Millar, 2009).

Figure 3.1 shows the pattern for one health-outcome measure, Potential Years of Life Lost (PYLL). PYLL is calculated by selecting an arbitrary age as a typical life expectancy and counting, for any death that occurs before that age, the years between age at death and the arbitrary life expectancy as a "potential year of life lost." In its calculations, the Organisation for Economic Co-operation and Development (OECD) measures life years lost before age 70 (PYLL70).[24]

Over the decade 1994–2004, PYLL in Canada declined from 4,236 per 100,000 population to 3,365, an average improvement (decline) of 2.3 percent per annum. Improvement is occurring in practically every country in the OECD, but some countries have exhibited a faster rate of decline than Canada. Countries with substantially greater room to improve could be expected to do so at a faster rate, but some countries with a similar initial rate of PYLL have also improved at a faster rate than Canada. Australia, for example, starting at 4,095 PYLL per 100,000 population, had a faster improvement rate at 2.7 percent per annum, as did Switzerland, which started at 4,220 with an average decline of 3.5 percent per annum.

Pritchard and Wallace (2011) compared the rate of improvement in mortality for both adult populations (those aged 15–74) and older populations (55–74) across a range of Western nations. Both measures are related to PYLL as they ignore deaths at older ages. Over the period from 1979–81 to 2002–04, adult mortality rates in Canada dropped by 35 percent and older mortality rates by 36 percent, in contrast to the somewhat better performance in the United Kingdom (39 and 40 percent, respectively) and the worse performance in the United States (26 and 27 percent). Pritchard and Wallace argued that the ratio of improvement in mortality rates (reduced deaths) to the health-expenditure share of gross domestic product is a measure of the

## FIGURE 3.1
## Potential Years of Life Lost (to age 70) per 100,000 population, selected countries, 1994–2004

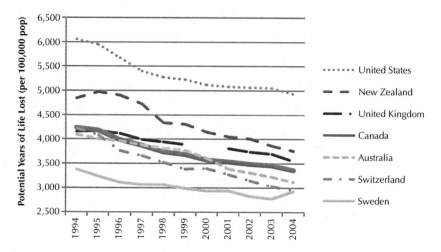

Source: OECD (2010b) Health Data.

cost-effectiveness of a country's health system. Using their measure, Canada ranked 11th out of 19 countries on the older adult ratio (1:841) compared with the United Kingdom at 2nd (1:1,490) and the United States at 17th (1:515). Canada's performance on reducing adult deaths relative to health spending was similar (1:324 compared with the United Kingdom at 1:557 and the United States at 1:205).

The decline in PYLL is not solely attributable to improvements in health care: some is also due to improved incomes and other environmental factors (Ford & Capewell, 2011; Harper, Lynch, & Smith, 2011). Some causes of mortality are amenable to medical care interventions, some to health policy or public health interventions, and some to neither (Castelli & Nizalova, 2011). Nolte and McKee (2008) estimated that the death rate from causes amenable to medical care in Canada in 2002–03 was about 22 percent of the all-cause death rate. Large gains in life expectancy are thus more likely to occur from reductions in death rates from causes of death that are not identified as primarily amenable to medical intervention.

Cross-national studies of health expenditure have shown that additional health expenditure results in life expectancy gains only for lower-income countries; above a certain national income level, there is relatively little gain, although additional expenditure may reduce the variability in the distribution of average age at death (Schoder & Zweifel, 2011). Joumard, Hoeller, et al. (2010) have estimated that a 10 percent increase in health care spending would increase life expectancy by only three to four months in the average OECD country.

But improvements in life expectancy and PYLL can and have been made: in Canada, for example, death rates for causes amenable to health care improved about 14 percent over the five-year period from 1997–98 to 2002–03, while death rates for other causes improved about 8 percent (Nolte & McKee, 2008). As Pritchard and Wallace (2011) pointed out, different countries have different rates of improvement in health outcomes, and so international comparative data can be used to establish targets for further improvement (Katz, Glazier, & Vijayaraghavan, 2009).

The Conference Board of Canada, for example, in a report published in 2004, the year of the Athens Olympics, ranked countries as gold, silver, or bronze performers and published "medal tallies" on overall results, health status, non-medical factors, and health outcomes. In overall results, countries ranked from Switzerland (weighted medal count of 37) to the Olympic host country, Greece, ranked 24 with a weighted medal count of 18. Canada was described as "middle of the pack," ranked 13 with a weighted count of 27. Canada ranked equal 5th on health status, equal 15th on non-medical factors, and equal last (20th) on health outcomes (PYLL measures, disease-specific mortality rates).

Armstrong's (1990) concept of "Arcadian normals" can be used to establish stretch improvement goals based on comparative data. Using this approach, cause-specific mortality (or PYLL) in any region or country can be compared with the best experience in comparator areas (or population groups) to measure gaps in achievement and establish realistic health-improvement targets (Danaei et al., 2010, set population group-specific targets; see also Petrie, Tang, & Rao, 2009; Ring & O'Brien, 2007). Table 3.1 shows such an approach for Canada and other similar countries for the eight major causes of PYLL70 (and all causes). All-causes data are provided for all countries, but data for each cause are provided only for Canada and for those countries that have better performance (defined as the three with the lowest PYLL rates) for those causes.

Canada does not have the lowest (or even third-lowest) rate for any of the selected causes. The table highlights the difference between Canada's PYLL and the countries with the lowest and third-lowest all-cause PYLL, and the lowest and third-lowest PYLL for each of the selected causes.

Iceland has the lowest all-cause PYLL rate (2,681 per 100,000 population), 80 percent of Canada's. Iceland has almost a ten-year lead on Canada in health improvement: its PYLL rate in 1994 was marginally better than Canada's position today.

It may be argued that the country with the lowest PYLL either for all causes or for any of the selected causes is an anomaly and so does not provide a reasonable basis for an achievable goal for Canada, and that a softer target, say third-best performance, should be established. The three countries with the lowest all-cause PYLL are Iceland, Sweden (2,929 PYLL rate), and Switzerland (2,952 rate). Switzerland's rate is 88 percent of Canada's.

**TABLE 3.1**
**Potential Years of Life Lost (to age 70) per 100,000 population, selected countries, selected causes, 2004**

| | All causes | External causes | Perinatal conditions | Malignant neoplasms | Congenital anomalies | Diseases of circulatory system | Diseases of digestive system | Endocrine and metabolic diseases | Diseases of nervous system |
|---|---|---|---|---|---|---|---|---|---|
| Australia | 3,122 | | | | | | | | |
| Austria | 3,499 | | | | | | | | |
| Belgium | 3,587 | | | | | | | | |
| Canada | 3,365 | 892 | 342 | 823 | 179 | 422 | 104 | 104 | 106 |
| Czech Republic | 4,338 | | | | 88 | | | | |
| Denmark | 3,718 | | | | | | | | |
| Estonia | 7,876 | | | | | | | | |
| Finland | 3,974 | | | 681 | | 364 | | | |
| France | 3,611 | 652 | | | | | | | |
| Germany | 3,360 | | | | | | | | |
| Greece | 3,394 | | | | | | 74 | 44 | 82 |
| Hungary | 6,583 | | | | | | | | |
| Iceland | 2,681 | | 101 | 705 | 69 | | 21 | | 70 |
| Ireland | 3,533 | | | | 79 | | | 34 | 42 |
| Luxembourg | 3,392 | 519 | | | | | | | |
| Netherlands | 3,103 | | | | | | | | |
| New Zealand | 3,761 | | 164 | | | 390 | 51 | | |
| Norway | 3,206 | | | | | | | | |
| Poland | 5,638 | | | | | | | | |
| Slovak Republic | 5,481 | | | | | | | | |
| Slovenia | 4,297 | | | | | | 74 | 44 | |
| Spain | 3,304 | | | | | | | | |
| Sweden | 2,929 | | 147 | 720 | | 333 | | | |
| Switzerland | 2,952 | 664 | | | | | | | |
| United Kingdom | 3,553 | | | | | | | | |
| United States | 4,934 | | | | | | | | |
| Minimum | 2,681 | 519 | 101 | 681 | 69 | 333 | 21 | 34 | 42 |
| Canada's potential against column minima | 684 | 373 | 241 | 142 | 110 | 89 | 83 | 70 | 64 |
| 3rd best | 2,952 | 664 | 164 | 720 | 88 | 390 | 74 | 44 | 82 |
| Canada's potential against 3rd best | 413 | 228 | 178 | 103 | 91 | 32 | 30 | 60 | 24 |

Source: Compiled by author with data from OECD (2010b) Health Data.

The concept of Arcadian normals is based on analysis of cause-specific mortality (or premature mortality). Using this as a basis, and setting a reasonable target as the third-best peer performance, the United Kingdom's PYLL from external causes (suicide, road trauma) is 664 per 100,000 population, three quarters of Canada's 892 per 100,000 rate.

If Canada were able to achieve the United Kingdom's PYLL rate for external causes, Norway's for perinatal conditions, and Sweden's for malignant neoplasms,[25] it would reduce the Canadian all-cause rate by 509 PYLL per 100,000 population, taking the all-cause rate to 2,856 per 100,000 population (85 percent of the current rate), the second-lowest rate after Iceland (assuming the other countries did not make commensurate improvements as well). The countries selected for comparison are not too dissimilar from Canada to make such targets unreasonable and consigned to the impossible bucket.

An alternative to setting targets based on international comparative Arcadian normals is to examine variation within Canada where different provinces (and territories) exhibit different outcomes in terms of health status, health utilization, and non-medical environmental factors (Arah & Westert, 2005; Manuel, Creatore, Rosella, & Henry, 2009). Table 3.2 shows provincial and Canadian all-cause PYLL75 for selected causes.

**TABLE 3.2**
**Potential Years of Life Lost (to age 75) per 100,000 population, by province, selected causes, 1999–2001**

| | All causes | Malignant neoplasms | Circulatory diseases | Respiratory diseases (excluding infectious and parasitic diseases) | Unintentional injuries | Suicides and self-inflicted injuries |
|---|---|---|---|---|---|---|
| BC | 4,879 | 1,405 | **735** | 148 | 869 | 348 |
| AB | 5,236 | **1,303** | 807 | 163 | 915 | 495 |
| SK | 5,812 | 1,483 | 952 | 223 | 1,028 | 412 |
| MB | 6,106 | 1,584 | 1,041 | 197 | 903 | 410 |
| ON | 4,755 | 1,505 | 823 | **146** | **471** | 258 |
| QC | 5,324 | 1,844 | 876 | 168 | 550 | 586 |
| NB | 5,334 | 1,622 | 982 | 210 | 804 | 466 |
| NS | 5,397 | 1,827 | 1,040 | 216 | 596 | 292 |
| PEI | 5,606 | 1,705 | 1,265 | 226 | 897 | 317 |
| NL | 5,620 | 1,872 | 1,243 | 167 | 676 | **251** |
| YT | 6,514 | 1,571 | 928 | 212 | 1,066 | 686 |
| NT | 6,397 | 1,268 | 460 | 182 | 1,510 | 791 |
| NU | 13,070 | 1,365 | 981 | 476 | 1,711 | 4,585 |
| Canada | 5,102 | 1,574 | 854 | 162 | 640 | 394 |
| Improvement opportunity | 718 | 271 | 119 | 16 | 169 | 143 |

Note: Note the different basis for calculating Potential Years of Life Lost. For Canadian statistics, obtained from Statistics Canada, premature mortality is assumed to occur in any death before age 75.

Source: Statistics Canada, CANSIM Table 102-0311, "Potential Years of Life Lost, by Selected Causes of Death and Sex, Population Aged 0 to 74, Three-Year Average, Canada."

Canadian all-cause PYLL75 rate is 5,102[26]; the range is from 4,755 in Ontario to 6,106 in Manitoba and 13,070 per 100,000 population in Nunavut. For each of the five causes, the lowest PYLL is in boldface. For malignant neoplasms, Alberta's rate of 1,303 PYLL per 100,000 population is 271 per 100,000 below the Canadian rate. If each province and territory were able to achieve the PYLL rate of the best performing province in these five causes, the all-cause PYLL rate (assuming independence of the selected causes) would improve by 718 PYLL per 100,000 population, to about 85 percent of its current level.[27]

Given the trend lines shown in Figure 3.1, improvement of this kind could occur naturally over time: additional purposive action would be required to speed up the improvement in PYLL. But of what kind? What interventions will yield the best results in terms of improved health? Addressing this question requires analysis of the determinants of ill health.

### Distributional effects

The analysis here has so far focused on averages, and this chapter commenced with a claim about the "average Canadian." Most measures of health status, including life expectancy and PYLL, are not evenly distributed with significant disparities by gender, occupation, income, location, and ethnicity (Raphael, 2009). Aboriginal people suffer particular deprivation, with life expectancies for First Nation and Inuit people five to 14 years less than other Canadians (Smylie, 2009). Newly arrived immigrants tend to be healthier than the average Canadian, but lose that advantage over time (De Maio, 2010).

People resident in low-income areas of urban Canada have more than three times the rate of hospitalization for substance-related disorders and 20 percent higher rate of admissions for injuries for children (see Figure 3.2)

For a range of conditions residents of lower-income areas have higher hospitalization rates, and Statistics Canada data show that compared to males on low incomes, males on higher incomes can expect to live longer at birth (78.4 versus 75.2 years) and live longer in good health (70.5 versus 65.8 years), with differences also seen for females (life expectancy at birth: 82.5 versus 81.4 years; health-adjusted life expectancy 72.3 versus 69.1 years).[28] Similar differences have been found in studies of specific diseases (Lipscombe et al., 2010) and using occupation as a measure of socioeconomic disadvantage (Mustard et al., 2010). Not only is socioeconomic status associated directly with poorer health outcomes, but there is also increasing evidence that the degree of inequality in a society is associated with poorer health status (Kondo et al., 2009; Wilkinson & Pickett, 2010; Xi, McDowell, Nair, & Spasoff, 2005).[29]

Although income differential gradients for mortality amenable to intervention with improved medical care or public health interventions have declined over recent decades, "there seems to be considerable unrealised potential of public health for further reducing health disparities in Canada"

**FIGURE 3.2**

**Rate ratios (lowest versus highest income terciles of residence, urban Canada) for selected causes of hospitalization, 2003–2005**

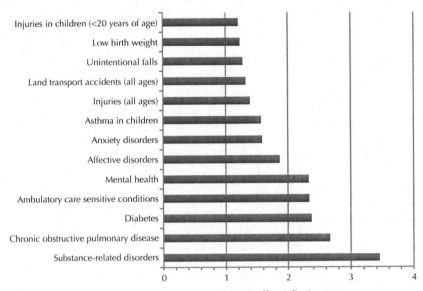

Rate ratio of hospitalization rates
(lowest versus highest third of population by average income of residence)

Note: All differences between high- and low-income areas reach statistical significance at 95 percent level.

Source: Canadian Institute for Health Information (2008b), *Reducing Gaps in Health: A Focus on Socio-economic Status in Urban Canada.*

(James, Wilkins, Detsky, Tugwell, & Manuel, 2007, p. 292). This is an understatement: Canada's performance has deteriorated over the last decade on critical policy fronts relevant to the social determinants of health (Bryant, Raphael, Schrecker, & Labonte, 2011).

So where does this lead in terms of policy responses? Buried deep in the 2004 First Ministers' statement on the future of health care was this recognition and commitment:

> All governments recognize that public health efforts on health promotion, disease and injury prevention are critical to achieving better health outcomes for Canadians and contributing to the long-term sustainability of Medicare by reducing pressure on the health care system.... Governments commit to accelerate work on a pan-Canadian Public Health Strategy. For the first time, governments will set goals and targets for improving the health status of Canadians through a collaborative process with experts. The Strategy will include efforts to address common risk factors, such as physical inactivity, and integrated disease strategies. (Health Canada, 2004, "Prevention, Promotion and Public Health" section)

There were indeed discussions with experts: The Canadian Public Health Association, "with the guidance of a Federal-Provincial-Territorial Government Working Group," produced a discussion paper in early 2005 "to assist senior decision makers and other interested Canadians to contribute in an informed way to the development of Pan-Canadian public health goals." The discussion paper identified the standard terminology to be used (goals, objectives, targets, indicators, strategies), obviously working within the conventional paradigm of establishing measurable goals and targets. Consultations were held throughout Canada.

What was produced was a set of "goals," no targets, a rather anodyne document entitled *Public Health Goals for Canada*, ambitiously but inappropriately subtitled "a federal, provincial and territorial *commitment* to Canadians" (emphasis added). The document includes broad, hortatory statements such as "every person receives the support and information they need to make healthy choices."[30] The Senate Subcommittee on Population Health thought that there was still some place for the *Goals* document and in a recent report recommended that "the Health Goals for Canada agreed upon in 2005 be revived and guide the development, implementation and monitoring of the pan-Canadian population health policy" (Senate, 2009, p. 23).

Although every province has developed a set of health goals and targets, they have a sorry history in terms of any continuing impact on policy (Williamson, Milligan, Kwan, Frankish, & Ratner, 2003). However, measurable goals and targets do have a purpose, if only as part of an accountability mechanism and to guide actions of multiple stakeholders.

*Consistent with the language of the 2004 First Ministers' statement, a pan-Canadian set of goals and targets for improving the health status of **all** Canadians should be developed by governments to cover the period of the next Accord. Once developed, each province should publish its own goals and targets, consistent with the national goals and targets, and report progress against those targets. Regional health authorities and other organizations should also consider the development of goals and targets consistent with the national goals and targets.*

Publishing goals and targets will set directions, but there will be no movement or improvement without action, and action requires allocation of resources. There is evidence that increasing public health spending yields improvement in health outcomes (Mays & Smith, 2011), and so published goals and targets need to be supported by implementation plans at national, provincial, and local levels.

## Creation of health and ill health

Some 45 years ago, then Canadian minister of National Health and Welfare, Marc Lalonde, released an eponymous report entitled *A New Perspective on the Health of Canadians* (Lalonde, 1974), which adopted public servant Laframboise's (1973) concept of four "health fields" that impact on health: human biology, environment, lifestyle, and health care organization. Developed internally within the Ministry with little external consultation (McKay, 2000), 11 of its 76 pages explicitly addressed the role for the federal government in improving health with unpublished internal government notations linking strategies to each of the four domains (scientific method, legislation, persuasion, and reorganization, respectively).

The Lalonde Report was hailed in the public health community[31] as one of the first government reports to acknowledge the government role in promoting health and the importance of factors other than medical care in improving health (Evans, 2002). The report, however, was stronger on rhetoric and analysis than as a stimulus for action, having little measurable impact on policy change (Evans, 2002; Hancock, 1986).

Thinking and research have evolved since Lalonde, stimulated in part by work of Evans and Stoddart (1990) distinguishing the physical and social environments, genetic endowment, and the individual response (in terms of both behaviour and biology), and by the development of a global health promotion movement with regular World Health Organization–sponsored global conferences on health promotion that issue declaratory statements and calls for action.[32]

Not all of the factors identified by Lalonde or Evans and Stoddart have (or should have) equal weight. Mouse model analysis suggests that genetic endowment may not be as critical as once thought; research has shown that the lifespan of a population of genetically identical mice is the same as that of a heterogeneous population, implying that genetic variation is not associated with a different lifespan (Carnes & Olshansky, 2001; Carnes, Olshansky, & Grahn, 1996). The role of the physical environment, a traditional focus of public health, has been somewhat neglected in the post-Lalonde resurgence in public health (Collins & Hayes, 2010), despite the potential to harness social interest in environmental issues to address what Masuda, Poland, and Baxter (2010) call "environmental health justice."

Evans and Stoddart (2003) acknowledge that a weakness of their original model is that it did not emphasize interacting effects: for example, the impact of the physical environment is mediated by the socioeconomic environment or the family. The physical environment may determine *available* food choices, but these are generally mediated through culture and family (Jackson, 1985; Richard, Gauvin, & Raine, 2011) and influenced by friendship networks (Fletcher, Bonell, & Sorhaindo, 2011). Felitti et al. (1998) have demonstrated that abuse or living in a dysfunctional household in childhood contributes directly to prevalence of so-called lifestyle conditions in adulthood: obesity, smoking, depressed mood.

Recognition of the interdependence of the factors impacting health has important consequences for health policy: It makes little sense to talk about some diseases being caused by "lifestyles" without recognizing that the choices available to individuals and families are constrained by their social, economic, and physical environments (Korp, 2008; Leichter, 2003). To determine relevant policy actions, decision makers must have clarity about the pathways of disease causation and the theoretical perspective underlying epidemiological studies (Graham, 2004; Krieger, 2001; Whitehead, 2007).

The recognition that the social and economic environments impact health status increases the complexity of developing policies to improve both average health status and its distribution. To the extent the causes of ill health are created outside the purview of *health* policy makers, health improvement strategies need to be multisectoral and enlist wider groups of stakeholders (Brownson, Haire-Joshu, & Luke, 2006). This may require new approaches to governance, balancing expert advice and engagement of citizens in whole-of-government structures (WHO Europe, 2011a). Although there has been a resurgence of epidemiological and public health practitioner interest in "social determinants," the focus has primarily been on proximal determinants and interventions rather than broad-scale macro-determinants such as taxation and urban planning policies (Putnam & Galea, 2008), or the economic, political, and cultural determinants to use Muntaner and Chung's (2008) categorization.

As was shown above, there are significant differences in health status by income. Addressing income inequality would improve health status, but the best means to do so are highly contested and the evidence base for interventions is weak or at least badly presented (Petticrew, 2007; Petticrew, Whitehead, Macintyre, Graham, & Egan, 2004; Whitehead et al., 2004). At the broadest level, political choices and events (democracy, regime instability, transition from communism) impact average health status and its distribution (Beckfield & Krieger, 2009; Catalano et al., 2011; Franco, Álvarez-Dardet, & Ruiz, 2004; Klomp & de Haan, 2009; Safaei, 2006). Political factors, such as voter priorities in a democracy, constrain policy action (Fox, 2006). Government spending, and hence potential health provision, is impacted by electoral cycles (Potrafke, 2010). The economic environment impacts mental health (WHO Europe, 2011b).

Addressing socioeconomic and environmental factors may be cost-effective (Kershaw et al., 2010; Milstein, Homer, Briss, Burton, & Pechacek, 2011): many strategies to redress health inequalities have been implemented around the world (Beach et al., 2006; Braveman, Egerter, & Williams, 2011; Collins & Hayes, 2010; Lurie, 2002; Mackenbach & Bakker, 2002) and methods to raise health issues in a whole-of-government context have been developed (Cole & Fielding, 2007; Kickbusch, 2010; Oxman et al., 2010; Snowdon, Potter, Swinburn, Schultz, & Lawrence, 2010) and implemented (Kearns & Pursell, 2011; Puska & Ståhl, 2010).

Action on socioeconomic and environmental factors requires action outside the health sector, but the health sector can facilitate this by stimulating coalitions and providing evidence of the real impact of environmental factors on health outcomes. The United States Centers for Disease Control and Prevention publishes a regular disparities report,[33] and the United States Department of Health and Human Services has published a toolkit to facilitate local action on disparities (National Partnership for Action to End Health Disparities, n.d.). Alberta Health Services also published a report on disparities in health outcomes within Edmonton (Predy et al., 2008).[34] As a first step toward building coalitions, *provinces and regional health authorities should publish regular reports on disparities in health outcomes.*

## Addressing causes

If Medicare is to be kept sustainable, the place to start is to reduce ill health, preventing both disease and consequent curative expenditure. Not every preventive intervention is socially efficient (an issue discussed further below), and so priorities need to be set. Rose (1985, 2001) contrasted two different preventive strategies: to focus on "high risk" individuals (the high-risk or targeted strategy) or to focus on shifting the burden of illness in the whole population (the population strategy). Both involve addressing causes, but the targeted strategy focuses on the causes of individual *cases* (and those cases are the ones that are targeted), whereas the population strategy focuses on the causes of *incidence*, attempting to shift the average population experience, and the causes of *causes*, focusing on changing underlying determinants. The relative cost-effectiveness of the two strategies will depend on factors such as incidence, cost and accuracy of case-finding, the cut-off point for determining the high-risk population, and the incidence of any adverse effects of the interventions (Ahern, Jones, Bakshis, & Galea, 2008; Zulman, Vijan, Omenn, & Hayward, 2008).

Unless carefully designed, a population strategy may inadvertently worsen health inequalities, as higher-income groups receive and adapt to population-wide messaging (or interventions) while lower-income groups adapt more slowly or miss out altogether (Frohlich & Potvin, 2008). This has been the experience of some interventions: tobacco reduction being the most notable example, where the decline in smoking prevalence has been greatest among higher socioeconomic status groups. However, it is not inevitable (McLaren, McIntyre, & Kirkpatrick, 2010), and population interventions can focus on shifting both the average (mean or median) and the distribution (Benach, Malmusi, Yasui, Martinez, & Muntaner, 2011).

Swerissen and Crisp (2004) distinguished four levels of health promotion interventions: individual level, organizational, community action, and institutional change (see Table 3.3).

**TABLE 3.3**
**Typology of health promotion interventions**

| Intervention level | Intervention strategies |
|---|---|
| Individual | Focus on information, modelling, education and training to promote individual change in knowledge, attitudes, beliefs, and behaviour about health risks, such as smoking, eating, and physical activity |
| Organizational | Focus on organizational change and consultancy to change organizational policies (rules, roles, sanctions, and incentives) and practices that produce changes in individual risk behaviour; greater access to social, educational, and health resources that promote health |
| Community action | Focus on social action and social planning to create new settings (organizations, networks, partnerships) to produce change in organizations and redistribute resources that affect health |
| Institutional change | Focus on social advocacy to change legislative, budgetary, and institutional settings that affect community, organizational, and individual levels of social organization |

Source: Swerissen and Crisp (2004).

A focus on the individual level involves the least challenge to existing power structures and is most consistent with a view that the principal causes of ill health are in the "lifestyle" domain, to use the language of the Lalonde Report. There are also parallels with Rose's dichotomy: organizational, community action, and institutional change interventions are almost inevitably about changing incidence, although strategies to change incidence might also focus on individual-level behaviour change (e.g., education campaigns to reduce smoking). Targeting high-risk individuals almost by definition focuses on the individual level.

The different levels of intervention differ in terms of their sustainability. Programs focused on the individual can be implemented quickly but might require ongoing resources to be sustained. Organizational, community action, and institutional change initiatives may take longer to implement, but once implemented may be self-sustaining as a program ("program sustainability" is Swerissen and Crisp's [2004] term). Interventions at the different levels also differ in terms of their impact. Swerissen and Crisp (2004) argue that programs targeted at the individual level have a low impact on behavioural outcomes, especially if the socioeconomic environmental factors that contribute to adoption of the behaviours are not addressed. In contrast, interventions at the other levels can have a high impact on individual behaviour (e.g., banning smoking in workplaces or restaurants). None of this analysis suggests that one level of intervention is best as each has its strengths and weaknesses (e.g., institutional change interventions take longer to implement and are likely to encounter significant opposition). What this does show, though, is the importance of focusing at multiple levels.

## Influencing obesity

The prevalence of obesity continues to increase in Canada: from 15.8 percent of the adult population in 2005 to 17.1 percent in 2007–08, a statistically significant increase (Public Health Agency of Canada & Canadian Institute for Health Information, 2011). The prevalence of obesity in Canada varies by region, income, and race. Obesity was estimated to cost the Canadian economy $4.6 billion in 2008, up from $3.9 billion in 2000 (Public Health Agency of Canada & Canadian Institute for Health Information, 2011).

The worldwide increasing prevalence of obesity (Finucane et al., 2011) is the current century's favourite health *cause célèbre*. A PubMed search of articles with the word *obesity* in the abstract or title revealed about 100,000 articles; about 4,000 of those were added in the 1970s, 7,500 in the 1980s, 15,000 in the 1990s, and 53,000 in the last decade. The acceleration of interest continues with more articles added since 2010 than in the 1990s.

The increased prevalence has been described as an epidemic (Starky, 2005), a pandemic (Spanier, Marshall, & Faulkner, 2006), a crisis (Dyment & Bell, 2008), and a tsunami (Anand & Yusuf, 2011). But there are also skeptics, such as Chiolero and Paccaud (2009, p. 568) who colourfully refer to the "obesity epidemic booga booga." Behind the hyperbole, there is a real issue: the prevalence of obesity has been increasing although there are signs of a plateauing (Rokholm, Baker, & Sørensen, 2010). Obesity increases the risk of mortality (Abdullah et al., 2011) and morbidity (Luo et al., 2007; Visscher & Seidell, 2001), and increases first-order direct and indirect health-care costs (Katzmarzyk & Janssen, 2004; Michaud, Goldman, Lakdawalla, Zheng, & Gailey, 2009; Withrow & Alter, 2011). Whether reducing obesity actually reduces net health costs in the long term is a moot point (van Baal et al., 2008), but the increased prevalence of obesity alone could reverse the secular trend of increasing life expectancy and lead to a decline in life expectancy in the United States (Manton, 2008; Olshansky et al., 2005; Reither, Olshansky, & Yang, 2011).

As obesity is essentially determined by the balance between physical activity and caloric intake (Bleich, Cutler, Murray, & Adams, 2008), obesity is often quickly framed as the result of individual "lifestyle" choices (Korp, 2008) or indeed as a "sinful behaviour" (Barry, Brescoll, Brownell, & Schlesinger, 2009), with consequent policy prescriptions focusing on changing that behaviour (Adler & Stewart, 2009). But food intake is influenced by supply and advertising (Swinburn et al., 2011) and by environmental factors, especially the social environment, including the social environment in childhood (Felitti et al., 1998). Obesity spreads in social networks (Christakis & Fowler, 2007; Cohen-Cole & Fletcher, 2008; Fowler & Christakis, 2008;

Trogdon, Nonnemaker, & Pais, 2008), suggesting that it exhibits some of the characteristics of a (socially) communicable disease, to the extent that obesity and poor fitness could be labelled as contagious (Carrell, Hoekstra, & West, 2011). In a sense this is not surprising for as Fowler and Christakis (2008, p. 1404) point out, "People are interconnected, and so their health is interconnected."

Wansink (2002, p. 90) appropriately laments the "lost lessons from World War II" when famous social scientists Margaret Mead and Kurt Lewin led action research to change *family* eating patterns in order to change United States' food consumption. A recent systematic review of dietary and physical activity interventions (Greaves et al., 2011) reaffirmed the importance of the social environment, concluding that

> interventions to promote changes in diet and/or physical activity in adults with increased risk of diabetes or cardiovascular disease are more likely to be effective if they a) target both diet and physical activity, b) involve the planned use of established behaviour change techniques, c) *mobilize social support*, and d) have a clear plan for supporting maintenance of behaviour change. (p. 10, emphasis added)

The physical environment also impacts both intake and activity, to the extent that some environments can be described as "obesogenic" (Giskes, Van Lenthe, Avendano-Pabon, & Brug, 2011). Land use affects obesity (Frank, Andresen, & Schmid, 2004), and so smart urban design can encourage people to walk (Durand, Andalib, Dunton, Wolch, & Pentz, 2011). Community engagement strategies should be part of local obesity prevention strategies (King, Gill, Allender, & Swinburn, 2011).

The Canadian Population Health Initiative of the Canadian Institute for Health Information, and the Institute of Nutrition Metabolism and Diabetes of the Canadian Institutes of Health Research, convened a "policy round table" in 2003 to identify actions to address obesity in Canada. Although there was a strong "more research is needed" flavour to the proceedings (Canadian Population Health Initiative, 2003), the round table recognized that causes of obesity are multifactorial and proposed actions in schools, urban design and transport, and industry. The Canadian Heart Health Strategy and Action Plan (2009) has also taken a multisectoral approach identifying the importance of creating "heart health" environments.

Despite this recognition of the importance of multisectoral action, to date, Canadian policies to address obesity have focused on lifestyle interventions (Alvaro et al., 2011). These policies should be supplemented to create a more balanced portfolio (Hawe & Shiell, 1995) involving strategies to address the causes of causes (to use Rose's language) and the other levels of interventions in Swerissen and Crisp's framework. A range of legislative and policy interventions is feasible in Canada (Eisenberg, Atallah, Grandi, Windle, & Berry, 2011).

There is increasing interest around the world in using economic incentives (such as taxes and subsidies) to influence the quantity and type of food intake (Gortmaker et al., 2011; Leicester & Windmeijer, 2004; Madore, 2007; WHO Europe, 2006), including use of incentives on both consumers and providers (van Rijnsoever, van Lente, & van Trijp, 2011). As Bhattacharya and Sood (2011) point out, this "is a complicated and controversial topic, filled with tradeoffs, and an area where uninformed tinkering with public policy can have unexpected and in some cases undesirable results" (p. 155).

Canada has already dipped its toe into the water in this arena with the lifestyle-oriented Children's Fitness Tax credit (von Tigerstrom, Larre, & Sauder, 2011). The research evidence on the efficacy of economic incentives on food intake is somewhat mixed (Cash & Lacanilao, 2007; Snowdon et al., 2010); for example, incentives to increase fibre may result in increased sugar and fat intake (Nordström & Thunström, 2009). The argument for a targeted tax on sugar-sweetened beverages is stronger (Brownell et al., 2009), partly because there is a clear dose-response relationship between additional intake and body mass index (Mattes, Shikany, Kaiser, & Allison, 2011). *The Canadian Health Services Research Foundation should be tasked to review the evidence on the use of tax incentives to promote public health objectives, including the case for a targeted tax on sugar-sweetened beverages.*

In addition to the health-promoting benefits of targeted taxes, the additional tax revenue would help to improve the long-term sustainability of public sector health care.

Changing tax policy will not be easy: the stakeholders involved in the production and distribution of sweetened beverages will likely react in line with the expected impact on consumption (Brownell & Warner, 2009). However, public opinion has shifted on taxation of cigarettes and regulation of smoking environments, and public support could be garnered for changed tax policies related to sugar-sweetened beverages.[35] To gain public support, activists and decision makers need to promote metaphors that emphasize the environmental influences on food consumption and combat the "sinful behaviour" metaphor (Barry et al., 2009), and overcome those interests and factors that have led Canada's obesity policies down the mono-causal, individual "lifestyle" path (Alvaro et al., 2011).

### Reducing smoking

In parallel with similar trends around the world, there has been a remarkable decline in tobacco smoking rates in Canada, from around 25.2 percent of the population smoking in 1999 to 17.5 percent in 2009 (Reid & Hammond, 2011). Unfortunately this rate of decline is not continuing, with the rate in 2008 (17.9 percent) not statistically significantly different from the 2009 rate.

Although there is little evidence to suggest that the remaining smokers are "hard core" smokers, less likely to quit, tobacco control policies should not be "more of the same" (Chaiton, Cohen, & Frank, 2008).

Tobacco consumption varies by education (6 percent of university graduates were daily smokers in 2009 versus 19 percent among people who did not complete secondary school). New smokers are young, with smoking prevalence declining from around 20 years of age. About one sixth of all deaths in 2002 in Canada were attributable to smoking, leading to over half a million life years lost (Baliunas et al., 2007).

The social context of smoking is increasingly recognized (Poland et al., 2006), and tobacco control is one field where there has been a strong take-up of regulatory (including economic) interventions to reduce smoking prevalence. Legislative interventions, such as banning smoking in public places, have reduced smoking and exposure to second-hand smoke (Callinan, Clarke, Doherty, & Kelleher, 2010; Naiman, Glazier, & Moineddin, 2011). Similarly, in terms of economic interventions, both subsidies to quit (Reda, Kaper, Fikrelter, Severens, & van Schayck, 2009) and increased taxes have been shown to be successful in reducing smoking (DeCicca & McLeod, 2008). Despite this, increasing tobacco tax is somewhat controversial because of the impact of high taxes on smuggling and contraband tobacco (Breton, Richard, Gagnon, Jacques, & Bergeron, 2006; Galbraith & Kaiserman, 1997; Gruber, Sen, & Stabile, 2003), the regressivity of increased tobacco taxes (Gospodinov & Irvine, 2009), and a possible link between higher tobacco taxes and obesity (Sen, Entezarkheir, & Wilson, 2010).

Revenues from a legal settlement with tobacco companies in the United States have been used to fund tobacco control programs that have been successful in reducing smoking (Farrelly, Pechacek, & Chaloupka, 2003; Wakefield & Chaloupka, 2000). California is the stand-out example in North America in terms of implementing a successful comprehensive tobacco control program, achieving smoking prevalence of 13.3 percent in 2008 (compare Canada's 17.9 percent in that year), increasing smoking cessation (Messer et al., 2007), and reducing daily cigarette consumption (Al-Delaimy et al., 2007) and smoking-related mortality (Barnoya & Glantz, 2004; Fichtenberg & Glantz, 2000). Comprehensive cancer control programs are still yielding benefits (Rochester et al., 2010), and new strategies to reduce smoking prevalence are being implemented regularly. Canada's approach to cigarette-labelling control may now be falling behind more aggressive approaches being taken in other countries such as Australia (Freeman, 2011; Miller, Quester, Hill, & Hiller, 2011; Mir et al., 2011). *Federal, provincial, and territorial leaders should commission an evaluation of the existing Canadian Strategy for Cancer Control and recommend how it might be enhanced to reduce smoking prevalence further.*

## What are viable interventions?

Obesity and tobacco consumption are, of course, not the only critical public health issues. The field of public health is a dynamic one, and what is conventional wisdom about appropriate public health interventions changes as new knowledge and new technologies emerge (the future for screening provides a case in point, see Esserman, Shieh, & Thompson, 2009) and potential legislative interventions become viable (Wong, Pawson, & Owen, 2011).

What should be the criteria used in setting priorities for health promotion interventions in the future? Consistent with a focus on sustainability, at least one criterion should be value for money: that the costs of the intervention are worth the benefits.[36] Although at first blush it might seem obvious to assume that "prevention is better than cure" as prevention "has an aura of omnipotence and good sense" (Gérvas, Starfield, & Heath, 2008, p. 1997), not every preventive intervention is cost saving, or indeed meets reasonable cost-effectiveness thresholds (Russell, 2009). Prevention is a slippery concept: what was seen as a risk factor to be prevented a decade ago is seen as a disease to be treated today (Starfield, Hyde, Gervas, & Heath, 2008).

There are challenges to the use of standard cost-effectiveness criteria based on robust high-level evidence in public health (Kelly et al., 2010), but there is now an extensive literature evaluating the cost-effectiveness of preventive interventions (Rush, Shiell, & Hawe, 2004) or, at least, their financial impact (Aldana, 2001). Certainly, economic evaluation has a place in setting priorities for public health interventions (Banta & de Wit 2008; Grosse, Teutsch, & Haddix, 2007; Phillips et al., 2011; Shiell & McIntosh, 2006; van Gils, Tariq, Verschuuren, & van den Berg, 2011).

A registry of over 2,500 cost-effectiveness studies exists that includes information on prevention.[37] Cohen, Neumann, and Weinstein (2008) showed that the distribution of cost-effectiveness ratios (cost per quality-adjusted life year) for preventive interventions was similar to that for treatment interventions: as with treatment interventions, preventive interventions could be cost-saving (*Haemophilus influenzae* type B vaccination of toddlers, one-time colonoscopy screening for colorectal cancer in men 60–64 years old), could cost small amounts for each quality-adjusted life year (screening newborns for medium-chain acyl-coenzyme A dehydrogenase deficiency), or could be quite expensive (screening all 65-year-olds for diabetes as compared with screening 65-year-olds with hypertension for diabetes) or indeed a waste of money.

In a major Australian study, Vos, Carter, et al. (2010) identified a range of interventions that were cost-effective in the Australian context. These were further subdivided into interventions with a "large" impact on population health in terms of disability-adjusted life years prevented, and interventions with a "moderate" impact. The most cost-effective interventions were an increase in tobacco tax; an increase and restructuring of alcohol taxation to impose a volumetric tax above the current excise on spirits; an unhealthy foods tax; mandatory salt limits on processed food; more widespread use of three blood-pressure-lowering drugs to replace current practice; polypill to replace current practice (see Dabhadkar, Kulshreshtha, Ali, & Venkat Narayan, 2011); laparoscopic gastric banding (body mass index >35); and widespread introduction of an intensive SunSmart program. These nine initiatives were estimated to cost around A$3 billion to implement, but yield savings of over A$11 billion and lead to over 1 million disability-adjusted life years prevented.[38] Most of these cost-effective interventions are at the institutional level in Swerissen and Crisp's (2004) framework and aimed at whole-population change in Rose's (1985) framework.

The RAND Corporation performed a similar, but less comprehensive, exercise for the United States, concluding that increasing provision of five preventive services (influenza and pneumococcal vaccinations and screening for breast, cervical, and colorectal cancer) would increase health expenditures but achieve significant improvements in life years saved (Bigelow, Fonkych, Fung, & Wang, 2005). The Scottish government has also engaged in a similar process and commissioned a study of cost-effectiveness of interventions to address health inequalities in early years (Hallam, 2008).

Goldsmith, Hutchison, and Hurley (2006) undertook the only comparable Canadian study, reviewing 672 economic evaluations of possible preventive interventions, but they still described their study as a "starting point." Nevertheless, they suggested that the following five interventions have sufficient robust and consistent economic evaluations that they should be recommended for universal implementation:

- varicella (chicken pox) vaccination
- colorectal cancer screening using fecal occult blood testing
- needle exchange programs
- community water fluoridation
- day care or preschool programs

Although cost-effectiveness studies in any country can be a useful guide to decision making, cost structures vary between countries and what might be seen as cost-effective at a particular ratio of costs to benefits based on an international study may not achieve the same cost/benefit ratio in Canada (Goeree et al., 2011). Further, not every preventive intervention has been subject to economic evaluation, and this is especially the case for interventions tackling "upstream determinants of health—those in the social, physical and economic environments in which people live and work" (Shiell & McIntosh, 2006, p. 30). Economic evaluations of preventive interventions for some conditions (e.g., mental and behavioural origin) tend to be underrepresented compared to disease burden (van Gils et al., 2011). All this suggests that further work is needed, building on the work of Goldsmith, Hutchison, and Hurley (2006), before the full panoply of policies necessary to improve public health can be developed. A "spending smarter" strategy (Flood, Stabile, & Tuohy, 2008c) thus requires more information to be viable.

*The Public Health Agency of Canada should commission a comprehensive economic evaluation of potential policies to improve health status (and its distribution) in Canada and ensure that the evaluation is updated every five years.*

Consistent with its history, the *Canada Health Act* currently privileges physician and hospital services. The Act includes provision for "extended health care services … as more particularly defined in the regulations," but the requisite regulations have never been promulgated. The "extended health care services" experience gives both a positive and a negative precedent for a further change to the Act: to include "cost-effective preventive services" within the ambit of the Act.[39] In order to overcome the negative precedent (no regulations to clarify the definition), the initial legislative change could either incorporate words to the effect that cost-effective preventive services are those determined by the Public Health Agency of Canada (or some acceptable joint federal-provincial body) or leave the definition vague (as is the case with medical and hospital services). Specific preventive interventions should not be included because Goldsmith, Hutchison, and Hurley's (2006) list should be expected to evolve over time as additional studies are undertaken. Despite the difficulties of phrasing, incorporating recognition of preventive interventions within the scope of the *Canada Health Act* would have important symbolic benefits in raising the status and profile of this area.

*The Canada Health Act should be amended to include "cost-effective preventive interventions" as part of required insured services.*

# Word cloud: Building the primary care foundation

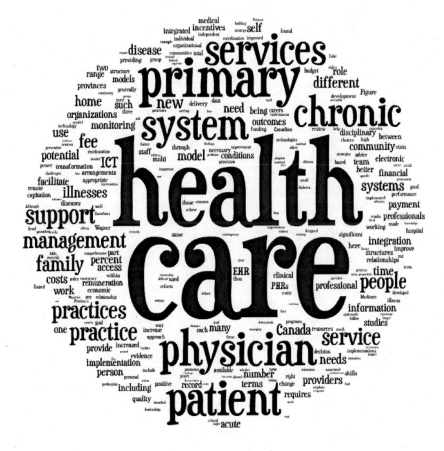

In this chapter I propose the following policy initiatives:

- Provinces should develop (or continue) programs to support quality improvement initiatives in primary care—including family practices—aimed at addressing access.
- Health Canada jointly with the Conference of Deputy Ministers should convene a regular conference of provincial telephone advisory services to facilitate exchange of information about new services being implemented by telehealth providers across the country.
- Provinces should review home care provision to ensure optimal use is being made of remote monitoring and other technologies that can enable and support community dwelling for at-risk people, including those with chronic diseases; where indicated provinces should invest in the infrastructure to allow new remote-monitoring models to be implemented.
- The federal government should make available a personal health record platform for all Canadians; all provinces should work with Health Canada to facilitate populating the personal health record with provincially held data.
- The federal government, as part of the next Accord, should provide support to the provinces to enable the transformation of primary care. Provinces should consider integration of home care and other community services with new (transformed) multidisciplinary primary care practices.
- Provinces should review their primary care funding arrangements to ensure that funding streams are adequate to allow collaborative team practice.
- Provinces should review the structure of their payment arrangements for family physicians to ensure that they incorporate the right set of incentives for care of patients with chronic illnesses including the ability to support self-management, community-level interventions, and the optimal division of labour.
- Provinces should give consideration to shifting responsibility for physician services budgets to regional health authorities.
- Provinces should give consideration to pilot programs of primary care budget holding and to the alternate policy direction, development of integrated care organizations.

# CHAPTER 4

# BUILDING THE PRIMARY CARE FOUNDATION

Make a mental picture of the health system. More than likely you thought of a hospital, and certainly most media imagery is of these high-tech citadels. But most Canadians' experience of health care is of the primary care system. In 2007–08 an estimated 22,098,339 people, 79 percent of Canadians, visited a physician.[40] In the same year, there were 2,778,445 hospital discharges, about one tenth the number of people visiting a doctor.[41] Unfortunately, neither data source is "pure": physician visits, which include visits to specialists, are estimated from a community survey about the number of people visiting a physician, and the hospital data are based on the number of discharges, but these are the best data available.

The primary care system is not only important because of the volume of interactions: a good primary care system can make a big difference to the health of the population, the functioning of other "downstream" parts of the system, and costs of health care (Engström, Foldevi, & Borgquist, 2001; Kringos, Boerma, Hutchinson, van der Zee, & Groenewegen, 2010; Starfield, Shi, & Macinko, 2005). Furthermore, primary care is equity enhancing (Rasanathan, Montesinos, Matheson, Etienne, & Evans, 2011; Sanders, Baum, Benos, & Legge, 2011).

Starfield (1992) defined primary care as

> the means by which the two goals of the health services system—optimization of health and equity in distributing resources—are balanced. It is the basic level of care provided equally to everyone. It addresses the most common problems in the community by providing preventive, curative, and rehabilitative services to maximize health and well-being. It integrates care when more than one health problem exists, and deals with the context in which illness exists and influences people's responses to the health problems. It is care that organizes and rationalizes the deployment of all resources, basic as well as specialized, directed at promoting, maintaining and improving health. (p. 4)

This is a normative and aspirational statement: more a goal than a reality in Canada today. But a good primary care foundation is essential for the functioning of the whole health care system. Investing in primary care should therefore be a priority for health system development.

The four main reviews of the literature on primary care over the last decade (Engström et al., 2001; Friedberg, Hussey, & Schneider, 2010; Kringos et al., 2010; Starfield et al., 2005) have shown a consistent pattern of findings from numerous studies:

- There is a positive association between the proportion of health care resources allocated to primary care and public health outcomes; for example, on comparing different states in the USA, an increased availability of primary care doctors was found to be significantly associated with lower mortality rates.[42] Similar results have been shown for other health status measures.
- There is a positive association between the adequacy of features of primary care and the provision of preventive services.
- Primary care provision seems to offset some of the effects of (neighbourhood) income inequality.
- Increased supply of primary care physicians was associated with lower total cost of health services.

In an international comparative study, Macinko, Starfield, and Shi (2003) showed that stronger primary care systems were associated with better health outcomes (e.g., prevention of premature mortality), after controlling for economy-wide indicators (e.g., GDP per head, physicians per head). This study judged primary care in Canada as marginally above the mean score in terms of strength of primary care (United Kingdom and Denmark rated 18 or 19 in each of three years; United States and France rated in the range of 1 to 3; Canada rated in the range of 8 to 11.5).

Not all Canadians have an identified family physician (about 15 percent do not), and not all family practices provide the comprehensive care seen as a hallmark of primary care. There are consequences of poor access to primary care for the whole system in terms of increased use of emergency departments (22 percent increase over a two-year period) and emergency hospital admissions (32 percent increase over two years; Glazier et al., 2008).[43]

Medicare has not overcome all the problems of access to medical care in Canada. It dealt with financial barriers—a critical achievement and a necessary, but not a sufficient, step.[44] Further, the challenges facing the health care system now are not the same as those faced when the struggle for Medicare was being fought. Sixty years ago, infectious diseases were still significant, and the acute model (a person gets sick, is treated, gets better, all in short order) was the common pattern of care. Alongside that went fee-for-service as the payment mechanism, designed to reward discrete episodes of treatment. The common pattern of care is no longer one of disconnected acute episodes: chronic illnesses are now seen in everyday practice, with no corresponding evolution of the payment model.

Thirty years ago, Terris (1984, p. 327) declared that the Lalonde Report (1974) marked the beginning of a "second epidemiologic revolution," a revolution that in his mind was going to lead to the "conquest of some of the most important non-infectious diseases" in the same way that the "first epidemiologic revolution conquered infectious diseases." Unfortunately, there is no evidence yet that the conquest is complete. The predominant causes of death are deaths from chronic diseases, and the prevalence of chronic disease is increasing. For example, the age-standardized prevalence of diagnosed hypertension in Canada increased from 12.9 percent in 1998–99 to 19.6 percent in 2006–07 (Dai et al., 2010), and the prevalence of diabetes in adults increased from 6.4 percent in 2002–03 to 8 percent in 2006–07 (Public Health Agency of Canada, 2009).

The more chronic conditions a person has, the greater his or her health care use: a person with three or more chronic conditions has about three times the number of health care visits per year (see Figure 4.1).

**FIGURE 4.1**
**Rate of total health care visits in the past 12 months per 1,000 seniors, by age and number of reported health conditions**

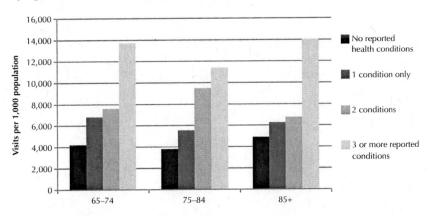

Source: Canadian Institute for Health Information (2011), *Seniors and the Health Care System: What Is the Impact of Mulitiple Chronic Conditions?* A report on findings of the 2008 Canadian Survey of Experiences with Primary Health Care.

Patra et al. (2007), in work done for the Ontario Chronic Disease Prevention Alliance and the Ontario Public Health Association, estimated the annual total direct and indirect health care costs for selected chronic diseases in Canada at over $112 billion dollars (2005 dollars, see Table 4.1).

About two thirds of the total was attributable to indirect costs (short- and long-term disability and premature mortality). The high proportion of indirect costs reflects the nature of chronic disease: short- and long-term disability is an inherent part of the condition. It also provides the basis for calls to action because the costs of chronic disease fall not only on those who have these conditions (in terms of pain, reduced mobility); there are also the economic costs of lost productivity and premature mortality to be addressed. People with diabetes who have complications, for example, are twice as likely not to be in the labour force and have 72 percent of the income of people without diabetes (Kraut, Walld, Tate, & Mustard, 2001).

Table 4.1 also highlights the significant costs associated with mental illness, with total economic costs almost twice the cost of cancers. Mental health costs are primarily driven by indirect costs, a measure of the consequences in terms of dislocation to jobs and daily living of those affected. Mental health services in Canada need reinvigorating and redevelopment (Senate, 2006), and the measures proposed in this chapter relating to chronic illness are important first steps in that regard (Andrews, 2000).

**TABLE 4.1**
**Estimated economic costs of selected chronic diseases in Canada, $million (2005 dollars)**

|  | Direct health care costs ($M) | Indirect costs ($M) | Total ($M) |
|---|---|---|---|
| Cancers | 4,433 | 13,475 | 17,909 |
| Musculo-skeletal | 4,903 | 15,739 | 20,641 |
| Cardiovascular | 7,619 | 13,024 | 20,643 |
| Diabetes | 4,234 | 5,632 | 9,866 |
| Mental illness | 10,469 | 23,389 | 33,858 |
| Respiratory disease | 3,868 | 5,665 | 9,533 |
| Total | 35,526 | 76,924 | 112,450 |

Source: Patra et al. (2007).

A health system designed for an era when infectious diseases were the major challenge will require reform to address the new and emerging needs. Decter (2007) argued,

> The reality of our time is that we are living longer, much longer, than previous generations. Yet, we are living longer not in perfect health, but with an array of chronic diseases such as diabetes, asthma, heart disease, arthritis and others. Managing those diseases well is the major challenge facing aging Canadians. Helping us manage these chronic diseases is the major challenge facing the Canadian health system. (p. xi)

## The challenge of chronic disease management

It could be argued that chronic care is different from acute care. The focus of acute care is diagnosis and definitive, time-limited treatment. Chronic disease management requires a focus on symptom management (Muenchberger & Kendall, 2010), and a longitudinal relationship, emphasizing continuity of care and trust-building (Tarrant, Dixon-Woods, Colman, & Stokes, 2010).

The principal method of paying for physicians in Canada is still fee-for-service payment, a model based on an implicit assumption that health care is a series of independent visits (or services) that should attract separate payments. Because people with chronic disease require continuity of care, a different form of reimbursement may be appropriate for physicians (an issue addressed further below).

Care of people with chronic disease also requires a team approach, drawing on the skills of a range of different health professionals (Tieman et al., 2006), and this appears to be at variance with contemporary practice. Schoen et al. (2007) reported that 30 percent of Canadians with a family doctor responded that their doctor or someone from their doctor's practice only sometimes, rarely, or never helps them coordinate care from other doctors/places.

Primary health care services in many parts of Canada have responded to these changed needs with innovative new service models,[45] but as Macgregor (2007) highlighted, there are significant gaps between the desirable standard of service provision for people with chronic conditions and the services generally available to them (Table 4.2).

**TABLE 4.2**
**The gap between needs and services for people with chronic illnesses**

| *What we think people with chronic conditions need:* | *What they often get in Canada (despite many pockets of excellence):* |
|---|---|
| Long-term, trusting relationships with a small group of people | Short-term, episodic care from people they may not know and who may not know them |
| Consistent, competent, comprehensive services | Inconsistent, incomplete services |
| Convenient, readily accessible services | Delays and inaccessible services |
| Good quality, secure health records | Minimal records, often missing when needed |
| Partnerships, and nourishment of self-management capability | Increased anxiety, and decreased confidence in the health care system |

Source: Macgregor (2007).

## System reorientation

Addressing the needs of people with chronic illnesses requires a transformation of the health system: although the rhetoric of "person-centred care" is now common, the reality is still far from that. Descriptions of the health care system often start with services available, rather than the needs of the person and his or her caregivers. Planning for the health system of the future has to start with the needs of individuals at the centre, and recognize the impact of proximal and distal environments. Figure 4.2 illustrates a way of conceptualizing the health system especially relevant in the context of care of people with chronic illnesses.

Putting patients at the centre emphasizes the individuality of each person, in terms of his or her biology, behaviour, culture, and values. Although everybody has the potential of being a patient in the immediate future, most people are healthy and want to live productive lives. Health in this sense is a "resource for living," and the health care system should support that; Breslow (2004, 2006) referred to this reorientation as the "third revolution" in health care.[46] Patients, their caregivers, and the primary care system are situated within contexts of specialty support, of community and global impacts. These broader environments affect the primary care system and the incidence of ill health, and so prevention efforts (as argued in the previous chapter) have to be multisectoral and must address issues in these wider environments (Brownson et al., 2006; Milstein, Homer, Briss, Burton, & Pechacek, 2011). The relationships between the broader environment and the health sector are reflexive: the health sector also needs to be cognizant of its impact on the physical environment and embrace "green" approaches to building design, energy consumption, recycling, and waste management (Lynch, 2011).

In Chapter 2, I proposed the following goal for the health system: *The right person enables the right care in the right setting, on time, every time.* A critical word here is *enables.* Individuals with chronic illnesses can become experts on their own conditions; the goal of the health system should be to support them in that. Not every person with chronic illnesses will be an Internet-savvy, independent learner. But the skills necessary for self-management can be taught, and people so taught have improved health outcomes whether taught in traditional face-to-face groups (Lorig et al., 1999) or via the Internet (Lorig, Ritter, Laurent, & Plant, 2006). Enabling self-management and thus empowering the person with chronic diseases, and his or her family/caregivers, is core to a patient-centred health system.

Teaching self-management should not be thought of as something that can be done by the family physician, alongside everything else, in a single patient consultation. It requires a systematic approach, with specific, articulated goals developed collaboratively (Battersby et al., 2010; Lawn et al., 2009). Not every family practice will have the skills, interest or resources to do this, which highlights the need for a system, rather than individual practice, reorientation (Oelke et al., 2009). The same argument applies to enhancing prevention in areas such as falls prevention, which involves interventions

# FIGURE 4.2: The patient at the centre of the health system

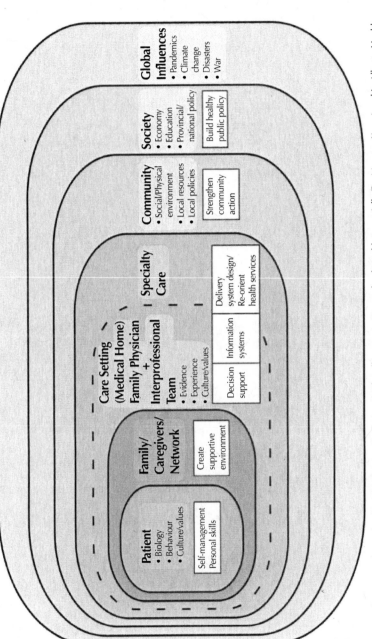

Source: This portrayal was developed following discussions with colleagues in Queensland Health (especially Dr. Maarten Kamp) and in Alberta Health Services (Heather Toporowski and Dr. Richard Lewanczuk). Our discussions drew on the work of Dr. Linda Meurer and others (from the Medical College of Wisconsin, see http://cgea.net/CGEA%20Poster%20A%20Population-based%20Model.pdf, retrieved 15 August 2011), who in turn drew on Gruen, Pearson, & Brennan (2004). Tannahill (2008) has a somewhat similar diagram, which he terms the "health improvement onion." Weaknesses in this portrayal remain mine.

at multiple levels (Freedman et al., 2006). Family practices should be able to draw on a wide range of resources to support them in their role of supporting their patients.

Oxley (2009), drawing on work by the French Inspection Générale des Affaires Sociales, found that chronic disease management interventions have better outcomes when

- providers are more integrated (e.g., in the United States' Veterans Health Administration or the Kaiser Permanente system);
- other health care personnel such as nurses, social workers, or pharmacists are integrated into the care process and follow-up; and
- programs encourage patients to change their behaviour through patient education and self-help.

Management of chronic illnesses requires a higher degree of attention to coordination of care. Powell Davies et al. (2006) reviewed 80 studies that examined interventions to improve coordination in primary care: 65 studies used health outcomes from coordination as endpoints, and 55 percent of these showed improved health outcomes (see Figure 4.3, "all

**FIGURE 4.3**
**Proportion of studies of coordination reporting positive outcomes by type of outcome and strategy type**

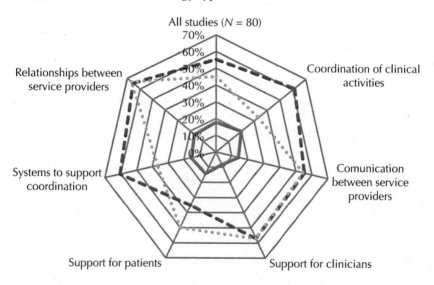

Source: Data from Powell Davies et al. (2006, p. 24).

studies" radius); 31 studies used patient satisfaction as an endpoint, with 45 percent showing improvements; and 28 studies looked at economic outcomes, but only 5 (18 percent) showed improvements. A variety of strategies can be pursued to improve coordination of care. Powell Davies et al.'s (2006) systematic review examined six types of strategies (in Figure 4.3 each designated as a separate radius), and the results for each strategy were similar to the overall study conclusions. The majority of strategies generally had positive results for health outcomes and patient satisfaction, but a positive impact on recorded economic outcomes (e.g., cost of care) was much less likely to be found.

## Wagner's chronic care model

Wagner et al. (1999) have advanced a comprehensive and multifaceted approach to system redesign appropriate for management of chronic illnesses, known as the chronic care model,[47] that is now the *lingua franca* of chronic disease management (McColl & Dorland, 2007). The model has been extensively implemented and evaluated, and implementation yields moderate beneficial effects on health outcomes (Bodenheimer, Wagner, & Grumbach, 2002a, 2002b; Tsai, Morton, Mangione, & Keeler, 2005).[48] Implementation of the Wagner model requires a system transformation, rather than establishing new specialist provider organizations for people with chronic illnesses. The latter approach appears to be less effective in management of people with chronic illnesses (Coleman, Austin, Brach, & Wagner, 2009).

The focus of Wagner's chronic care model is a "productive interaction" between an "informed, activated patient" and a "prepared, proactive practice team"; both sides of this interaction require support to be effected. In Wagner's model, support comes both from the community (in terms of resources, policies, and self-management support) and from the health system, involving improvements to the organization of health care, delivery system design, decision support, and clinical information systems.

A patient with chronic illness lives with it 24/7, and often so too does the patient's partner, family, or caregivers. Going back to the health system goal, *the right person enables the right care in the right setting, on time, every time,* the "right person" will often be a family member or other caregiver. Most care needs of a person with chronic illnesses are met within the family/caregiver home environment (Chappell, McDonald, & Stones, 2008). The role of the partner/family/caregiver is thus to create a supportive environment for the person with chronic illnesses: to make the home safe for walking around and other activities of daily living (showering, eating), and to assist with medication management and health monitoring. Helping to create a supportive environment is an important function of the health or community services system, for example, by potentially supporting home modifications or providing assistance to the caregivers, including respite care (Chappell & Hollander, 2011).

Effective self-management is more difficult in vulnerable populations and those with low health literacy (Clark et al., 2008), and supporting self-management in those populations will require tailoring of programs and interventions. In the absence of that, "chronic illness care will fall well short of desired outcomes" (Clark et al., 2008, p. S317).

The outer ellipses are relevant here too: communities that are stronger in terms of their social capital have lower use of family physicians (Laporte, Nauenberg, & Shen, 2008). Enhanced community-level prevention opportunities need to be developed. It should be as easy for a family physician to "prescribe" participation in an exercise group as it is to prescribe medication. Exercise group prescriptions of this kind have been shown to be effective in increasing walking (Isaacs et al., 2007; Lamb, Bartlett, Ashley, & Bird, 2002; Leijon, Bendtsen, Nilsen, Ekberg, & Stahle, 2008).

Besides being better care, a greater emphasis on an "enabling" or "supporting" role for the health system, rather than simply a "providing" role, is also more sustainable into the long term. As the prevalence of chronic illnesses increases, without changes to the contemporary service model, workforce requirements will increase as will costs of employment. An emphasis on supporting self-management and creating supportive environments will allow each health professional to manage a greater number of patients. Many of the ongoing care needs of people with chronic illnesses under a new model will be met by people with a narrower skill set such as health care aides, allowing other health professionals to manage an increased number of patients.

Importantly, these shifts require purposive action and support. It is not a case of the health system off-loading responsibilities onto partners, families, or caregivers. Without training in self-management, and without support to caregivers, this new approach.will fail, with resultant additional downstream costs in terms of health care utilization.

Obviously not all care needs can be met in the home, through self-management and by caregivers. Especially for people with chronic illnesses, the skills and knowledge of the primary care team are essential to support ongoing monitoring and management, deal with destabilization of the chronic illnesses, and manage acute episodes. But the primary care team of the future will be different from the historical model. The avuncular, solo practice family physician is no longer a sensible image of contemporary family practice or a viable model for the future.[49]

The skills and knowledge of the family physician need to be complemented by skills and knowledge of other professionals: nurses and nurse practitioners (often already part of family practices), professionals skilled in managing mental illness, physical therapists, dietitians, and others. Primary care teams have to work as teams, where the person with the best match of skills to the patient's problem takes the lead, where group discussion is used to bring evidence and multidisciplinary talent and experience to both individual care and addressing system issues (Taplin, Galvin, Payne, Coole, &

Wagner, 1998), and where the team is trained to function as a team (Thomas, 2011). A new range of services will need to be made available in the community including intensive case management for people with a history of high use of hospital emergency departments, self-management support, and improved support for people with chronic mental illness.[50]

A health system oriented to managing chronic illness will be structured to support longitudinal care and coordinated care, and professionals would be appropriately remunerated for that. Managing care over time is facilitated by patients having a relationship with a single provider and the converse, providers having responsibility for a panel of patients. Remuneration arrangements for physicians should encourage this longitudinal responsibility (discussed further below), and the development of "patient registers" in family practice to facilitate recall and reminder systems appropriate for management of chronic conditions (Steele et al., 2010).

Family practices and primary care teams need to be accessible to their patients to deal with acute problems that arise, and obviate use of more expensive health system resources such as hospital emergency rooms, or services that do not provide continuity of care such as "medi-clinic" type services. Email consultations can help here, although patients perceive practices that provide telephone support as more accessible (Haggerty et al., 2008). Both alternatives have a positive impact on the environment through reduced travel to appointments. Quality improvement initiatives, with an emphasis on reducing the delays for appointments with primary care providers,[51] can also demonstrably improve availability (Solberg, Hroschikoski, Sperl-Hillen, O'Connor, & Crabtree, 2004) and quality of care (Herring, 2009; Wagner et al., 2001).

All of this illustrates that improving access requires action at multiple levels of the health system: there is no magic wand that can bring about immediate and costless improvements in access. One strategy to improve access is thus to support local initiatives and local change efforts. Some provinces already have programs in place that allow physicians and other primary care team members to stand back from their daily activities, analyze the current practices in an open and trustful environment (Lanham et al., 2009), and develop and implement improvements. *Provinces should develop (or continue) programs to support quality improvement initiatives in primary care—including family practices—aimed at addressing access.*

### The role of information systems in system reorientation

Information and communication technologies (ICTs) have the potential to transform the way health care is experienced in the future. But as the OECD (2010c) has pointed out, the promise and the reality diverge:

> Today the range of possible applications of information and communication technologies in the health sector is enormous. The technology has progressed

significantly and many estimate that ICT implementation can result in care that is both higher in quality, safer, and more responsive to patients' needs and, at the same time, more efficient (appropriate, available, and less wasteful).... In the past few years, however, there has been a significant and growing debate internationally about whether or not these much touted benefits and savings can be gained or, indeed, even measured. Despite the promise they hold out, implementing ICTs in clinical care has proven to be a difficult undertaking. More than a decade of efforts provide a picture of significant public investments, notable successes and some highly publicised costly delays and failures. This is accompanied by a failure to achieve widespread understanding of the benefits of electronic record keeping and information exchange. (p. 11)

Health care may be little different from other industries: ICT implementation in many industries involves a significant divergence from forecast (or promised) performance to actual, with low rates of reported success, driven in part by poor forecasting of costs, time to complete, and potential functionality (Eveleens & Verhoef, 2010).

ICT adoption in health care is often championed by zealots (health ICT departments and enthusiastic clinicians), and this advocacy sometimes sounds as if ICT implementation is an end in itself and (immeasurable) benefits would automatically flow. This sort of "magical thinking" (Diamond & Shirky, 2008) has been evident for the last few decades. It is important to emphasize that ICT is an *enabler* of the clinical process and ICT adoption is one strategy to achieve improved clinical care: ICT is a tool, not a goal (Diamond & Shirky, 2008).

Many ICT implementations have prioritized the acute hospital environment. The technology and ubiquitous communications infrastructure necessary to facilitate implementations that crossed organizational boundaries (and especially acute to primary care boundaries) was slow to develop and to implement. These new technologies are now available and have potential to respond to contemporary challenges such as continuity in chronic disease management. Returning to our ellipses in Figure 4.2, judicious adoption of ICT can be used to support self-management and thus help to reposition primary care. Three particular applications of ICT have real transformative potential: remote monitoring, electronic personal health records, and Health 2.0.

### Telehealth

Support needs to be immediately accessible to caregivers when they need guidance and advice, and this is most efficiently done through telephone advisory services.[52] Sometimes called telenursing (Goodwin, 2007), telephone advisory services use computerized decision support algorithms, coupled with nursing skills, to provide triage and advice (Purc-Stephenson & Thrasher, 2010). Although patients who are able to speak to their family physician for urgent advice report higher satisfaction (Howard, Goertzen, Hutchison, Kaczorowski, & Morris, 2007), compliance with advice from telephone advisory services is good (Kempe et al., 2006; Marklund et al., 2007) and these services substitute for physician after-hours visits (Bunn, Byrne, & Kendall, 2004; Dunt, Wilson, Day, Kelaher, & Gurrin, 2007; Grandchamp & Gardiol, 2011). Telephone advisory services are taking on a broader range of functions, including supplementing the call-receipt functions with call-outs to follow-up patients (Wennberg, Marr, Lang, O'Malley, & Bennett, 2010) or functioning as part of preventive programs (Cantrell & Shelley, 2009; Rothemich et al., 2010). *Health Canada jointly with the Conference of Deputy Ministers should convene a regular (every second year) conference of provincial telephone advisory services to facilitate exchange of information about new services being implemented by telehealth providers across the country.*

## Remote monitoring

Remote monitoring (telehealth, remote patient management) aims to support people to remain independent in their own homes by use of monitoring technologies, either automated (e.g., sensing type and extent of movement) or through patient self-management (e.g., vital signs monitoring). Technologies may be completely automated using interactive voice recognition (Schneider et al., 2011), or health personnel may call patients. These technologies are generally designed to facilitate exception-based interventions when reported data trigger action by crossing predetermined thresholds. An extensive range of technologies is now available for use in remote monitoring, and "Smart home" programs have been developed in a number of countries (Chan, Campo, Estève, & Fourniols, 2009). Although there is some overlap in the studies included in recent systematic reviews of remote monitoring, the conclusions are cautiously positive for specific conditions and more generally, and in terms of economic analyses.[53]

The systematic reviews almost invariably call for further research. The field is developing rapidly and there is currently a "lack of national and international consensus on terminology, classification or taxonomy of devices, products or service models" (Martin, Kelly, George, McCreight, & Nugent, 2008, p. 5), no standardization of what remote-monitoring elements should be provided for which specific groups of patients (Dang, Dimmick, & Kelkar, 2009; Maric, Kaan, Ignaszewski, & Lear, 2009), and uncertainty about the best way to implement telecare and integrate it with local service delivery systems (May et al., 2011).

Remote monitoring has been described as a "disruptive technology" that has the potential to overturn existing power relationships in health care (Sinha, 2000). User needs are not always taken into account in the design of new remote-monitoring programs (Chan et al., 2009), symptomatic of what Milligan, Roberts, and Mort (2011, p. 353) describe as "an industry that has tended to be dominated by a 'technology-push' rather than engaging with the needs and experiences of older people themselves." Again, the focus has been on the technology or devices rather than how they might be used in practice to enhance self-management.

Consistent with characterization as a disruptive technology (Christensen 1997; Christensen, Grossman, & Hwang, 2009), more widespread adoption of remote monitoring will be challenging:

> Its use relies upon a reorganization of care processes that include physiologic monitoring, protocol driven decision support, newly defined roles for clinical and nonclinical providers, and telecommunications that place patients at a distance in space, and frequently time, from the providers of their care. It also relies on a disruption of the usual business model for care of chronic disease, shifting some responsibilities to the patient and nonclinical providers; reducing use of and revenues for emergency departments, hospitals, and skilled nursing facilities; and producing a net reduction in the total cost of care for chronic disease. (Coye, Haselkorn, & DeMello, 2009, p. 127)

*Provinces should review home care provision to ensure optimal use is being made of remote monitoring and other technologies that can enable and support community dwelling for at-risk people, including those with chronic diseases; where indicated provinces should invest in the infrastructure to allow new remote-monitoring models to be implemented.*

### Personal health records

The electronic health record (EHR) is the Holy Grail of health ICT initiatives, imbued with miraculous powers to improve health care efficiency and quality. Greenhalgh, Potts, Wong, Bark, and Swinglehurst (2009) summarize this vision of a technological utopia:

> According to many policy documents and political speeches, they will make health care better, safer, cheaper, and more integrated. Lost records, duplication of effort, mistaken identity, drug administration errors, idiosyncratic clinical decisions, and inefficient billing will be a thing of the past. (p. 730)

EHR implementation is often implicitly seen as a necessary foundation for wider application of ICT in the health sector (Bower, 2005; Shekelle, Morton, & Keeler, 2006), including introduction of clinical decision-support systems that improve practitioner performance (Garg et al., 2005), although the extent of improvement may in some cases be only marginal (Romano & Stafford, 2011). However, this is an area of linguistic confusion. The following meanings are used here: an *electronic medical/health record* is an electronic repository of health information owned by a medical practice (electronic medical record) or other health facility or service (electronic health record) for storage of its information (Häyrinen, Saranto, & Nykänen, 2008); in contrast, a *personal health record* (PHR) is an individual's record, often partly populated by data drawn from an EHR, to which the patient has access and can add information.

Tang, Ash, Bates, Overhage, and Sands (2006, p. 121) describe the differences:

> While EHR systems function to serve the information needs of health care professionals, PHR systems capture health data entered by individuals and provide information related to the care of those individuals. Personal health records include tools to help individuals take a more active role in their own health. In part, PHRs represent a repository for patient data, but PHR systems can also include decision-support capabilities that can assist patients in managing chronic conditions. Most consumers and patients receive care from many health care providers, and consequently their health data are dispersed over many facilities' paper- and EHR-based record systems.

Once implemented, EHRs can provide the mechanism for a range of service-enhancing capabilities including electronic decision support. The literature on EHRs and their implementation is immense. Greenhalgh et al. (2009) identified 24 systematic reviews, covering hundreds of primary studies, from a range of disciplinary backgrounds. Their conclusion contrasted the assumptions underpinning the most recent ICT implementation in the United Kingdom with their findings from the literature:

> The (UK program) appeared to be built on six assumptions, that the EHR (1) is primarily a container for information about the patient; (2) can be integrated seamlessly and unproblematically into clinical work; (3) will increase the effectiveness and efficiency of clinical work; (4) will drive changes in how staff interact with the patient and one another; (5) should replace most, if not all, forms of paper record, which are old-fashioned and limited; and (6) the more comprehensive and widely distributed it is, the more value it will add. Much of the literature covered in this review suggests, conversely, that (1) the EHR may be alternatively conceptualized as an "itinerary," "organizer," or "actor"; (2) seamless integration of different EHR systems is unlikely because human work will always be needed to bridge the model-reality gap and recontextualize knowledge for different uses; (3) while secondary work (audit, research, billing) may be made more efficient by the EHR, primary clinical work is often made less efficient; (4) the EHR may support, but will not drive, changes in the social order of the workplace; (5) paper will not necessarily disappear, as it offers a unique level of ecological flexibility (although workable paperless systems have been developed in one or two centers); and (6) smaller, more local EHR systems may often (though perhaps not always) be more efficient and effective than larger ones. (p. 767)

The summary of UK assumptions is probably equally valid for Canadian ICT implementations. Although there are some outstanding counter examples,[54] Canada is a laggard in EHR implementation, with a number of identified weaknesses in strategy implementation (Office of the Auditor General, 2010; Rozenblum et al., 2011). ICT investment has often been viewed as discretionary or focused on maintaining existing systems. Big visions for national EHRs, requiring significant investment, have failed to be delivered. But consistent with Greenhalgh et al.'s (2009) findings, EHR progress is probably more likely to be via slow, steady, and small incremental implementations, rather than these grand plans and national strategies.[55]

Although EHRs provide an important foundation, PHRs have more direct and obvious impacts on health care processes. The transformation of the health care system necessary to support patient self-management will be facilitated by PHRs. Further, because of the access to the additional information that PHRs will bring to patients, there will be a consequential enhanced ability of patients to take a more active role in managing their condition.

The current state of PHRs is evolving as new applications are developed and implemented. Applications to remind people about medications, or to track and estimate medication adherence, for example, by comparing expected time to refill prescriptions with actual repeat time (Schneeweiss & Avorn, 2005), would be simple to develop. These applications could have a significant benefit in terms of increased medication adherence, which has been shown to be associated with a reduction in overall health systems costs (Encinosa, Bernard, & Dor, 2010; Roebuck, Liberman, Gemmill-Toyama, & Brennan, 2011; Stuart et al., 2011). If patients expect access to PHRs, this may put pressure on physicians and other health providers to adopt EMRs/EHRs as feeders into PHRs, thus in turn helping to accelerate EMR/EHR implementation.

The evidence-base of some implementations is weak (Goldzweig, Towfigh, Maglione, & Shekelle, 2009), but PHRs are at the early stage of development and the potential to improve the patient centredness of many implementations exists (Reti, Feldman, Ross, & Safran, 2010). A number of health systems have recognized the importance of PHRs and other "patient focused" ICT applications in patient empowerment and have commenced implementations or pilots, often using platforms developed by corporate giants, such as Microsoft's HealthVault (Do, Barnhill, Heermann-Do, Salzman, & Gimbel, 2011; Liao, Chen, Rodrigues, Lai, & Vuong, in press; Steinbrook, 2008).

In Canada, the Romanow Report (Commission on the Future of Health Care, 2002) recommended "establishment of personal electronic health records for each Canadian" (p. 76). More recently, Alberta Health Services (2009) has also explored the implications of PHRs. Importantly, the context of Alberta Health Services' exploration was a service-improvement focus, rather than an ICT application-driven approach. Specifically, Alberta Health Services' goal was phrased as ensuring "access to a personal electronic health record for anyone with diabetes, which will include their personal care plan and allow them to monitor and track their condition, within 18 months." It was expected that PHRs would be available to the whole population over time. The approach also started with an intent to operate over multiple settings and with multiple users, incorporating new generation technology to escape from the institutional orientation of existing systems.

PHRs have the potential to be truly transformative: reducing duplication of tests and investigations, providing an electronic underpinning and support for patient self-management, and facilitating a shift in power from provider to consumer.

Although adoption of consistent information-transfer standards can help to address portability, there is a potential role for the federal government in providing a common expression of Medicare in twenty-first-century terms through a national PHR platform. Existing federal ICT funds could be re-prioritized to achieve this goal.

*The federal government should make available a personal health record platform for all Canadians; all provinces should work with Health Canada to facilitate populating the personal health record with provincially held data.*

## Health 2.0

The Internet is transforming many aspects of social interaction and has the potential to do the same in health care (Laing, Hogg, & Winkelman, 2004). Following Hughes, Joshi, and Wareham (2008), Health 2.0 can be defined as "the use of a specific set of Web tools (blogs, Podcasts, tagging, search, wikis, etc.) by actors in health care including doctors, patients, and scientists, using principles of open source and generation of content by users, and the power of networks in order to personalize health care, collaborate, and promote health education."[56] Web 2.0 technologies can facilitate a "location independent" health system where patients anywhere can obtain assistance and advice from any other web user or web-accessible provider.

A characteristic of Web 2.0 is its decentralized (or democratic) nature; people can post contributions regardless of their scientific expertise. This creates two bases for tension in Health 2.0: patients may follow accurate advice obtained from the web without involvement of their health care providers, or they might follow inaccurate advice (Hughes et al., 2008). However, patients find these tools valuable (Frost & Massagli, 2008), and health-related Web 2.0 sites are mushrooming (Swan, 2009). The decentralized nature of Health 2.0 means that coordinating or directing roles for government or health services are not viable. Nevertheless, health providers should encourage use of these sites, host them where feasible, and help patients to evaluate the accuracy of information gained from websites, blogs, social networks, and the like. Providers can also make use of the feedback potential from the sites (Adams, 2011).

## Aligning organizational structures and financial incentives

The Canadian health care system as we see it today is the clear descendent of the health system of 60 years ago, familiar to Tommy Douglas and his colleagues when they developed the Saskatchewan antecedents of Medicare. The health issues then were not the same as they are today (Houston, 2002), nor are the treatments. Remuneration levels for physicians have improved (Duffin, 2011), but the primary care structures of relatively small, autonomous, family physician practices, operated on a private basis with fee-for-service reimbursement, have been a constant. Not that physicians necessarily want to maintain fee-for-service as the principal remuneration model: alternative models of reimbursement are growing both in terms of number of physicians and proportion of physician remuneration (Wranik & Durier-Copp, 2009).[57]

Tommy Douglas saw the introduction of Medicare and the removal of financial barriers to access as being the first of a two-phase reform process. The second phase was to include change to the delivery system, including primary care restructure through an emphasis on group practice (Douglas, 1979).

Transforming primary care to reposition it so it better addresses contemporary health needs has implications and impacts beyond primary care. The relationships between family practice, community services, and acute care all need to change.

So what needs to be done? In brief, the organizational structures of care delivery need to be changed to facilitate better care coordination and minimize information loss or discontinuities as patients pass from one health professional or service to another, and the financial incentives on providers and organizations have to be aligned with the new models. Organizational structure choices involve two dimensions: size and disciplinary nature of practices ("delivery structure"); and whether practices have broader responsibilities beyond primary care ("scope"). There are therefore three main axes where transformation might occur. Figure 4.4 shows examples of possible service delivery choices aligned on each axis. There are a total of 60 possible combinations (4x5x3), some more realistic than others. The points on the axes are not organized so that the outermost point is unequivocally better than the other points.

### Delivery structures

The first dimension where transformation is taking place is in delivery structure. Traditionally, primary medical care was delivered in physician-owned solo practices. Over the last few decades, average practice size has increased, and by 2007 most (50.7 percent) of physicians were in a group practice.[58] Whether this transformation has gone far enough is a moot point: smaller practices are less likely to support elements of a new model of care associated with best practice chronic disease management (Rittenhouse et al., 2011). Care of people with chronic illnesses requires access to a range of professions, and in 2007 almost one quarter of family physicians worked in multidisciplinary practice settings (23.5 percent). Most (74 percent) family physicians did not have formal arrangements with specialists with whom they collaborated.

**FIGURE 4.4**
**Dimensions of structural transformation in primary care**

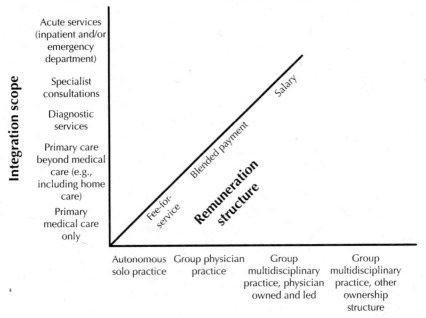

**Delivery structure**

Two alternatives for multidisciplinary practice settings are shown, distinguished by ownership. This is a contentious area, as many physicians jealously guard their autonomy and role as "leader" of the health care team (McColl & Dorland, 2007), and physician ownership of practices might be seen as essential for this. However, alternative ownership models exist, in Canada and elsewhere, including ownership by universities, health services, and private corporations. Community health centres, with local boards of directors, are another model of multidisciplinary practice that typically emphasizes a broad approach to primary care, including concern for social determinants of health (Albrecht, 1998; Hutchison et al., 2001; Hutchison, Levesque, Strumpf, & Coyle, 2011). Different ownership models are associated with different practice patterns, for example, in take-up of clinical preventive services (Provost et al., 2010).

Multidisciplinary practice is used here neutrally, but there is a range of different ways in which multidisciplinary working can occur. Boon, Verhoef, O'Hara, and Findlay (2004) array team working along a continuum from the weakest model ("parallel" working, where each professional works side by side in a common setting), through consultative, collaborative, coordinated, multidisciplinary, and interdisciplinary models to integrative practice with "a seamless continuum of decision-making and patient-centred care and support."

Multidisciplinary involvement is essential in enabling good care for people with chronic conditions, and increasingly that is being provided from within the primary care practice. But the move from a primary medical care delivery structure to a multidisciplinary one involves challenges and adaptations by all concerned. Bélanger and Rodríguez (2008) identify four key challenges in implementing new multidisciplinary practice models:

- the need for investment of time and resources in team building
- development of locally appropriate working structures and shared goals
- development of clear roles and effective communication mechanisms
- agreement on power sharing

The latter two points are particularly apposite. In an environment where different professionals have different sets of skills, knowledge, and expertise, shared leadership—"the law of the situation" as Follett (1926) would describe it—is critical. But how does shared leadership work? Who is accountable (professionally and/or legally) for the work undertaken? Physicians often feel that they have ultimate legal accountability and in many cases expect a "task assigning role relationship"[59] in working with other professionals, where other professionals are accountable to them. Other health professionals also value their autonomy and want a "task initiating role relationship"—to exercise their independent professional judgment within different accountability structures, expecting physicians to refer patients to them.

Physicians also may have a particular conceptualization of what a team means, and how it works, that is at variance from the views of other team members:

> For most of us, the model of teamwork is baseball, where a collection of well-paid superstars are judged by personal performance with occasional situational collaboration, like a double play. We accept the football model of teamwork, where one individual directs an unquestioning cadre of supporters with special skills toward the goal line, only when we are the quarterbacks heading a team of non-peers. But where in medicine do we follow a basketball model of teamwork, in which a collection of peers appropriately takes responsibility as dictated by the situation, then relinquishes it in a similar manner? That sort of teamwork is critical to the effectiveness of many organizations, yet it does not fit the psychological makeup of most physicians. (Mayer, 1999, p. 16)

In small work settings, especially in physician-owned practices or in smaller, rural communities, informal relationships and employer-employee relationships help to minimize conflicts. But in larger practices, and where staff may be seconded from other organizations, clarity of roles, relationships, communication mechanisms, and power is essential. Negotiating these new roles will be difficult (Solberg et al., 2004). It will take time (Bélanger and Rodríguez's first point above), trust and respectful relationships (Lanham et al., 2009), and acknowledgement of the potential for "reciprocal learning" (Leykum et al., 2011). As Nutting et al. conclude,

> Transformation to team-based care requires that primary care physicians and other health professionals envision new roles for themselves and that practices incorporate new paradigms of how best to care for patients. Both of these challenges are more difficult than anyone had imagined. (2011, p. 441)

Although such challenges add to the pressures already underway on family physicians (Beaulieu, Rioux, Rocher, Samson, & Boucher, 2008), multidisciplinary practice has to be the future for primary care in an era of chronic disease. Coordinated and comprehensive care requires close working relationships (College of Family Physicians of Canada, 2009), best promoted by co-location and working with a defined group of patients.[60] All the adaptation will not fall on primary medical care: other health providers will also need to adapt.

Adequate home care is critical to a system designed to support people with chronic illnesses (Tsasis & Bains, 2009), and expansion of services and transformation is required here, too. The need for close working relationships between home care providers and family physician practices has long been recognized. There are incremental steps that can be taken here:

- Work of home care staff can be organized to strengthen the relationships between groups of staff and particular family physician practices.
- Home care staff could be co-located with practices.
- Home care staff could be seconded to practices.
- Home care staff could be employed by practices.

Consideration might also be given to changing the roles of home care staff. Should home care staff follow patients under their care into acute settings when the patients have acute episodes? The home care staff might continue to provide the care they previously provided for their clients in the home setting. This sort of initiative would facilitate continuity of care between hospitals and home care, including ensuring continuity of medication management (Bell et al., 2011), and home care staff are probably more able and likely to act as patient advocates in the acute setting.

Strengthening links with (transformed) primary care practices will facilitate a more community-based orientation to care: Wagner's chronic disease model relies on supportive communities (for resources, policies, and self-management support). Stronger and more activated communities[61] also allow community-based preventive strategies, such as walking groups to encourage exercise. Integrated primary care services, providing home care and other services, will not only facilitate continuity of care but also increase the visibility of primary care in the community and thus help to remind communities of the availability of primary care services. As people become more oriented toward primary care services, they will be less likely to turn to hospitals. Primary care services could thus evolve from atomized, small, discrete services to services reaching whole communities. This could also foster local action to address the social determinants of ill health.

Nutting et al.'s (2011) evaluation of implementation of "medical homes" found that

> transformation is more than a series of incremental changes.... To become medical homes, practices need to see themselves as organizations that apply the four pillars of primary care to the needs and preferences of patients in their communities, rather than as organizations that process patients for the convenience of physicians. As collaborative care teams are established and services are better coordinated across the larger health care neighborhood, structures and processes within practices need to encompass a broader set of proactive, population-based, integrated activities for patients, groups of patients, and eventually entire defined populations. For most practices, this represents a major paradigm shift. (p. 441)

These transformational shifts will not occur overnight, or without support. In addition to change-management support, new physical investment may be required. *The federal government, as part of the next Accord, should provide support to the provinces to enable the transformation of primary care. Provinces should consider integration of home care and other community services with new (transformed) multidisciplinary primary care practices.*

Development of teams in primary care requires funding streams to support the new team members. Primary care teams have the potential to be cost saving (Roblin, Howard, Becker, Adams, & Roberts, 2004) and provide services equally acceptable to consumers as traditional physician delivery with similar outcomes (Mundinger et al., 2000). These funding streams can be special (capitated) grants to family practices, secondment arrangements of health authority employees, or access to independent funding arrangements (akin to alternate relationship plans) for new classes of professionals (e.g., nurse practitioners).

*Provinces should review their primary care funding arrangements to ensure that funding streams are adequate to allow collaborative team practice.*

### Remuneration structure

Remuneration choices are, as Grogan (2011, p. 643) points out, not simple technical choices but also political and "philosophical":

> Under any insurance scheme, public or private, the payer must determine how to best structure provider payments. This question at first blush appears quite mundane. Indeed, payment policy is often discussed in highly technical terms.... Such discourses suggest the answer is difficult to find but ultimately lies deep in a data set if only it can be unearthed. Of course if we pause and look again, we realize that a host of important philosophical questions underlie this deceptively simple question about payment.

Preferences for particular modes of remuneration (such as fee-for-service) can be held quite strongly with heated and vocal opposition to attempts to change remuneration structure. This may be one reason why change occurs so slowly in this area. However, as Fuchs (1998, p. 60) points out, it is a "common mistake to think that the behaviour of physicians can be understood only in terms of their desire to maximize income." Fuchs lists other motivators as peer approval, patient approval, and providing quality care; Allard, Jelovac, and Léger (2011) add altruism as a factor. Physicians are also influenced by work-family/leisure trade-offs.

Notwithstanding these other motivators, income and financial reward influence physician behaviour. Financial incentives on providers work! And how those financial incentives are structured can facilitate good models of practice or inhibit them (Allard et al., 2011; Chaix-Couturier, Durand-Zaleski, Jolly, & Durieux, 2000; Conrad & Christianson, 2004; Gosden et al., 2001; Greß, Delnoij, & Groenewegen, 2006; Sarma, Devlin, Belhadji, & Thind, 2010). Remuneration design involves choices along three dimensions:

- the source of information as remuneration can primarily rely on characteristics of the patient (e.g., capitation systems), the provider (e.g., in salaried arrangements), or the interaction/service provided under fee-for-service;
- the breadth of the payment (how much bundling); and
- the number of categories (Ellis & Miller, 2008).

There are a limited number of ways of combining these dimensions and paying for primary care, and family physicians in particular. Robinson (2001, p. 149) provocatively summarizes the state of the evidence:

> There are many mechanisms for paying physicians; some are good and some bad. The three worst are fee-for-service, capitation, and salary. Fee-for-service rewards the provision of inappropriate services, fraudulent upcoding of visits and procedures, and the churning of "ping-pong" referrals among specialists. Capitation rewards the denial of appropriate services, the dumping of the chronically ill, and a narrow scope of practice that refers out every time-consuming patient. Salary undermines productivity, condones on-the-job leisure, and fosters a bureaucratic mentality in which every procedure is someone else's problem.

Fee-for-service is particularly inappropriate in primary care dominated by chronic illnesses. By its very nature fee-for-service rewards episodic care, rather than a long-term-care relationship with a person with chronic illnesses. Fee-for-service remuneration can also act as a disincentive to the use of other health professionals such as nurse practitioners (DiCenso, Bourgeault, et al., 2011). When Medicare was first designed, it incorporated the then dominant funding method for physicians: fee-for-service practice, and that has remained. Fee-for-service rewards output, but there is increased questioning of whether this goal should be the principal one pursued, as "flat of the curve medicine" or diminishing marginal returns from additional health care activity become more prevalent (Weinstein & Skinner, 2010).

In contrast to standard fee-for-service, other remuneration methods with different incentive effects can lead to improved health outcomes. For example, Tu, Cauch-Dudek, and Chen (2009) showed that capitated physicians had better results in terms of management and control of hypertension compared to salaried or fee-for-service physicians. In Ontario, Glazier, Klein-Geltink, Kopp, and Sibley (2009) found comprehensiveness of care better and emergency department visits fewer in enhanced fee-for-service practices compared with capitation. Kantarevic, Kralj, and Weinkauf (2011) found that enhanced fee-for-service achieved better productivity than the standard fee-for-service approach.[62]

It is for these reasons that "blended payments" are increasingly recognized as the appropriate structure for remuneration in primary medical care (Grignon, Paris, & Polton, 2002, 2004; Léger, 2011; Naccarella et al., 2008; Nasmith et al., 2010; Simoens & Giuffrida, 2004). Initially, blended payments involved a mix of the three main types of reward systems: fee-for-service, capitation, and salary. Fee-for-service, for example, might be retained for care out-of-hours, capitation components to measure practice size, and salary to provide a base guarantee. Initially, practices may have autonomy in adopting their proportion of funding from each source, but where evidence is strong, payment policy should follow and incent the desired payment mix. Transition to blended payments needs to be managed carefully because in Ontario implementation appeared to lead to windfall gains to physicians (Glazier & Redelmeier, 2010).

*Provinces should review the structure of their payment arrangements for family physicians to ensure that they incorporate the right set of incentives for care of patients with chronic illnesses including the ability to support self-management, community-level interventions, and the optimal division of labour.*

Increasingly, remuneration structures and blended payments involve some form of pay-for-performance (P4P), either on the individual family physician or more commonly on the family practice. Under pay-for-performance arrangements, financial incentives can be structured to reward achievement of specified targets (such as the proportion of patients in practice who have been immunized). But the more comprehensive the targets are, and the more they reward all aspects of desirable practice, the more complex the blended payment arrangements become, and the more difficult they are to administer and to describe to those affected (Robinson, Shortell, Casalino, & Rundall, 2004). P4P relies on good measurement of the indicators being rewarded (and appropriate risk adjustment); there are weaknesses here (Nicholson et al., 2008), and so implementation obstacles for P4P abound (McDonald, White, & Marmor, 2009).

The theory underpinning P4P is sound, and there is certainly evidence that P4P arrangements lead to improvements in health processes or outcomes[63] and that physicians see merit in use of some indicators (Burge, Lawson, & Putnam, 2011). However reviews of P4P studies are still showing mixed results (see Table 4.3).

**TABLE 4.3**
**Conclusions of systematic reviews of pay for performance**

| Study | Conclusion |
|---|---|
| Town, Kane, Johnson, and Butler (2005, p. 237) | The evidence hints that small rewards will not motivate doctors to change their preventive care routines. |
| Petersen, Woodard, Urech, Daw, and Sookanan (2006, p. 265) | Five of the six studies of physician-level financial incentives and seven of the nine studies of provider group–level financial incentives found partial or positive effects on measures of quality. One of the two studies of incentives at the payment-system level found a positive effect on access to care, and one showed evidence of a negative effect on access to care for the sickest patients. |
| Rosenthal and Frank (2006, p. 151) | The empirical foundations of pay for performance in health care are rather weak. Among the health care studies … reviewed, many of those with the strongest research designs yielded null results with only two positive findings. |
| Christianson, Leatherman, and Sutherland (2008, p. 305) | The findings regarding the impact of purchaser P4P initiatives on quality measures are somewhat equivocal. |
| Tanenbaum (2009, p. 718) | The scholarly literature on P4P in health care offers little evidence that paying providers to meet specific performance indicators significantly improves the quality of care. |
| Conrad and Perry (2009, p. 365) | Properly designed, selective financial incentives can improve quality of health services on the dimensions of structure, process, and outcome. |

Note: P4P = pay for performance.
Source: Author's review of published studies. Conclusions are direct quotes.

New models of P4P are emerging that address some of the weaknesses of earlier models (Rosenthal, 2008). P4P will therefore have a continuing place in physician (or practice) reimbursement (Naccarella et al., 2008), but it should not be relied on as the sole strategy to drive improvement in primary care.

## Getting there from here

Who gets what is the stuff of politics, and so remuneration policy could be expected to be highly contentious. Physicians and physician organizations value "professional control" almost above everything else (Blishen, 1969). The founding bargain of Medicare had as its objective "to find a way of combining publicly supported universal coverage with the true essentials of professional freedom" (Taylor, 1978, p. 323). In reality, this meant that "organised medicine was able to improve the economic position of its members even while it preserved the contractual system of remuneration and private practice, protected the role of physicians at the centre of the healthcare system, and prevented major changes to primary healthcare" (Marchildon & Schrijvers, 2011, p. 222).

Not only did fee-for-service payment continue as the dominant payment mode, "professional freedom" was further operationalized as a requirement that payment levels and relativities be negotiated with the profession. The *Canada Health Act* enshrines this requirement for negotiations but goes further to enhance the power of professional organizations by requiring provinces to establish arbitration processes

> for the settlement of disputes relating to compensation through, at the option of the appropriate provincial organizations ... conciliation or binding arbitration by a panel that is equally representative of the provincial organizations and the province and that has an independent chairman; and that a decision of (such) a panel ... may not be altered except by an Act of the legislature of the province. (s. 12 (2)(b) and (c))

This cession of power is an example of the "profession-state accommodation" that now characterizes the Canadian health care system (Tuohy, 1999). The original fee negotiations were about fee levels, with volume unconstrained and not part of the negotiating frame. With the economic crunch of the early 1990s, provinces have adopted various forms of expenditure caps, either on individual physicians or on spending on physicians in total (Barer, Lomas, & Sanmartin, 1996; Hurley & Card, 1996; Katz, Charles, Lomas, & Welch, 1997).

Although differential fee rises for different items or different specialties had always been part of fee negotiations, the global expenditure caps introduced a new zero-sum dynamic into fee negotiations. Consistent with the "professional freedom" basis of the profession-state accommodation, intraprofessional distribution of fee increases was generally ceded to the professional associations, leading to significant intraprofessional conflicts (Katz et al., 1997). This in turn stimulated some interest in moving away from fee-for-service payment as the dominant payment mode:

> Some Canadian physicians now see fee-for-service payments as a hindrance to attempts to resolve economic disputes between physicians. Linking incomes to the volume of care discourages individual physicians from taking responsibility for total costs. These economic incentives may aggravate poor physician relations by producing unstable conditions that may increase work but decrease incomes. In contrast, capitation and vertical integration may decrease friction within the profession in two ways. First, capitation could limit wide variation in levels and growth of physician incomes and increase the stability of the hourly

workweek. Second, vertical integration across health sectors might provide physicians an opportunity to limit expenditures for hospitals, laboratories, and pharmacies while maintaining physician incomes. (Katz et al., 1997, p. 1428)

However, the shift from fee-for-service has been glacially slow, and any carve out from the global physician services budget to establish new alternate payment plans needs to be endorsed by the relevant provincial physician organization. Although shifting the arena for intraprofessional fee disputes to one managed by the profession itself has some political benefits, it also has downsides. The interests of the profession and government/health system/ public are not necessarily coincident. If the health system is to be reoriented toward primary care, that has the corollary of a reorientation away from specialist care. The cohesive interest of a minority group of stakeholders can be easily harnessed (Easton, 1979) and can be used to block proposals for redistribution (e.g., ophthalmologists in British Columbia successfully blocked fee reductions for cataract operations; see Katz et al., 1997).

Responsibility for negotiations on the funder side is usually vested in the provincial ministry of health, with regional health authorities as a possible second-tier partner. After the negotiations are concluded, budget responsibility remains with the ministry. In turn this means that priority setting within a regional health authority does not encompass physician services' expenditure, limiting choices and potentially excluding sensible trade-offs between physician and non-physician (e.g., nurse practitioner) expenditure, and acute medical versus preventive interventions. *Provinces should give consideration to shifting responsibility for physician services budgets to regional health authorities.*

Although enlightened leadership in physician associations may accept the need for system reorientation, such leadership cannot be guaranteed in every province, every year. Even if it could, the leadership may not be able to ensure that the broad membership of the physician association endorses a negotiated reform proposal. On the other side of the negotiation table, the desire to conclude an agreement may lead to a focus on the big issue of the size of any remuneration lift, sidelining discussions on structural change to remuneration to facilitate system reform.[64]

The structure of remuneration is one of the critical policy levers that drive reform of the health care system. The Canadian accommodation, where use of this lever is attenuated by passing through physician organization processes, potentially weakens and slows the necessary system reorientation.

## Integration model

Primary care is not an island unto itself. It is a gatekeeper or gate opener to a range of other services including community services (such as home care), diagnostic services, specialist medical services, and acute services. A good relationship between primary care and these other services is critical to the provision of high quality and efficient health care. Many authors have argued the benefit of integration across the care continuum of primary care services, specialist services, and hospital services, and there are many different models for integration (MacAdam, 2008). Ham (2010, p. 81) for example recommends, as one of the ten characteristics of a high-performing health system, that "care should be integrated to enable primary health care teams to access specialist advice and support when needed." "Integration," and related terms such as "coordination," "continuity," and "partnerships" can, however, have a number of meanings (El Ansari, 2011). Singer et al. (2011) reinforce this pointing out that organizational integration and integration of care are two distinct concepts. Integration of care is difficult, especially if it involves more powerful strategies such as funds pooling or common assessment processes (Leutz, 1999, 2005); this is also why Figure 4.4 shows a continuum of options. Challenges to integration are many (Armitage, Suter, Oelke, & Adair, 2009), with few reported successes, possibly because the evaluation task is difficult (Bravo, Raiche, Dubois, & Hebert, 2008). Further, organizational integration is neither necessary nor sufficient to achieve integrated care. Organizational incentives and restructuring is only one of the strategies that might be pursued to improve integration of care.

Softer strategies to facilitate integration include co-location, discussed above in regard to home care but relevant to a range of services: co-locating specialist physicians on a visiting basis in larger primary care services would have a range of benefits (including ease of secondary consultations for other health professionals and easier physical access for patients) and would be a visible demonstration of moving toward a primary care–led model of service delivery. Co-location of specialist services would also facilitate family physicians' working to their top scope of practice.

Most provinces have moved part way toward integrated structures with the development of regional health authorities that typically incorporate hospital and community services. However, physician services typically remain outside these structures, in autonomous practices. A number of provinces have established regional groupings of primary care practices.[65] This approach has merit as a reform direction by itself (Naccarella et al., 2008; Russell, Hogg, & Lemelin, 2010; Scott & Hofmeyer, 2007), as well as providing the potential for integration with the acute sector. Further, as proposed above, *provinces should consider integration of home care and other community services with new (transformed) multidisciplinary primary care practices.*

But organizational integration, as contemplated in the development of integrated care organizations, goes beyond multidisciplinary practice to integrate primary and acute care; this step has generally not been taken in Canada to date.

Ham (2010, p. 79) identified as another characteristic of a high-performing health system that "priority is given to primary health care." Given the political profile of acute health services, and the career trajectories of the leadership of many health systems, it is unlikely that organizational integration would by itself achieve the system reorientation necessary.

Organizational integration naturally evolves to include development of some elements of managed care, use of guidelines, second opinion review and so on. Physicians generally view these tools unfavourably, especially when imposed exogenously (Deom, Agoritsas, Bovier, & Perneger, 2010). But the norms of practice developed within some high-performing integrated systems in the United States (Kaiser Permanente, Geisinger), which emphasize the role of the physician group in managing its own performance (Paulus, Davis, & Steele, 2008; Weber & Joshi, 2000), seem to overcome some of the traditional antipathy to these approaches.

The alternative to organizational restructure as a means of coordination is the use of financial levers to achieve integration and responsiveness of downstream services to primary care. Use of financial levers requires the ability to specify the desired outcomes, or what is to be purchased (Williamson, 1975, 1986), and this is increasingly possible for all aspects of health care.

New policies in United Kingdom rely on the use of financial levers to transform the health system (Roland & Rosen, 2011). Under the most recent proposals, much of the budget of the National Health Service will be controlled by primary care organizations that will purchase ("commission" is the term used in England) downstream services.[66] Putting budgets in the hands of the primary care system certainly has the potential to increase responsiveness of downstream services, as well as putting incentives on the primary care organizations to be more judicious in their referrals.[67] However, the evidence from the English experience with "commissioning" is mixed (Le Grand, Mays, & Mulligan, 1998; Mannion, 2011).

In a Canadian context, budgets could be held by individual practices, by organizations of practices, or by new, multidisciplinary organizations created for this purpose.

It is not necessary that all referral services be treated in the same way; the third axis of Figure 4.4 highlights the different choices that might be made if a budget-holding model were to be pursued. At its simplest, the primary care organization or practice could assume responsibility for other aspects of primary care such as home care. Moving beyond primary care, the next step might be for budget holding for diagnostic services including diagnostic imaging and laboratory testing.

Introduction of budget holding by primary care organizations would be a dramatic demonstration and commitment to system reorientation; however, it would disrupt existing power structures and for that reason alone could prove difficult to implement. In addition there are considerable technical issues that would need to be addressed as part of implementation. For example, choices would need to be made about who would be the budget holder (individual practices or larger groupings), and different choices here would yield different incentive effects. Small entities would probably not have the skill sets required to manage budget holding. Reasonable budgets would need to be established, taking into account the mix of patients for which the primary entity is responsible.

Experience in other countries can inform the choices that might be made here; even in the United States where capitation has been in place for many years, there is still room for improvement in the design of the capitation or risk-adjustment systems (Frogner, Anderson, Cohen, & Abrams, 2011). To the extent that there is inadequate risk adjustment, a capitation system can be exposed to moral hazard, adverse selection, and gaming (Arrow, 1963).

Nevertheless, budget holding has the real potential to drive creation of a much more responsive, primary care–led health system. *Provinces should give consideration to pilot programs of primary care budget holding and to the alternate policy direction, development of integrated care organizations.*

## Where to next?

The need to invest in, and change the shape of, primary care is well recognized. A number of provinces have started that process (Hutchison et al., 2011). But progress is uneven. Hutchison et al. (2011, p. 282) conclude their review of primary care transformation in Canada with faith that laggard provinces "will likely follow the leaders, each in its own way and in its own time." They trace the stimulus for the transformation to actions taken at the national level in the early 2000s. The slow progress of reform in some provinces (which were exposed to the same stimuli) suggests that the existing mechanisms to facilitate policy transfer are not working, hence the proposals in this chapter for a stronger federal role in providing an electronic patient record platform and funding to facilitate transition to the new models.

# Word cloud: Ensuring access to (the right) drugs, technologies, and innovations

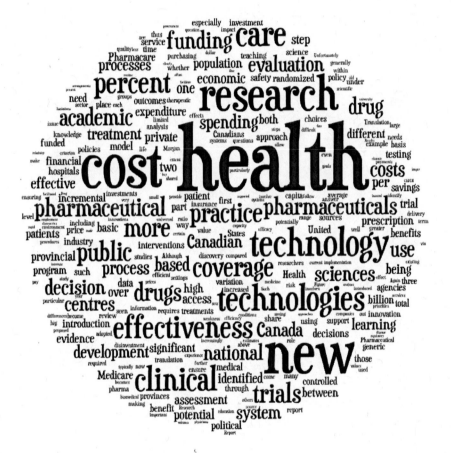

In this chapter I propose the following policy initiatives:

- Prescription pharmaceuticals should be an insured service under Medicare. Federal, provincial, and territorial leaders should, as soon as possible, commission an independent study of the most practicable way of introducing prescription pharmaceuticals as an insured service under Medicare, and consider that report as part of the negotiations of the 2014 Accord renewal.
- The Canadian Institutes of Health Research should assess on a regular basis the impact of funded health research.
- Each academic health sciences centre should identify its relative strengths and publish its research priorities, level of research investment, and outcomes of research at least every three years.
- Academic health sciences centres should review their teaching practices to identify the extent to which they reflect and encourage inefficient practice. Academic health sciences centres should document, and publicize to their students, how the centres' research leads to improvements in efficiency in the delivery of care.
- Academic health sciences centres should plan to become the centres of learning health care systems.
- Federal, provincial, and territorial leaders should task and fund the Canadian Agency for Drugs and Technologies in Health to establish the capacity (and advisory processes) to undertake a rolling program of reviews of potentially obsolescent health technologies. Provincial health technology assessment agencies should develop complementary programs for evaluation of disinvestment opportunities.

CHAPTER 5

# ENSURING ACCESS TO (THE RIGHT) DRUGS, TECHNOLOGIES, AND INNOVATIONS

The health sector environment is one of rapid change, especially in available drugs and technology to use in treatment. One would think that it would therefore be adept at responding to this environment and exhibit dynamic efficiency (Ghemawat & Ricart I Costa, 1993). At the treatment level this is true. But at the systems level, structures and policies have been slow to adapt. The most notable instance of this is that Medicare is still limited to its two initial components: hospital and medical services. There has been no expansion of the definition of "comprehensive" care to include pharmaceuticals and home care, despite a myriad of reports recommending this. Mechanisms to evaluate new technologies are also inconsistent across the country. If health care in Canada is to be sustainable, then it needs to ensure that the right investments are being made, and that new technologies (including drug technologies) are being appropriately evaluated prior to their introduction. Unfortunately, this is not currently happening.

### Expanding coverage for pharmaceuticals

At its foundation, Medicare did not make explicit provision to eliminate financial barriers to access to pharmaceuticals outside hospitals. As a result, provinces have highly variable programs of addressing drug coverage, with differences in groups eligible for subsidies, in copayments, in whether there is any safety net or maximum copayment, and in premiums (Gagnon, 2010). People with significant chronic conditions and pharmaceutical needs may face financial hardship to pay for care, relocate to ensure better long-term coverage, or be admitted or stay longer in hospitals simply to obtain drug treatment under hospital Medicare coverage.

In 2009 pharmaceutical expenditure accounted for about one sixth of total health expenditure, disproportionately from private sources, with private expenditure comprising almost two thirds (62 percent) of pharmaceutical expenditure compared to less than one third of total health expenditure.[68] The private share of pharmaceutical expenditure is split evenly between insurance and out-of-pockets. About 6 percent of the public share is from the federal government, with almost all the public share balance from provincial government sources.

The pharmaceutical share of total health spending has grown markedly over the past 25 years from 9.5 percent in 1985 to 16.4 percent in 2009, with public funding taking an increased share of pharmaceutical spending (29 percent to 38 percent), but even so, pharmaceuticals have taken up an increased proportion of total private spending (27.5 percent to 34.1 percent). High private shares of expenditure can lead to financial barriers to access, especially given the uneven distribution of illness and pharmaceutical use. About 10 percent of Canadians did not fill prescriptions or skipped doses in the previous year because of cost problems (Schoen et al., 2010). The Kirby Report (Senate, 2002a) supported "the view that no Canadian should suffer undue financial hardship as a result of having to pay health care bills" and went on to assert that "it is essential that this principle be applied to prescription drug expenses" (p. 125).

Hanley and Morgan (2009) found that 5 percent of the population accounted for almost half of ambulatory prescription use. These high users were more likely to be older, female, and low income than the rest of the population.

Patterns of spending on pharmaceuticals differ across Canada with an almost 50 percent variation in per capita (total) spending (see Figure 5.1). Canadian average spending was $893 per head, ranging from $714 in British Columbia to $1,057 in Nova Scotia. The public share of spending ranged from 29 percent in Newfoundland and Labrador and in New Brunswick to 47 percent in Saskatchewan, with territory public shares being over 50 percent.

Although some of the difference in per capita (total) spending is driven by differences in the age and gender of the provincial population, even after standardizing for those factors, residents of British Columbia spent 27.6 percent less per head than the Canadian average (see Figure 5.2). This difference was primarily driven by lower prescription volumes (30 percent less than Canadian average) and a different pattern of pharmaceutical prescribing (choosing different therapeutic classes and different choices within therapeutic classes), yielding an 8 percent lower weighted effect, although these effects were partly offset by larger average prescription sizes (Gagnon, 2010). The main drivers for the differences between provinces are prescription volumes and size. In only one province (Newfoundland and Labrador) did the combined price and therapeutic class effects account for more than a 10 percent variation in per capita spending.

## FIGURE 5.1
## Per capita spending on pharmaceuticals, 2009, by province, source of funding and type of pharmaceuticals

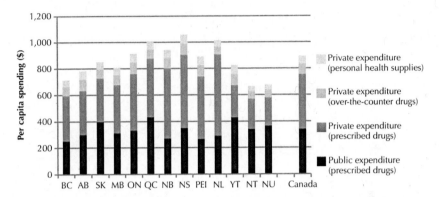

Source: Canadian Institute for Health Information (2010a), *Drug Expenditure in Canada 1985 to 2009.*

## FIGURE 5.2
## Source of variation in per capita total spending on pharmaceuticals, 2007

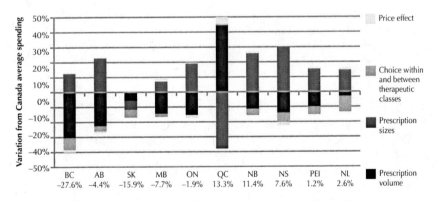

Source: Derived from Gagnon (2010, Table 2.1).

Quebec spends just over 13 percent more on pharmaceuticals than would be expected given its demography, with a significantly greater number of prescriptions (45 percent), partly offset by smaller sizes of each prescription (38 percent). This significant variation in patterns of use (prescription volumes especially) shows there is unfulfilled potential for interprovincial learning in strategies to influence prescriber behaviour and control of pharmaceutical expenditure generally (Chafe et al., 2011; Pomey, Forest, Sanmartin, De Coster, & Drew, 2010). Even though price variation is small, there is also the potential to harness the combined purchasing power of all the provinces (Law & Morgan, 2011) as part of the development of a more equitable pharmaceutical system for Canada.

Pharmaceutical policy generally covers three main elements: ensuring safety and efficacy, ensuring equitable access, and ensuring responsible prescribing. Canada, nationally, is still missing the last two elements, despite a commitment in the 2004 Health Accord to address this. Pharmaceutical policy is often supplemented by industry development policies promoting pharmaceutical manufacture or industry-funded research, with the two potentially in conflict (Lehoux, Williams-Jones, Miller, Urbach, & Tailliez, 2008; Vandergrift & Kanavos, 1997). Again, Canada does not have national policies in this area, but several provinces have developed industry-support programs.

Gagnon's (2010) conclusion of the overall Canadian position on pharmaceutical provision is sobering:

- We spend more per capita on drugs, the costs of which are growing faster than elsewhere.
- Our public plans are inequitable because they do not provide suitable coverage to a large portion of the population.
- The meagre industrial benefits in the biopharmaceutical sector are totally out of proportion with the money given by Canadians in various privileges to the industry.

He goes on to argue for the establishment of a national Pharmacare program. Gagnon's model incorporates first-dollar coverage, citing Tamblyn et al.'s (2001) study of the effect of copayment changes in Quebec that found increased adverse events and emergency department use following increased copayments for pharmaceuticals. Gagnon's proposed national Pharmacare involves a combination of balancing elements, including more efficient purchasing and assessment processes for inclusion of pharmaceuticals into the coverage formulary. Hollis and Law (2004) showed that a single national formulary of itself would be cost saving. The Common Drug Review processes in place go part way toward this (Morgan, McMahon, & Mitton, 2006) but inefficiencies remain, principally because of intraprovincial variation (Tom Noseworthy, personal communication, 7 August 2011).

Canada pays more per unit for both patented medicines and off-patent items compared to comparable countries (other than Switzerland, home of many Big Pharma companies), paying around 10–15 percent more for patented drugs than France, Italy, and the United Kingdom and more than twice what Sweden pays for generic drugs (see Table 5.1).

**TABLE 5.1**
**Average relative unit prices for pharmaceuticals, compared to Canada, adjusted using market exchange rates**

| | Canada | France | Italy | Germany | Sweden | Switzerland | United Kingdom | United States |
|---|---|---|---|---|---|---|---|---|
| Patented drugs, 2010 | 1 | 0.90 | 0.87 | 1.2 | 0.98 | 1.03 | 0.86 | 1.91 |
| Generic drugs, using pharmacy acquisition cost, 2008 | 1 | 0.73 | 0.7 | 0.62 | 0.42 | 1.12 | 0.54 | 0.57 |

Source: Patented Medicine Prices Review Board (2011a, 2011b).

There is clear room for improvement in prices paid: Canada's regulatory regime for generic manufacturer access seems designed to inflate prices (Hollis, 2010). Non-price mechanisms, such as support for evidence-based therapeutic choices (Morgan, 2004) and review of "off-label" use of drugs (Wyatt & Black, 2011), should also be part of an efficient policy mix. Other writers have identified other desirable innovations to get better value for Canada's public pharmaceutical expenditure. Grootendorst and Hollis (2011), for example, come to the following conclusions:

- Bulk purchasing and reference pricing policy have numerous advantages for all Canadians compared to the practice of best price policies by some provinces.
- Innovation in important clinical areas can be encouraged and accelerated using approaches such as a pay-for-performance reward model, subsidizing the costs of pharmaceutical research and development (both basic research and clinical trials), and considering all sources of value in health technology assessment.
- Reimbursement of generic drugs using a sliding scale and granting a royalty to the first generic firm would allow market forces to set the price of generic drugs and promote timely generic competition. The use of tendering can also effectively drive generic price down.[69]

Addressing appropriate use of pharmaceuticals will be challenging. Canadians, for example, are exposed via television to United States' direct-to-consumer advertising of therapeutic products (and diagnostic tests), which leads to increased take-up of advertised products in ways that may be inconsistent with professional guidelines (Price, Frank, Cleary, & Goldie, 2011).

Gagnon (2010) estimates that his proposal for a universal Pharmacare program with no copayments is likely to increase pharmaceutical utilization by 10 percent. However, he also identified offsetting savings from reduced dispensing fees, more rigorous listing processes (modelled on the processes used in British Columbia), and reduced administrative and purchasing costs from economies of scale. Pharmaceutical pricing in many provinces is also used as part of industry policy, to attract and retain either research or manufacturing capacity. If industry support were eliminated, and the other identified savings strategies implemented, Gagnon estimates that introduction of universal Pharmacare would lead to savings of around $10.7 billion, around 42 percent of current pharmaceutical expenditure.

Gagnon (2010) identified three other scenarios for national Pharmacare implementation, involving different industry development policies; all scenarios involve net cost savings ($2.7 billion to $4.5 billion). Even if some of Gagnon's estimates are incorrect, it is probably safe to assume that a national Pharmacare system could be introduced in a sustainable manner.

An alternative design has been advanced by Busby and Robson (2011) who proposed social insurance to support the Ontario drug benefit program, although this model will not garner the savings that Gagnon (2010) identified as flowing from a national approach. Morgan and Willison (2004) have identified other options for catastrophic coverage, as did the Kirby Report (Senate, 2002a).

Implementing Gagnon's first-dollar coverage approach would entail significant redistribution of funding from private to public sources, and potentially from provincial to federal spending. Gagnon (2010) recognizes these difficulties in implementation:

> Let's not be naive: establishing a national, universal drug plan providing first-dollar coverage is not a simple matter. Government funding, even when lower than comparable private spending, is often extremely difficult to justify publicly. A national Pharmacare program will have to find a balanced approach to ensure coherence across the country while respecting provincial health jurisdictions. But these are not insurmountable obstacles. Quite the contrary. A clear policy backed by real political will would allow all Canadians to have equal and universal access to the best treatments available, while generating substantial savings over the current plans. The analysis in this report shows that the only hindrance to establishing a fair, effective drug insurance program is political apathy, not economic or cost restraints. (pp. 68-69)

It is not just "political apathy" that would militate against adoption of Gagnon's proposals but significant opposition from vested interests, especially those who benefit from existing arrangements that produce higher prices (Evans, 2010), as well as ideological opposition to any proposals to increase public funding.

However, there may be ways to make national Pharmacare more politically feasible. A significant portion of private spending on pharmaceuticals is mediated via employment-related (private) insurance arrangements, a cost to businesses that provide this coverage as part of their employment benefits. By reducing these employment costs, a national Pharmacare scheme could (marginally) improve the competitiveness of Canadian employers in certain industries the same way Medicare does (Monk, 2008), and thus potentially offset industry vested interests.

In 2009, Canadians spent about $25.4 billion on prescribed medications, of which $11.4 billion was from public sources, $9.4 billion from private sources via insurers, and $4.6 billion as out-of-pockets. A potential modification of Gagnon's model would be to see prescription medication become an insured service under Medicare, establishing a national formulary and purchasing system. Private insurance for prescriptions would no longer be necessary (saving the public $9.4 billion), and provincial "prescription" premiums would be introduced to generate approximately $9.4 billion, leaving provision for copayments. This would still represent a significant expansion of public funding and of federal standardization, but the increased public sector role would come with a funding source and be at no net cost to the public (although there would be distributional effects).

There would be other options of a similar kind. The premise here, though, is that the absence of systematic coverage of pharmaceuticals is a significant weakness for the Canadian health care system and needs to be remedied. Whatever the model adopted, a national Pharmacare program should be introduced. The historical legacy of a Medicare that simply focused on physicians and hospitals should no longer continue to define the nationally consistent health care program.

The 2004 *10-Year Plan to Strengthen Health Care* (Health Canada, 2004) recognized that "the founders of Medicare a half-century ago established the principle of equity of access to hospitals and doctors' services for all Canadians. First Ministers agree that no Canadians should suffer undue financial hardship in accessing needed drug therapies." But the relevant section, entitled "National Pharmaceuticals Strategy," only included a commitment for further study of issues of access: "to develop, assess and cost options for catastrophic pharmaceutical coverage." Gagnon's (2010) analysis shows that a national pharmacare program can be introduced in a fiscally responsible way. What is now required is detailed work on whether Gagnon's model should be introduced or whether some other model should be preferred. Further action on this issue beyond the 2014 Accord is not warranted.

*Prescription pharmaceuticals should be an insured service under Medicare. Federal, provincial, and territorial leaders should, as soon as possible, commission an independent study of the most practicable way of introducing prescription pharmaceuticals as an insured service under Medicare, and consider that report as part of the negotiations of the 2014 Accord renewal.*

### Research and innovation

The year 2010 was the centenary of the publication of Flexner's trans-formational review of medical education in North America (Flexner, 1910; Kirch, 2010; Markel, 2010). Flexner's model of a scientific basis for medical education and practice has created a legacy of complex relationships and tensions between the organizations responsible for academic preparation of physicians (and other health professionals) and those with primary respon-sibility for clinical service delivery.

For the health system to achieve dynamic efficiency, it must embrace—and be structured to facilitate—worthwhile innovation. It must exhibit a cul-ture that encourages "efficiency-enhancing" innovations, not just advanced medical technologies (Lambooij, Engelfriet, & Westert, 2010). Across multiple research themes or pillars (biomedical; clinical; health systems and services; and social, cultural, environmental and population health research), it must be prepared to experiment, fail, and where successful, disseminate findings.

Research investments need to be prioritized alongside other investments, and metrics that have been developed to measure research impact can assist in this process (Canadian Academy of Health Sciences, 2009). A developing evidence base about the returns from investments in health research indi-cates that these returns are positive, but not exceptional (Buxton, Hanney, & Jones, 2004; Health Economics Research Group, 2008). *The Canadian Institutes of Health Research should assess on a regular basis the impact of funded health research.*[70]

### *Academic health sciences centres*

Innovation in health care evolves along at least three pathways: innovation in basic science, development of new technologies, and learning in clinical practice (Morlacchi & Nelson, 2011). A critical vehicle for health research in Canada for all three, and particularly the third, is the health service–uni-versity partnership, sometimes called an academic health sciences centre. Dougherty and Conway (2008) have identified three translational steps[71] in the research process and associated key activities:

- Translation step 1: from basic biomedical science to clinical efficacy knowledge. This involves testing what care works.
- Translation step 2: on to clinical effectiveness knowledge. This involves testing who benefits from the discovery.
- Translation step 3: on to improved health care quality and value, and population health. This requires research to evaluate how to deliver high-quality care reliably and in all settings.

It is thus only after translation step 3 that benefits of discoveries are accessible and shared across settings. The type of research required is different for each of the translation steps. Translation step 2, for example, requires outcomes and comparative effectiveness research. Translation step 3 requires research to support the key activities at this step: measurement and accountability of health care quality and cost; implementation of interventions and health care system redesign; and scaling and spread of effective interventions. Academic health sciences centres should play a critical role in all "translation" steps, not just within their own walls but reaching out to affect practice more widely. Unfortunately, this is not occurring to the extent required.

For biomedical research to have an impact, it must be a "superior innovation" (Lehoux et al., 2008), applied in clinical practice and evaluated in different settings. But in getting beyond translation step 3, there is many a slip between bench, bedside, and a patient's following a prescribed treatment regimen (Glasziou & Haynes, 2005). It is hard to get research findings universally adopted because practice innovation does not occur automatically via osmosis: purposive, multilevel interventions are necessary (Grimshaw et al., 2001).

At the broadest level, the two partners in academic health sciences centres espouse shared goals of clinical service, teaching, and research. The three goals are interlinked, of course, as the core of the partnership is clinical research and teaching[72] that rely on clinical services, but there are natural differences in emphases and priorities between a service organization and a university. These need to be acknowledged, and formal and informal processes need to be in place to address role conflict and conflicts over priorities. Collaboration is also facilitated where the partners agree on where they are going (vision and goals). *Each academic health sciences centre should identify its relative strengths and publish its research priorities, level of research investment, and outcomes of research at least every three years.* Such regular reporting, which could be in the form of a paper report, website, or presentation to staff or the community (or a mix of these), will assist in keeping goals aligned between teaching hospitals and medical schools and in focusing the research endeavours of academic health sciences centres on their comparative strengths.

Universities are prestige or status-maximizing organizations (Garvin, 1980; Slaughter & Leslie, 1997), and academic health sciences centres are probably in the same mould. The knowledge-generation activities of the basic biomedical sciences confer very high prestige (with associated financial rewards if translational step 1 is completed), but research status somewhat declines along each step of the transformational pathway. Academic health sciences centres, despite their rhetoric about being *loci* of translation, place greater emphasis and make greater investments in the early rather than later steps of this process. The pursuit of innovation attracts status and rewards but the hard slog of getting new, beneficial treatments into practice everywhere is not seen as a high-value task. However, this is where the largest returns to the population occur. The triennial research report proposed above could also highlight contribution to Dougherty and Conway's (2008) translation step 3, ensuring take-up of new, evidence-based treatments into practice.

Academic health sciences centres have a critical role in the creation and shaping of the future workforce. Professional values are transmitted in this environment through a "hidden curriculum" in apprenticeship-like clinical placements (Karnieli-Miller, Vu, Holtman, Clyman, & Inui, 2010). Students learn from both positive and negative observations. Much of a student's experience is gained in major academic health sciences centres, which may prioritize learning opportunities over efficient practice. As Fuchs and Milstein (2011) point out,

> Academic health centers are typically slow to adopt cost-saving innovations in care delivery because they may conflict with, or be perceived as conflicting with, the centers' research and education missions. Because many medical educators believe that resident learning requires some tolerance of inefficiency, they rarely prioritize teaching cost-effective clinical practice—a reality that has important consequences for the entire health care system. Young physicians learn primarily by doing or watching others do. They can't learn how to practice cost-effective medicine if it's not being practiced where they're being trained. The problem is exacerbated by accrediting teams for graduate medical education that leniently audit the teaching of the two competencies most likely to improve cost-effectiveness: "systems-based practice" (reflecting an understanding of how patient care relates to the overall health system) and "practice-based learning and improvement." (p. 1986)

The adverse impact of teaching needs on clinical practice can occur in a host of ways.[73] *Academic health sciences centres should review their teaching practices to identify the extent to which they reflect and encourage inefficient practice.*

Academic health sciences centres also need to demonstrate that efficient practices are valued and prioritized locally. Accordingly, *academic health sciences centres should document, and publicize to their students, how the centres' research leads to improvements in efficiency in the delivery of care.*

### Issues in contemporary approaches to drug development

Academic health sciences centres are also key venues for knowledge creation. The escalating costs for individual therapies (e.g., HIV, orphan drugs/ rare diseases, metabonomics) have focused policy attention on the rates of cost growth for this sector. What is seldom considered are the more fundamental processes of discovery and testing of new pharmaceuticals, and their sustainability.

Most science is targeted at discoveries one disease at a time. This paradigm may be increasingly inappropriate as people with chronic disease often have more than one condition, and the antecedents of chronic disease may be shared (Olshansky, Goldman, Zheng, & Rowe, 2009). The next Kuhnian shift may come from a different approach to try to address multiple manifestations of illness simultaneously.

Even within the contemporary paradigm, the current approach has weaknesses. Stevens et al. (2011) have highlighted the extent to which the drug discovery process is reliant on basic, publicly funded bioscience research. Increasingly, universities and their publicly funded researchers are allowed and even encouraged to profit from the discovery process in which they participate, and this process is facilitated by co-located incubators and other research clusters (Cooke, 2003).

Typically, a new drug entity is discovered through basic scientific research using animal models for both efficacy and safety testing. Some phase 1 trials for dose estimation and safety assessment in humans are also undertaken by university-based researchers. From this point, the research takes one of two directions: either the researchers form a small start-up company to fund further testing using investor funds, or the discovery is purchased by big pharma for its own development (Stuart, Ozdemir, & Ding, 2007). When successful in further trials of a new chemical entity, the small start-up companies are bought by big pharma or enter alliances with big pharma, to the profit of researchers and/or universities (Hopkins, Martin, Nightingale, Kraft, & Mahdi, 2007).

The large clinical trials that regulators require to demonstrate efficacy and ensure public safety require additional investment, and are almost always undertaken by or on behalf of big pharma. Clinician enthusiasts are selected to recruit patients for phase 3 randomized controlled trials, funded to employ data managers and data collectors, and sometimes to undertake any additional testing or other procedures that are required solely by the clinical trial design. Such trials are generally limited to a highly specialized subpopulation of patients to limit sources of variation in outcome other than from treatment (or not) with the drug on trial (Järvinen, Sievänen, Kannus, Jokihaara, & Khan, 2011). Because of the high cost of following patients over time, follow-up time for patients enrolled in trials is generally as short as required by regulatory agencies, and the nature of the drug itself. Although now the "gold standard" for new technology evaluation, trials have their limitations:

> The randomized controlled trial (RCT) is a powerful tool that has provided the evidentiary basis for many of the advances of modern medicine. However, RCTs have, as currently executed, certain limitations. Although theoretically, one can answer, using an RCT, almost any question that can ethically be asked, one can answer only one or a few questions per trial. Unfortunately, there are an unlimited number of questions about the appropriate use of drugs and the outcomes of such use, and these questions evolve over time. At the same time, there is a decidedly limited universe of funding, patients, investigators, time, and resources available to conduct trials to answer these questions. And it is not always easy to know the right question to ask. (Woodcock, 2007, p. 165)

As we enter an era of "personalized medicine," new forms of evaluation will be necessary, for example to ensure that both the drug and the diagnostic marker are subject to rigorous evaluation in parallel (Hamburg & Collins, 2010).

Results of randomized controlled trials typically present measures of central tendency with the reasonable assumption that these represent the "average" patient (at least in terms of those selected into the trial). But each distribution has a dispersion as well, and so it can be quite likely that clinicians will notice a divergence between the experience of their patients and the results predicted by trials (Kelley & Kaptchuk, 2010). Results from controlled trials and population-based analyses can diverge quite significantly, challenging the external validity of the controlled trial. For reasons such as these, non-randomized methods, such as use of routine data sets and patient registers, are increasingly seen as an essential part of health technology assessment (Harvey, Rowan, Harrison, & Black, 2010).

This model of drug development and testing is expensive (Adams & Brantner, 2010), is coming under increasing criticism (Dickson & Gagnon, 2004; Suryawanshi, Zhang, Pfister, & Meibohm, 2010; Woodcock & Woosley, 2008), and is probably inadequate for evaluation in the next generation of "personalized medicine" drug development (Woodcock, 2007).

Pharmaceutical companies complain about the high costs of the process, and particularly about the regulatory and coverage requirements that they face.[74] Yet their profits over the last decade have been very high, because of a reliance on so-called "blockbuster" drugs. Big pharma has justified these profits as a reward for risk, and as an investment in the development of the next generation of drugs that is promised to follow. Criticism has been levelled at this argument, as many of the "new" drugs marketed by big pharma are in fact "me too" formulations of existing drugs that come at a high cost for testing, but add very limited clinical benefit (Angell, 2004; Lee, 2004). Fojo and Grady (2009) have suggested that clinical trials be limited to those that are designed (powered) to find cost-effective outcomes.

University priorities for appointment and support of faculty have become distorted by this new, "magic pudding" of pharma investment.[75] Breakthrough bioscience discoveries become the basis of the university's marketing to donors and potential students, giving these scientists a privileged place in the institution. "Breakthroughs" are often announced in the media well in advance of any marketing approval. Patients then complain about the long timeframes that these processes impose on their access to potential cures. Clinicians often share this impatience, but also have to deal with the downstream consequences of trial-and-error prescribing for patient groups (the elderly, children, pregnant women) typically excluded from clinical trials. Short-term follow-up of patients in clinical trials means that it is clinicians who often discover and must treat the unanticipated downstream effects of drugs and/or their interactions with other drugs.

Funders are nervous about escalating drug costs, and reluctant to allow access to drugs that are potentially ineffective, and worse, might be unsafe and expose them to criticism about inadequate safety regulation. Moreover, as drug discovery and testing becomes ever more specific to particular genotypes in the population, the randomized controlled trial becomes more difficult to conduct and to rely on to provide the evidence-base to regulate the safety of new pharmaceuticals (Frueh, 2009).

What is needed is a re-think of the process from "bench to bedside." The economic benefits of public investment in basic science should be shared across the entire population, not just among the universities currently engaged in a scientific "arms race" to sponsor the most promising bioscience researcher—and certainly should not add to the profits of investors in pharmaceutical companies who purchase only the successful outputs of scientific research, seldom bearing the costs of failure along the way (Kapczynski, Chaifetz, Katz, & Benkler, 2005). Pharmaceutical companies in part justify their large profits as return for the risk they have borne by investments in clinical trials. One approach to reengineering the risk equation would be to expand public funding of trials (Jayadev & Stiglitz, 2009); another is to improve assessment of "technology readiness" at earlier stages of the development life cycle (Mankins, 2009).

To the extent that randomized controlled trials define the academic health sciences centres in which they are conducted, these centres must at a minimum recover their costs to do so. Patients can become more active participants in the research process, as the HIV community has demonstrated. With this participation must come the willingness to participate in clinical trials of new agents or devices with largely unknown (animal-tested) risks. Risk-averse funders must be willing to back patients by funding clinical research, but also must be able to profit (or at least recoup losses) through risk-based funding arrangements with commercial sponsors.

## *A learning health care system*

Central to this reformed pharmaceutical development system is something the United States Institute of Medicine calls "the learning health care system."[76] Data about many interactions with the health system are already captured in computerized data collections. It is now possible to mine those collections to report on the experiences/outcomes of particular hospitals or practitioners in managing particular conditions or performing particular procedures. Relying on the potential of evolving health information technology, a learning health care system could identify and assemble sufficiently large trial populations across multiple health care settings/systems, based on genomic or other clinical markers (Schneeweiss & Avorn, 2005). Cohort studies derived in this way could be important precursors or supplements to randomized controlled trials. Creation of such capacity for learning from patient outcomes in everyday clinical care would not be economical for any single private company, thus requiring investment by public science and health care agencies.

Electronic templates for data collection on patients consenting to novel treatments could supplement the wealth of diagnosis and procedure information already being collected. Moreover, monitoring of longer-term outcomes becomes more feasible with electronic rather than paper- and telephone-based follow-up, as well as the identification of safety issues in more diverse populations over time.

The new data sets, especially linked data sets, are becoming important components of health research infrastructure. They have the potential to expedite knowledge creation in that researchers are using more intensively data that already exist rather than relying only on new data created especially for research purposes. Etheredge (2007) emphasized this speeding up by referring to the development of a "rapid-learning" health system. *Academic health sciences centres should plan to become the centres of learning health care systems (as described by the United States' Institute of Medicine).*

## Introduction of new technologies

Unlike in other industries, the introduction of new technologies in the health sector rarely reduces costs. Rather, new technologies are designed to enhance quality by reducing the side effects of existing treatments, by making it possible to treat previously untreatable conditions, and by increasing the chance of a favourable outcome in treatment (Cutler & McClellan, 2001). Introduction of new health technologies—alongside rising incomes, public health interventions, and a range of other factors—have certainly contributed to the historical decline in mortality rates (Cutler, Deaton, & Lleras-Muney, 2006). But all this comes at a cost. Smith, Newhouse, et al. (2009) estimated that technology change accounted for between one quarter and one half of the increase in per capita health spending over the 40-year period from 1960 to 2000 in a cross-section of OECD countries.

Not all new technologies are equally worthwhile: some are indeed "game changers" or "home run" technologies, which can range from being cost saving to quite expensive; others are cost-effective in some patient groups but not in others, and their average cost-effectiveness will depend on how the technology diffuses; yet others may be shown to have modest or uncertain effectiveness or to be not clinically effective once diffused into the real-world context. The relative prevalence of the latter two types of technologies (group dependent and modest/uncertain effectiveness) may account for the higher costs of health care in the United States (Chandra & Skinner, 2011).

Policy attention is increasingly being turned to strategies that will ensure that new technologies are worth their costs. Such policies involve the use of economic evaluations (such as cost-effectiveness analyses) and decision analytic approaches from health technology assessment to inform whether particular technologies (new pharmaceuticals, machines, or procedures) should be covered in health insurance or other funding models (Chalkidou et al., 2009; Petrou & Gray, 2011). There are challenges to the use of economic evaluation, including mistrust in the methods and lack of relevance, but these can be addressed (Neumann, 2005).

Health technology assessments are conducted by the Canadian Agency for Drugs and Technologies in Health (CADTH) at the national level (see Husereau, Boucher, & Noorani, 2010, for how CADTH prioritizes technologies to review), by funding agencies such as provincial governments (Tarride et al., 2008) and by regional health authorities or hospitals (Heller, Gemmell, Wilson, Fordham, & Smith, 2006; Lee, Marshall, Waddell, Hailey, & Juzwishin, 2003; Lettieri & Masella, 2009). Unfortunately, the processes adopted by the multiplicity of agencies in Canada are not structured to facilitate information sharing and avoidance of duplication of effort (Lavis et al., 2010), an issue identified in the Romanow Report (Commission on the Future of Health Care, 2002, p. 83).

Any resource allocation decision involves choices and trade-offs—about who might be treated with a new technology (and who won't), and about who will be paid for the new technology and how much. It is a quintessentially political process (Giacomini, 1999), working at the intersection of politics, ethics, economics, and science. There are two basic questions that need to be asked about new technologies: What is the nature of the evidence about the cost-effectiveness of the new technology? How much will introduction of the new technology cost?

### Evidence about cost-effectiveness

The first basic question posed above was not cast as a dichotomy: Is the new technology cost-effective? Rather, the phrasing adopted highlights the contingent nature of the cost-effectiveness decision and the evidence. Choice of comparators for cost-effectiveness studies involves judgments about the range of alternatives to be considered (including whether to compare new pharmaceutical interventions with preventive interventions). Choice of comparator can obviously affect the incremental cost-effectiveness ratio and hence listing decisions based on incremental cost-effectiveness (Clement et al., 2009) and can be inappropriately influenced by source of funding for the analysis (Lexchin, Bero, Djulbergovic, & Clark, 2003).

Valuation of benefits especially is an inexact science, leaving room for a potential disconnect between societal values as expressed through political decisions and those reported in academic studies (Brousselle & Lessard, 2011; Hankivsky et al., 2004). Although methods for cost-effectiveness analysis are increasingly standardized (Gold, 1996), valuation choices about benefits (or costs) can influence the benefit: studies funded by proprietary interests are particularly vulnerable to this risk (Polyzos, Valachis, Mauri, & Ioannidis, 2011).[77] Valuation of benefits will also be affected by different cost structures and practice patterns between countries (Goeree et al., 2011; Vemer & Rutten-van Mölken, 2011) and by differences in societal preferences (e.g., willingness to pay).

Often the evidence advanced in support of effectiveness is from randomized controlled trials. Although they are thought of as the "gold standard" for evaluation of new technologies (Kaptchuk, 2001), extrapolation of results from the controlled research environment to practice faces challenges: the groups selected into trials may differ from the typical patient seen in practice (Bayer & Tadd, 2000; Järvinen et al., 2011), and patients may be excluded from analyses because of failure to complete treatment (Stanley, 2007).[78] The types of patients who do not complete treatment may regularly be seen in practice settings. Introduction of a new technology may expand the patient groups considered suitable for treatment through "indication creep" (Djulbegovic & Paul, 2011), making it difficult to project demand for the new treatment (and hence costs), for example, the experience with robotic surgery (Makarov, Yu, Desai, Penson, & Gross, 2011).

Further, most new technologies have not been evaluated systematically in practice settings, in terms of their effectiveness or cost-effectiveness in routine practice. In these circumstances introduction of a new technology is sometimes supported to allow gathering good evidence (a process known as "access or coverage with evidence development"). There is some evidence that the public supports this approach (Chafe, Merali, Laupacis, Levinson, & Martin, 2010), and where it has been used, it has led to better informed decisions across the full range of possibilities: confirmation of, modification to, or discontinuation of coverage (Levin et al., 2011).

All this of course relies on demonstrated clinical effectiveness: a technology cannot be cost-effective if it is not clinically effective. Often, however, the incremental benefit from a new technology is very small (e.g., life extension measured in weeks), with uncertainty even surrounding those estimates. Buyx, Friedrich, and Schöne-Seifert (2011) have recently suggested that the first screen for health technology assessment should be achievement of a "minimum effectiveness threshold" to avoid some of the contentious issues surrounding economic evaluation.

But let us assume that the information is in and the studies are valid. Should the cost-effectiveness information then *determine* the coverage decision? The brief answer is no, regardless of whether or not the technology is shown to be cost-effective above a standard threshold.

### Evidence about affordability

Results of economic evaluations are commonly presented in terms of an "incremental cost-effectiveness ratio," the ratio of the marginal (or incremental) benefits to the marginal costs. Threshold ratios can thus be derived that give decision-making zones where interventions are seen as definitely cost-effective and should be funded, definitely not, and a grey zone between the two (Braithwaite, Meltzer, King, Leslie, & Roberts, 2008; Eichler, Kong, Gerth, Mavros, & Jönsson, 2004).[79]

Let us assume that our rule of thumb is that if an intervention costs less than $100,000 per quality-adjusted life year, we will fund it.[80] Prima facie, if a new intervention meets that criterion it is economically "worth it," at least compared to other previously funded interventions. This then becomes a built-in engine for cost escalation, albeit where benefits also escalate (Birch & Gafni, 2006). The costs of a coverage decision based on a favourable incremental cost-effectiveness ratio will vary depending on the number of people eligible for treatment with the new intervention and the cost of each treatment (offset by any savings from discontinued treatments).

And thus the second basic question posed above: How much will introduction of the new technology cost? If the incremental cost is low, and the introduction can be absorbed within the normal budget escalation envelope, the coverage decision will be simple. On the other hand, if the total coverage cost is high, decision makers will have to make significant choices about opportunity costs and affordability, or budget impact becomes another decision-making criterion (Garattini & van de Vooren, 2011; Neumann, 2005).

Consider now the opposite end of the cost-effectiveness continuum: where the cost of achieving an incremental benefit is high. Should this automatically preclude funding or coverage of the technology? Again the short answer is no. Explicit, hard thresholds have disadvantages; Coast (1997, 2001) suggests there is a "disutility" to the use of explicit rationing. Hard "go/no go" decisions may be particularly inappropriate in areas where knowledge is advancing rapidly (Graff Zivin & Neidell, 2010; Shechter, 2011). Such rationing decisions involve difficult choices, even more so when the individuals affected are able to be identified calling for different decision-making criteria (Russell, Greenhalgh, Burnett, & Montgomery, 2011).

Society clearly does not function as if it wants every decision to be based on economics (Buxton & Chambers, 2011). Other factors (love, values) often come into play. Ghemawat and Ricart I Costa (1993) provide a framework for this. They posited four different behavioural bases for choice with different consequential decision criteria: passive, leading to inactivity; active but mindless, with decisions based on routines; mindful and calculated, with cost-benefit analysis as the criterion; or mindful and uncalculated, with principle as the criterion. Following this framework, it could be argued that there are certain decisions that society wants to be "calculated" (possibly where the choices are about anonymous people and "statistical lives") and other decisions that society would want made on the basis of principles and values—decisions under the "rule of rescue" with identified lives might be an example. Certainly there is now a burgeoning literature on how to incorporate ethical considerations into economic evaluation and the ethics of use of economic evaluation in health care (Arellano, Willett, & Borry, 2011; Broome, 1999; Dranove, 2003; Hofmann, 2008; McKie, Richardson, Singer, & Kuhse, 1998).

### The appropriate place of economic evaluation

Economic evaluation thus has its limitations. Is it so inherently flawed that it has no place in managing the introduction (and discontinuation) of new technologies? Acceptability of economic evaluations might be strengthened by greater public involvement and transparency in assessments (Gagnon et al., 2011; Gauvin, Abelson, Giacomini, Eyles, & Lavis, 2010, 2011). Economic evaluation occurs within a political context that needs to be recognized (Goddard, Hauck, Preker, & Smith, 2006; Syrett, 2003), and so in the meantime a pragmatic approach recognizes that the incremental cost-effectiveness ratio should be an input into, rather than a determinant of, the decision-making process. The relativity to any threshold value needs to be supplemented by other considerations, including ethical analysis, as a separate stage in the decision process (Cleemput, Neyt, Thiry, De Laet, & Leys, 2011; Duthie & Bond, 2011; Tannahill, 2008).

At present there is a national agency (CADTH) involved in health technology assessment as well as agencies in the larger provinces. One weakness in Canada seems to be the ability of unevaluated new technologies to sneak in under the radar: a physician or other advocate sets up a "trial" supported by the manufacturer, demonstrates positive results in an observational study reported in the media rather than in peer-reviewed journals,[81] and then seeks routine ongoing operational funding.[82] Again, this links to political processes: rewarding guerrilla activity of bypassing any systematic priority-setting and economic evaluation by approving funding weakens the legitimacy and effectiveness of any systematic processes. In these circumstances, avoidance of short-term political pain comes at the expense of greater long-term financial and political pain.

Hospitals (or other delivery agencies) need to eschew demands from clinician-advocates to enter a "medical arms race" with nearby hospitals (Foote, 1992), bypassing provincial planning guidelines (Shortt, 1998), and develop their own local processes for management of technology implementation.[83] But funders, too, have a role in ensuring that delivery agencies have the incentive to manage. This in part requires moving funding from "global budgets" where everything can be negotiated and where there is no evidentiary basis for the adequacy or otherwise of the budget, to funding based on an efficient price for activity performed. This issue will be addressed further in Chapter 7.

Another weakness is that technological innovation is typically seen as additive, and disinvestment is relatively rare (Garner & Littlejohns, 2011). But there is a technology life cycle that should routinely incorporate reassessment of the technology's value (Joshi, Stahnisch, & Noseworthy, 2009). This failure to recognize the life cycle of technologies and to incorporate that into both economic evaluation and clinical policies is a significant weakness of the Canadian health care system but, concomitantly, provides an equal opportunity to enhance sustainability. Substantial savings could be made from disinvestment in obsolete technologies. Elshaug and Garber (2011), for example, identified potential savings in the United States of at least $450 million per annum from halving the use of just two procedures (vertebroplasty and kyphoplasty).

Economic evaluation requires assessment of a new technology against a comparator: the investment decision can thus also involve a disinvestment decision where the new technology clearly dominates the old. Levers to effect disinvestment include both administrative directives and financial incentives, the latter including either removing an item from a fee schedule or changing its price relativity. The ability to use the fee schedule in this way is facilitated by more direct health service/government involvement in setting fee schedule relativities, an issue discussed in the previous chapter.

Many new technologies do not clearly dominate old ones, but dominate for certain conditions or when specific indications are present, and the new technology is approved for use in these specific circumstances. Again administrative directives and financial incentive can be used here, but need to be coupled with monitoring of use of both the old and the new. Implementation of rapid-learning health system capacity (discussed above) can facilitate such monitoring and also can speed up evaluation of take-up and outcomes of both new and old technologies.

The range of existing technologies that have not been reviewed is large, and diagnostic and treatment technologies are potentially becoming obsolete on a daily basis. Systematic processes need to be put in place to identify potential technologies for review (Ibargoyen-Roteta, Gutierrez-Ibarluzea, Asua, Benguria-Arrate, & Galnares-Cordero, 2009) and to manage the review process (Elshaug, Watt, Moss, & Hiller, 2009; Mortimer, 2010). Another agency need not be established for this process. *Federal, provincial, and territorial leaders should task and fund the Canadian Agency for Drugs and Technologies in Health to establish the capacity (and advisory processes) to undertake a rolling program of reviews of potentially obsolescent health technologies. Provincial health technology assessment agencies should develop complementary programs for evaluation of disinvestment opportunities.*

# Word cloud: Supporting seniors' care needs

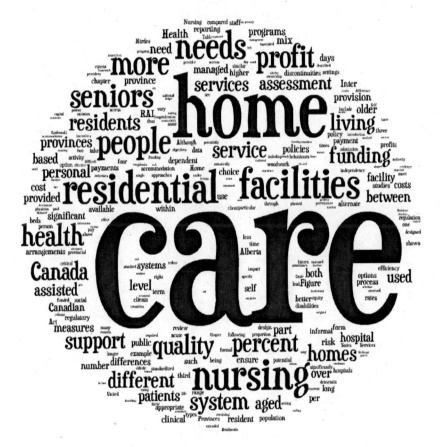

In this chapter I propose the following policy initiatives:

- Provinces should incorporate self-managed care as an integral part of their home care systems.
- Seniors' health care, whether provided in the home or in a residential aged-care facility, should become an insured service under the *Canada Health Act*.
- Provinces should review their home care provision to ensure that the full benefit of strong home care provision is available throughout the province.
- Provinces should explore introduction of public reporting of quality of nursing home care.
- Provinces should review their regulatory frameworks for seniors' care to ensure that they incorporate a best-practice mix of instruments. As part of this, the Canadian Health Services Research Foundation should be tasked and funded to support a review of current practice in Canada and experience internationally.
- Provinces should encourage and facilitate development of a broader range of accommodation options for seniors including an intermediate residential care option, assisted living.
- Provinces should ensure efficiency of residential care provision, and equity among providers, through the introduction of activity-based funding for residential care.

# CHAPTER 6

# SUPPORTING SENIORS' CARE NEEDS

As we age, we become frailer and our informal social supports (often through partners, husbands, wives) become more fragile. Our care needs often increase in fits and starts because of acute events (strokes, falls), but sometimes simply as a result of a slow continuous functional decline. But the service system, as currently structured, is poorly suited to respond. It is characterized by discontinuities—between hospitals and services outside those walls, between home care and residential care, between "health" and "social" care. These discontinuities affect both individuals and the system as a whole. Individuals may not get the service that is most appropriate for them. In the system, discontinuities may lead to inefficiency in that people sometimes remain in hospital, for example, when they would be better cared for in another location (Manzano-Santaella, 2010a, 2010b).

There is no national road map to address these issues and no coherent national policy framework for seniors' care. As Hirdes (2001) pointed out,

> Canada's universal, publicly funded health care system has not been designed in a way that established a uniform national approach to long-term care. Instead, the needs of the frail elderly are addressed through a policy mosaic that results in inequalities in access to services and differential burdens of care on family members. Moreover, the lack of a standardized health information system has made it difficult to compare the experiences of users of long-term care systems from province to province. (p. 79)

Relatively little is known about how the service system is structured to address seniors' needs: the language used to describe residential aged-care facilities differs from province to province (Berta, Laporte, Zarnett, Valdmanis, & Anderson, 2006; Hollander & Walker, 1998), and there is no complete national data collection about non-institutional care. Statistics Canada produces a report on residential care facilities[84] but even that is incomplete as it does not include information about the characteristics of residents in terms of their needs for care.

In 2008–09 there were about 2,200 residences for the aged providing care to more than 200,000 residents. The number of residents increased 3 percent over the previous year. Most residents (70 percent) are accommodated in larger facilities, with 100 beds or more, although such facilities comprise about one third of the number of facilities. About one third of facilities have fewer than 50 beds, accommodating 9 percent of residents. Just over half the facilities are owned by for-profit groups (55 percent), accounting for about 44 percent of the beds. Half the residents are 85 and over, a further fifth are 80 to 84 years old; 70 percent of residents are women.

There is an uneven distribution of beds across Canada: Prince Edward Island (with 14.2 beds per thousand population) has almost three times the 5.1 per thousand population provision in Alberta or the 5.2 in Quebec (Figure 6.1). One reason for the Alberta disparity is because of its younger population.

**FIGURE 6.1**
**Approved aged-care beds per 1,000 population (total and > 65), by province, 2009**

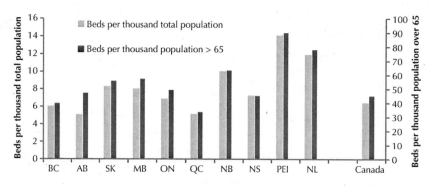

Source: Statistics Canada (2011), *Residential Care Facilities 2008/2009.*

In addition to older people in residential aged-care facilities, there are about 5,200 acute hospital beds occupied on any given day by "alternate level-of-care" patients, patients who no longer need acute care but remain in hospital awaiting residential care or home support.[85] Alternate level-of-care patients are older than other patients (median age 80 compared to 63). Although the median length of stay as an alternate level-of-care patient is 10 days, about 4 percent of these patients stayed more than 100 days. About one third of all alternate level-of-care bed days were taken up by people who had dementia, either as a main diagnosis or as a comorbidity. These patients stayed longer than other alternate level-of-care patients (median 23 days if main diagnosis of dementia and 16 days where dementia was a comorbidity).

Forty-three percent of patients who had been classified as alternate level of care were discharged to a long-term-care facility, 27 percent were discharged home with some support, and 12 percent died. Seventeen percent of former alternate level-of-care patients were readmitted within 30 days (compared to 12 percent of other patients), and in Ontario (the only province with available data) 27 percent of these patients had an emergency department visit within 30 days (22 percent for other patients).

The risk of residence in a residential aged-care facility is higher for a person with Alzheimer's disease or other dementia (9.33 times more likely than no condition), or with urinary incontinence (4.94 times more likely than no condition), for older people (85 or older 4.96 times more likely than 65–69), and for single people (7.59 times more likely than married people). Men are less likely to be in a residence than women (57 percent of risk for men with a severe disability relative to women).[86] Institutionalization risk of elderly patients admitted to hospital can be reliably predicted using standardized assessment tools (Noro et al., 2011), facilitating early intervention.

But most older people do not live in residential care settings; only 14 percent of people over 85 do so, for example. Among the oldest-old (people over 90), 60 percent of males and 53 percent of females live in a traditional home setting, the single, detached dwelling (Wister & Wanless, 2007). The dominant form of support for older people is (and should be) provided in the home, formally or informally: 42 percent of people over 85 received some form of in-home support in 2003 (Carrière, 2006). "Homes" may change over the life course as children leave the family dwelling, as "empty nesters" move into smaller dwellings, apartments, or seniors' complexes.

About 563,000 people received some form of support in their home in 2003, almost three quarters (72 percent) receiving care from "formal" sources, including government-subsidized health care or homemaker services, care purchased from private agencies, or care provided by volunteers (Carrière, 2006). Family and friends (informal sources) often supplemented formal care (15 percent of people received care from both formal and informal sources). Although official estimates of the proportion of home care that is provided privately are weak (Ballinger, Zhang, Hicks, & Gyorfi-Dyke, 2003), Coyte and McKeever (2001) estimated that in the late 1990s about 20 percent of formal home care was funded privately. The rate of growth of private funding is higher than that of public funding (Le Goff, 2004), so the private share may now exceed 25 percent.

Almost two thirds of home-support recipients were assisted with housework, with just under one third receiving nursing care in the home (see Figure 6.2). Home care can respond to a range of health, social, or personal needs and can involve an equally broad range of services (as shown in Figure 6.2, house work, nursing care, meals). Needs can be short term (e.g., following an acute episode) or ongoing. From a funder's perspective, the objectives of home care support might also vary from general support and prevention for people with chronic illness to preventing admission to hospitals or residential care facilities (Hollander, 1995). Home care has been shown to substitute for days in hospital (Hughes et al., 1997).

**FIGURE 6.2**
**Type of home support received by source, 2003**

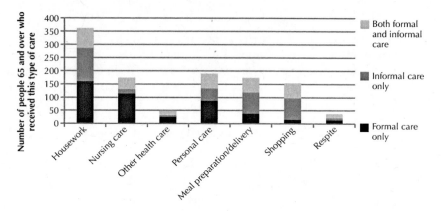

Source: Data are from Carrière (2006).

There are significant unmet needs for home care (Carrière, 2006; Wilkins, 2006). Although there was an increase in the number of people receiving government-subsidized home care between 1994–95 and 2003, the proportion of people over 65 in receipt of home care fell (22.3 percent to 19 percent), most notably because of reduced access to help with housework (Wilkins, 2006).

## Starting with home care

Seniors' needs can be arrayed on a continuum, from personal and social support needs related to activities of daily living (dressing and feeding) and instrumental activities (shopping, housework), through health care needs (wound care, monitoring).

Although the needs are continuous, as pointed out above the service system response is not, with disjunctions and discontinuities. The most obvious is the physical: different packages or elements of care are available in some buildings and not in others. The buildings go by different names in different provinces and sometimes within the same province. In this chapter the generic term "residential aged-care facility" will be used subdivided where necessary into "nursing home" (for facilities able to provide care for the most dependent residents) and "assisted living facilities."[87]

But there is another significant discontinuity: "When people leave hospitals, they are now understood to be leaving the protection of the principles involved in the *Canada Health Act*" (Armstrong & Banerjee, 2009, p. 13). This means different access to pharmaceuticals and different principles for payment, potentially stymieing continuity of care (MacAdam, 2008).

Reform of policies related to seniors' care needs to address these discontinuities. Seniors' care in Canada is overly focused on institutional provision,[88] and nursing homes are often seen as the flagships of the sector. Residential provision is able to function as a visible symbol of political commitment to seniors, and capital grants for nursing home construction are fungible political assets. In contrast, consistent with an emphasis on "the least restrictive alternative" posited as a value in Chapter 2, and putting the patient at the centre of the health system (Figure 4.2), policy about supporting seniors' care needs should start with ensuring a strong and effective system of home support, described in the Romanow Report (Commission on the Future of Health Care, 2002) as "the next essential service."

Branch (2001) identifies four components to developing home care policies:

- Who gets something?
- What do they get?
- Who pays?
- What impact does it have?

## Assessment and access (Who gets what and what do they get?)

Access rules—targeting or gatekeeping—are typically involved in any government service, and subsidized home care is no exception. The assessment process needs to start with clarification of program objectives: Is home care designed to prevent or delay residential care? Or is home care a social support service? Without clarity of objectives, it is more difficult to design assessment criteria with appropriate weightings for different types of risks to be averted, leading to confusion in program design, and exacerbating principal-agent problems in program administration (Weissert, Chernew, & Hirth, 2003). Assessment processes and classification systems vary across provinces (and sometimes within provinces) making interprovincial (or intraprovincial) benchmarking impossible.

A number of provinces are standardizing on the Inter-RAI[89] suite of tools, which provide an integrated system covering assessment for a range of settings (including home care and residential aged care). The Inter-RAI suite uses standardized sets of questions as part of the assessment, both to avoid duplication for clients being assessed for different settings and to ensure consistency in the way in which a particular issue is assessed (Gray et al., 2009). It has been adopted in a number of countries thus allowing international benchmarking (Hirdes, Ljunggren, et al., 2008). Implementation of the system in Canada was preceded by evaluation in Canadian settings (e.g., for home care; Poss, Hirdes, Fries, McKillop, & Chase, 2008). Home care assessment tools have also been shown to be good predictors of risk of residential care (Hirdes, Poss, & Curtin-Telegdi, 2008). An Inter-RAI–based tool has also been shown to be a sensitive and specific predictor of institutionalization or death for elderly people admitted to hospital (Noro et al., 2011).

The assessment process is not a simple one of applying a standard set of questions. It necessarily involves clinical judgments and assessments about the strength or fragility of informal networks of support (Egan et al., 2009), but standardization of approaches allows assessment to be undertaken by nurses with remote specialist physician support (Gray & Wootton, 2008).

Implementation of assessment standardization is not without difficulty, as Hirdes (2006) describes in these lessons from Ontario:

- The introduction of any standardized instrument is a major perturbation to the health care system, and requires appropriate resources and effective change-management processes.
- The availability of computerized information systems is a prerequisite to successful implementation.
- Education of clinicians, managers, and policy makers in the use of these instruments and the data they yield must be provided on an ongoing basis.
- Feedback is critical for all stakeholders. The data must be used to inform decision making at all levels of the health care system.
- Although the data can be used for many purposes, there must be a clear emphasis on clinical applications to sustain the use of data in daily care provision.

Assessment is not an end in itself, and there may be gaps and discontinuities following assessment. The services recommended following assessment might be personal care or health care. Depending on the structure of the support systems, the assessment process may lead to recommendations to the assessor's own (employing) agency or to other agencies for service provision or assistance. In an environment where priority setting is often required, service recommendations may not be effected within recommended time frames.

### Self-managed care

A characteristic of seniors' policy over the last decade, in Canada and elsewhere, has been enhancing choice. As Carlson (2010, pp. 191-92) puts it, "An inability to live safely at home no longer leads inevitably to the door of the local nursing home." Choice is available for many aspects of care: from what happens within a residential aged-care facility (allowing residents more choice and autonomy), to choices about available types of residential care (nursing homes, assisted living), to choices about whether at a particular level of disability a person can have enhanced home support to avoid moving to a residential facility, to the ability to control the way home services are provided (Colombo, Llena-nozal, Mercier, & Tjadens, 2011). Although originally focused on adults aged under 65 with disabilities (Glasby & Littlechild, 2009), this latter option, sometimes called "personal budgets" or "self-managed care," is now an established option in a number of European countries (Da Roit & Le Bihan, 2010; Lundsgaard, 2006; Timonen, Convery, & Cahill, 2006) and is being trialled in a number of provinces in Canada (Spalding, Williams, & Watkins, 2006). Essentially, these programs involve older people being given responsibility for a care budget, determined following client assessment, which they can use to purchase the services they need from the service provider of their choice. Ottmann, Allen, and Feldman (2009) distinguish two types of programs: "cash for care" and "self-directed care," the former focusing on the cash payment, the latter more on self-management. The term "self-managed care" will be used here to include both types of programs.

Self-managed-care programs have the potential to be much more tailored to the needs of the older person and his or her caregivers, and to introduce a high degree of flexibility and responsiveness into the care system.

There are a number of prerequisites for any form of self-managed care. First is a method of determining the budget for a particular client. This requires the introduction of standardized assessment approaches to ensure equity in resource allocation and negotiation with the client/caregiver about the resources to be provided (Rijckmans, Bongers, Garretsen, & Van de Goor, 2007). The assessment approach used should enable benchmarking of self-managed-care allocations with cost of services to similar clients in traditional home care or residential programs. Second, the budget must be adequate to meet the needs of those who want to be involved in self-managed care. Participants in these programs should neither be favoured over clients in standard seniors' care arrangements, nor subject to tighter resource availability. Third, services need to be available to be purchased from the allocated budgets, else the program is illusory and clients may have no effective choice, a particular risk for clients labelled as "difficult" by provider agencies (Egger de Campo, 2007). Fourth, there needs to be rules about accountability for spending public funds that balance the intent of giving flexibility with meeting public audit and accountability requirements. Finally, drawing on experience in the disability sector, self-managed care should be seen as more than simply service reform, but should be part of broader initiatives for capacity building and service development (Lord & Hutchison, 2003).

Self-managed-care approaches are not without risks and critics (J. Clarke, 2006; Keefe & Rajnovich, 2007; Vabø, 2006). Design of such systems need to take into account "moral hazard," where clients, not paying the full cost of services, might seek to consume more than they would otherwise. This has been termed the "woodwork effect," where clients or needs, which had not been apparent before system implementation, emerge from the woodwork. Formal and informal modes of care are, to some extent, substitutes (especially in aspects of personal care) that further heighten the risk of the woodwork effect. However, the empirical evidence suggests that the woodwork effect may be small (Meng et al., 2006) and does not crowd out informal caring (Daatland & Lowenstein, 2005).

Self-managed-care programs have different design attributes in different countries and are introduced into a particular regulatory and system context (Da Roit & Le Bihan, 2010). Different design attributes can mitigate potential moral hazard or woodwork effects, for example, through tight targeting (Grabowski, 2006). Caps on expenditure per client can also be used to ensure efficient use of resources.

*Provinces should incorporate self-managed care as an integral part of their home care systems.* Subject to favourable evaluations, such programs should expand as a proportion of seniors' support funding.[90]

### Copayments (who pays?)

Unlike the situation for hospital care, personal contributions abound in seniors' care. Copayments for physician services and hospitals are essentially prohibited because of the accessibility criterion of the *Canada Health Act.* The long title is an "Act relating to cash contributions by Canada and relating to criteria and conditions in respect of insured health services and *extended health care services*" (emphasis added). The Act's definition of extended care services includes both residential and home care. But beyond defining extended care, the Act imposes no obligations on provinces in this area, hinting and tantalizing but going no further.

Some level of copayment for extended care is not necessarily unreasonable, for as shown in Figure 6.2, home care includes personal care such as housekeeping and bathing. The same is true for residential aged-care facilities: part of the service there directly substitutes for a home (that would otherwise have been paid for by the resident as rent or capital), and for the food, light, and power that would normally be paid for by the individual. But some services—health care provided by nurses and other staff such as personal care workers—are not a substitute.

The question of "Who should pay?" is inextricably linked with what is provided, so it is better phrased as "Who should pay for what?" To the extent seniors' care substitutes for normal household expenditure, it should be paid privately. To the extent it is health care, there is little logic in establishing a payment dividing line between hospitals and residential care, or even home care where it is a substitute for long stays or prevents admissions. Different copayment requirements have the potential to create perverse incentives, where the marginal cost to the resident/patient may drive longer stays in hospitals, or distort service options (home care vs. residential care) to the detriment of system efficiency and equity. Provinces have recognized this logic and already provide subsidies to home care and residential care. Copayments for the *health component* of seniors' care should therefore be abolished to introduce consistency with other aspects of health care covered by the *Canada Health Act* and to reduce perverse incentives that may militate against use of home care. *Seniors' health care, whether provided in the home or in a residential aged-care facility, should become an insured service under the Canada Health Act.*

Rationalization of payment arrangements for the health component of seniors' care simplifies arrangements but still leaves significant complexity in funding. As a person becomes more dependent, the personal support components of care may differ from that experienced by people not so dependent. Take shopping for example. For people living independently, there is no payment for this service; it just costs time. But if this is provided as part of formal home support, there is a cost to the provider and thus an issue of who should pay. There is a similar issue for costs in residential care: the normal dwelling does not have the same services as a residential care facility and there may be an increment over ordinary housing costs; unlike in the home situation, food is prepared by paid staff and there is an incremental cost here too. For these sorts of reasons, it is appropriate that some personal costs be subsidized.

Subsidies (and differential copayments) will also be required to ensure equity. Canadians face significantly different copayments for residential care based on their province of residence, and income tests also vary (Fernandes & Spencer, 2010). Provincial copayment policies do not appear to take into account the differing cost of maintaining a reasonable standard of living across Canada (MacDonald, Andrews, & Brown, 2010). Mechanisms to assist in the transition from owning one's own home to purchasing accommodation in some form of seniors' accommodation (including assisted living or "lodges") also vary across Canada.

## The impact

Home care works! Integrated systems of home care for older people can reduce rates of institutionalization, reduce alternate level-of-care days in hospital, and save money (Béland et al., 2006; Grabowski, 2006; Hollander & Chappell, 2007; Johri, Béland, & Bergman, 2003; Low, Yap, & Brodaty, 2011; MacAdam, 2008). It is no surprise that aged-care clinicians support a rebalancing of the care system in favour of home and community care (Grabowski et al., 2010), and that contemporary policies in a number of countries emphasize "rebalancing care" toward home support and the "least restrictive alternative" (Johnston, Lardner, & Jepson, 2008).

Importantly, different definitions (or incidence) of costs do not change the fact that home care options are cost-saving relative to residential care. Costs to government, and total costs—that is, costs to government plus the costs of informal care at different levels—all show the cost advantage of home care (Chappell, Dlitt, Hollander, Miller, & McWilliam, 2004). Together, these findings also give comfort that, to the extent there is a "woodwork effect," it is offset by other savings.

Expansion of home care was supported by both the Kirby and Romanow reports (Senate, 2002a, Chapter 8; Commission on the Future of Health Care, 2002, Chapter 8), the latter describing it as "the next essential service" (p. 171).

*Provinces should review their home care provision to ensure that the full benefit of strong home care provision is available throughout the province.*

Home care, of course, is not only relevant to seniors' care: it has long been recognized as an important component of services for people with disabilities or mental illness and for those at the end of their lives. Increasingly palliative care is provided in the home (Brumley, Enguidanos, & Cherin, 2003). Home-based palliative care is associated with better symptom control and quality of life than inpatient hospice care (Peters & Sellick, 2006), and hospitalization and emergency department use is now seen as a measure of failure of palliative care (Earle et al., 2003). The above recommendation should thus be read broadly to include ensuring that home care provision is adequate for people with disabilities or mental illness and for people at the end of their lives.

## Residential aged care

Policy issues about residential care have parallels with home care; the need for assessment and the issues of copayments have been discussed above. There are differences of course, to some extent stemming from the fact that residents in nursing homes are more dependent (and vulnerable) than people who are able to remain at home, with residents in assisted living facilities falling between the two in both risk and independence. A critical difference relates to assuring quality.

### Assurance of quality in residential care

Residents in residential aged-care facilities are vulnerable. Many of them have cognitive impairment and need surveillance and regulatory systems to protect their interests. Unfortunately, the track record internationally is that regulatory systems for aged care are imperfect, often characterized by ritualism across a range of dimensions, for example, documentation ritualism where the facility gets the documents right and the care wrong, or rule ritualism where the regulator writes rules instead of solving problems (Braithwaite, Makkai, & Braithwaite, 2007). Regulatory failure leads to abuse and occasional scandals as the abuse is uncovered (Clough, 1999). At least in the United States, aged-care specialists see current regulatory regimes as in need of improvement (Mor, Miller, & Clark, 2010).

Contemporary regulation calls for a mix of graded enforcement, and rewards and incentives (Braithwaite, Makkai, & Braithwaite, 2007). This does not appear to be in place in all provinces.

Traditional inspection approaches to regulation can now be supplemented by quantitative measures derived from the assessment and reassessment process (Castle & Ferguson, 2010). For example, the Inter-RAI "changes in health, end-stage disease and symptoms and signs" (CHESS) score is an independent predictor of mortality (Hirdes, Frijters, & Teare, 2003); hospital admissions for potentially avoidable conditions can also be used (Walker, Teare, Hogan, Lewis, & Maxwell, 2009).

The Inter-RAI system incorporates specific quality measures across 12 clinically oriented domains: accidents, behavioural and emotional patterns, clinical management, cognitive functioning, elimination and continence, infection control, nutrition and eating, physical functioning, psychotropic drug use, quality of life, sensory function and communication, and skin care (Zimmerman, 2003). The incidence and/or prevalence of these can be used as part of the regulatory framework in a variety of ways: to target facilities for more regular inspections, as part of public reporting, or as part of rewards systems such as pay for performance. A similar set of quality measures is available as part of the Inter-RAI home care measurements (Dalby, Hirdes, & Fries, 2005).

Public reporting, via the Nursing Home Compare website,[91] is being used to drive quality improvement in nursing home care in the United States. Nursing home admission has different characteristics from acute admissions (generally more time to make a choice, less dependent on a treating physician's work locations), and so prima facie has better potential to be used as part of the consumer decision-making process. However, nursing home choice is a complex process (Castle, 2003), rational search is uncommon, and few consumers appear to use the website (Castle, 2009). Deborah Stone (2004), describing her own search for nursing home care for her mother, stated,

> It's fairy-tale magic, this market story with Wise Consumer as its hero, and it revolves around fairy-tale characters. I don't know any real people, especially frail elders, who are motivated or think much like *homo economicus*. (p. 192)

All this undermines the consumer sovereignty arguments for public reporting.

However, there are other arguments for public reporting. Nursing home managers regularly review the website quality scores and take action to remedy poor results, with homes with poorer quality more likely to take action (Mukamel et al., 2007). Taking action in response to poor scores was also more likely in competitive markets and where nursing home administrators perceived physician referrals would be impacted (Zinn, Weimer, Spector, & Mukamel, 2010). Actions taken include increasing the proportion of spending on clinical services (such as nursing time) versus hotel services (such as cleaning; Mukamel, Spector, Zinn, Weimer, & Ahn, 2010). There was an overall increase in quality in the few years after public reporting of quality measures commenced in 2002, particularly in the more competitive markets and for nursing homes where prior occupancy scores were low (Castle, Engberg, & Liu, 2007). There appears to be only limited evidence of perverse responses such as cream skimming by nursing homes to avoid residents who might predispose poorer scores (Mukamel, Ladd, Weimer, Spector, & Zinn, 2009).

There are differences between the nursing home markets in Canada and the United States, not least in the degree of market competition (more waiting lists for admission in Canada), so the impact of public reporting of nursing home quality might be mitigated. Nevertheless, *provinces should explore introduction of public reporting of quality of nursing home care.*

Public reporting alone will not suffice in terms of reforming residential care regulation. A range of other initiatives will be required: properly staffed long-term care ombudsman programs, for example, can be effective supplements to the more rule-based approaches to regulation (Estes et al., 2010).

Quality in seniors' care, and hence quality measurement, is not only about clinical dimensions of care. Especially in assisted living facilities, other domains such as preservation of independence and autonomy are critical. Greater independence in residential care has been shown to be associated with improved health status and reduced mortality rates (Rodin & Langer, 1977).[92] As with the need for health professionals to focus on *enabling* care in primary care settings (rather than simply "doing"), and promoting independence, so too in seniors' care. This may require the long and difficult process of engendering extensive culture change for staff and facilities (Miller et al., 2010). Existing nursing home regulation generally focuses on issues directly associated with resident safety and clinical measures, over-medicalizing the settings and tending to de-emphasize measuring promotion of independence. This approach to regulation may lead to increased costs of nursing home care.

Development of quality measures for assisted living facilities is not as advanced as for nursing home care, but Hawes and Phillips (2007) have proposed a framework including structure, process, and resident-focused outcome indicators.[93]

*Provinces should review their regulatory frameworks for seniors' care to ensure that they incorporate a best-practice mix of instruments. As part of this, the Canadian Health Services Research Foundation should be tasked and funded to support a review of current practice in Canada and experience internationally.*

## Private provision

Unlike hospital care, for-profit providers play a significant role in residential aged care in Canada, and there is regular questioning about whether for-profit provision is associated with poorer quality care (e.g., Jansen, 2011). The evidence on this issue is inconclusive. The literature in this area consists predominately of studies of experience in the United States, where the role, funding, and ownership of nursing homes is quite different from Canada. The most recent systematic review (Comondore et al., 2009), for example, reviewed 82 studies comparing for-profit and not-for-profit nursing homes. Only five studies used Canadian data, and two of these used staffing as a proxy for quality. In contrast, there were 74 American studies. The trend from Comondore et al.'s review favours not-for-profits:

> More studies had all statistically significant analyses showing higher quality in not-for-profit nursing homes than in for-profit nursing homes. Many studies, however, showed no significant differences in quality by ownership, and a small number showed statistically significant differences in favour of for-profit homes. (p. 13)

The Canadian literature is small and shows a similar, somewhat equivocal, picture (Table 6.1). There are three Canadian empirical studies of nursing

**TABLE 6.1**
**Conclusions of studies of association of profit status and quality in Canadian nursing homes**

| Study | Conclusion |
|---|---|
| Shapiro and Tate (1995) Manitoba, 1987–1991 | No statistically significant difference found in death rates between for-profit and not-for-profit nursing homes. For four of eight conditions studied, residents of for-profit nursing homes had higher rates of hospital admission than not-for-profits; for the other four there was no statistically significant difference. |
| Bravo, De Wals, Dubois, and Charpentier (1999) Quebec, 1996–1997 | Statistically significant difference between for-profit and not-for-profits on univariate analysis did not persist on multivariate analysis. |
| McGregor et al. (2006) British Columbia, 1996–1999 | Adjusted hospitalization rates for all outcomes were significantly higher at for-profit facilities compared with not-for-profit facilities attached to a hospital, and in many cases risk ratios were more than twofold higher. Adjusted hospitalization rates were higher for most outcomes at for-profit facilities compared with not-for-profit facilities amalgamated to a health authority, and significantly higher for three outcomes at for-profit facilities compared with not-for-profit multisite facilities. However, risk ratios at for-profit facilities compared with not-for-profit single-site facilities were the same for four outcomes, and significantly lower for urinary tract infections and decubiti/gangrene. |

home quality using outcome measures, with none drawing on data from the last decade. The most recent study (McGregor et al., 2006) went beyond the simple for "profit versus not-for-profit" comparison, examining subcategories of both types of providers.[94] The study found no differences among for-profit providers; however, there were differences among the various not-for-profit subcategories.

Facilities attached to a hospital (all of which were not-for-profit) perform significantly differently from other facilities (either for-profit or not-for-profit) in terms of admission rates. This suggests something else other than owner-ship status is at work here. The comparisons of for-profit with the other categories of not-for-profits used by McGregor et al. (2006) showed mixed results: regional health authority nursing homes performed better on five of the six hospitalization measures than for-profits, multisite not-for-profits performed better on three of the six measures, and for-profits performed better than single site not-for-profit facilities on two of the six measures (with no statistically significant differences on the other four measures). The evi-dence thus seems to preclude a clear conclusion about quality differences based on ownership.

### Expanding residential care options

Nursing homes are designed for the most dependent elderly. With 24/7 registered nurse coverage, these homes are prepared to deal with unstable patients. The residents often have complex clinical needs. Nursing homes are physically designed to meet these needs (for example, piped oxygen), leading to a culture that is often more clinical than home-like. One of the discontinuities in seniors' care has been the gap between facilities suitable for the most dependent and home care. Assisted living facilities are designed to fit into this gap, providing additional options for seniors between nursing homes and home care. Going by a variety of names, assisted living facilities attempt to create greater continuity of service options to match better the variation in needs of potential residents.

Table 6.2, adapted from Hernandez (2005), outlines resident needs along three dimensions: personal care, nursing care, and orientation/behaviours.

Nursing homes are organized to meet the care needs described in the third column, for all residents. But the reality is that not all residents have high care needs; some residents will have personal care needs described in the second column of the table, with nursing care needs in the first or vice versa. Assisted living facilities have more flexible staffing arrangements and are thus appropriate for a mix of residents with, on average, less complex care needs. The provincial regulatory frameworks for assisted living facili-ties in Canada are still evolving (Canadian Centre for Elder Law, 2008), and various "niche" categories of assisted living facilities have been created (e.g., focusing on dementia care). In fact, assisted living facilities form part of a continuum of residential aged care. Depending on their staff mix, these facilities could care for some residents whose personal care needs or whose orientation and behaviours are best described in the third column of Table 6.2, and whose nursing care needs fit within the second column.

**TABLE 6.2**
**Potential care needs in seniors' care**

|  | Basic | Intermediate | High |
|---|---|---|---|
| Personal care | Supervision, reminders and some assistance with bathing, dressing, and personal hygiene | Assistance with bathing, dressing and hygiene, plus limited assist with toileting, ambulation and eating assistance | Assistance with all activities of daily living includes regular incontinence care, transferring and feeding |
| Nursing care | Coordination with third party provider | Consultation, coordination, assessment, and regularly scheduled direct care (e.g., wound care) | 24/7 capacity for ad hoc reassessment of nursing care needs |
| Orientation and behaviours | Occasional reminders; infrequent behavioural interventions | Regular reminders, prompting, and direction; manage occasional episodes of disruptive or intrusive behaviours | Structured programming; behaviour plans to manage occasional, potentially unsafe behaviours |

Source: From "Assisted Living in All of Its Guises," by M. Hernandez, 2005, *Generations*, *29*(4), p. 20. Copyright 2006 by the American Society on Aging, San Francisco. Reprinted with permission.

Service delivery models in assisted living need not follow the traditional nursing home model where most of the care is provided by facility staff. Registered nursing care could be provided to residents in assisted living by visiting nurses. This model would enhance a home-like orientation, facilitate care continuity with previous residential arrangements, and allow for a more dependent mix in the assisted living facility.

Because assisted living facilities are a relatively new development in most provinces, there are many parts of Canada where seniors do not have the option for this lower intensity, less clinical accommodation. Because of the different staffing models in nursing homes (more staff per resident, greater proportion of registered nurses), this lack of choice for seniors is coupled with a less efficient service mix as residents who do not need to be in a nursing home are forced into that option if they can no longer remain at home.

*Provinces should encourage and facilitate development of a broader range of accommodation options for seniors including an intermediate residential care option, assisted living.*

### Funding residential care facilities

Funding arrangements for residential aged-care services across Canada differ substantially, both within provinces and between provinces.

Intraprovincial variation in funding policies has inevitably led to different facilities receiving different funding for treating patients at the same level of acuity. The situation in Alberta prior to the establishment of Alberta Health Services provides a case in point. Each of the previous regional health authorities developed their own funding formulas; most, but not all, used the Inter-RAI classification system. In some instances payments were facility specific as different facilities negotiated different arrangements for capital funding. There was a consequent lack of clarity about what the regional health authority (and subsequently, Alberta Health Services) was responsible for funding (e.g., care cost, accommodation cost).

When Alberta Health Services was established, it aimed to introduce consistent and equitable funding of care needs, using a standardized way of describing the acuity of residents: the Inter-RAI–based Resource Utilization Groups adopted as a Canadian standard by the Canadian Institute for Health Information.[95] Once residents had been assessed under the new system, it became possible to see the variation in health authority payments per resident (see Figure 6.3).

**FIGURE 6.3**
**Funding per weighted resident day, Alberta nursing homes (ranked lowest to highest), 2009**

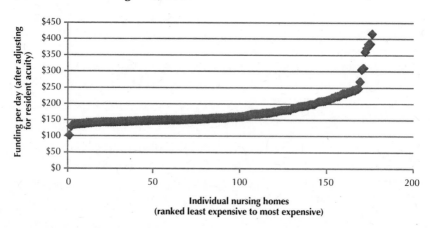

Source: Duckett, Sarnecki, and Kramer (2011).

There was a more than fourfold variation in cost per weighted resident day across the 180 nursing homes funded by Alberta Health Services. Implementation of activity-based funding in Alberta will lead to equalization of this funding over time, with the level of potential savings depending on the base level of funding per weighted day used.

There is no reason to believe that similar differences in funding do not exist in other provinces.

Efficiency (and equity) would be promoted by adoption of activity-based funding in every province. The design of activity-based funding policies may vary to take account of provincial differences (in, for example, how capital is funded), but should clearly specify what the provincial subsidy is for (care costs versus personal or hotel costs). These policies should be implemented through separate funding streams to ensure access for people with limited means, and accompanied by policies to ensure quality (see above).

Design of activity-based funding arrangements can also include pay-for-performance elements, potentially incorporating Inter-RAI type measures discussed above. Funding incentives could be introduced to encourage programs to reduce the likelihood of unnecessary acute hospitalizations (Grabowski, Stewart, Broderick, & Coots, 2008; Konetzka, Spector, & Limcangco, 2008).

*Provinces should ensure efficiency of residential care provision, and equity among providers, through the introduction of activity-based funding for residential care.* Smaller provinces could draw on the resources of larger provinces and the Canadian Institute for Health Information to facilitate this.

## Parallels for other groups

The focus of this chapter has been on seniors, partly because they are the largest population group who use home care and residential services, and partly to highlight that there are strategies that can be adopted which meet the dual objectives of ensuring system sustainability and improving choice/quality for older people. But the issues canvassed in this chapter are also of relevance to people with disabilities (physical, developmental, or psychiatric) who need home support, nursing, personal or behavioural care, or some form of supported accommodation. Again the service mix required to meet needs is often not available. There is inadequate choice, and institutional services may be the only option when a less restrictive alternative would meet the assessed needs and the person's preference. Worse still, younger people with disabilities may be accommodated in seniors' facilities because of the absence of an appropriate service mix in the geographic location.

While it may be practical to focus the policy reforms outlined in this chapter for the senior population initially, it is also important for the provinces and the federal government to take a critical and specific look at the policy impacts on people with disabilities. Ensuring that practices and policies do not push toward dependence and institutionalization is important for both sustainability and quality of life.

## The need for reform in seniors' care

The doomsayers' views about the crisis being created because of the aging of the population are typically based on naive linear extrapolation of the current utilization and service mix. These arguments were refuted in Chapter 2. But it is not the hypothesis of this book that this means no reform is necessary. There will be more older people. And the current mix of services and policies is not serving seniors well.

In Chapter 2 I articulated the following goal for the Canadian health care system: *The right person enables the right care in the right setting, on time, every time.* Addressing seniors' needs in the right setting is critical to the sustainability of the health care system.

What has been proposed in this chapter is a mix of strategies: some expansionary but some designed to drive efficiency both in terms of technical efficiency (activity-based funding) and social efficiency (more appropriate options for seniors, which might result in lower average costs). The expansionary and the efficiency policies should proceed side by side.

# Word cloud: Getting hospitals and acute care right

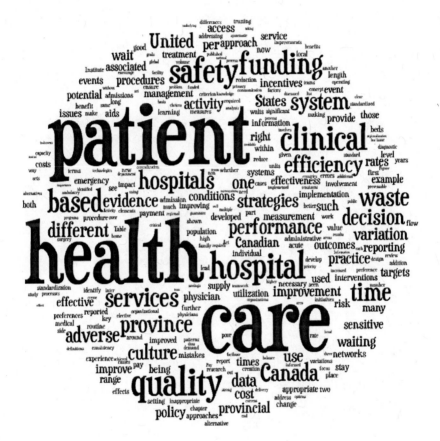

In this chapter I propose the following policy initiatives:

- The Canadian Patient Safety Institute should develop guidelines for incident-reporting systems and mechanisms to share lessons from incident reviews across Canada.
- The Canadian Institute for Health Information and provinces should develop feedback strategies to provide hospitals with information on hospital-acquired diagnoses.
- The Canadian Institute for Health Information should be tasked and funded to expand publication of data on variation in utilization rates across Canada.
- Provinces should fund health-care-provider access to a suite of patient decision aids and should encourage hospitals to use patient decision aids as part of their routine consent procedures for preference-sensitive conditions.
- The Canadian Institutes of Health Research should be tasked and funded to establish a research program to evaluate provincial (and regional) initiatives to address variation in utilization rates.
- Provinces should create and fund clinical networks to provide leadership in sharing good practice to improve access, quality, and sustainability of health care.
- The comprehensiveness criterion in the *Canada Health Act* should be amended to include an obligation on provinces to cover effective services, with a requirement that effectiveness be determined in a transparent way.
- Provinces should request clinical networks (when established) to review differences in intra- and interprovincial utilization rates. Networks should be invited to develop and/or update priority-setting criteria.
- Provinces should commit to adopting common definitions of waiting times for the full patient journey.
- Federal, provincial, and territorial leaders should agree on waiting-time targets for a broad range of services. Provinces should publish consistent data on achievement of these targets at least quarterly, and the Canadian Institute for Health Information should collate and publish these data at least annually.
- The 2014 Accord should expand the penalty provisions in the *Canada Health Act* to incorporate penalties for consistent failure to reach agreed waiting-time targets.
- Provinces should review current administrative structures to identify the potential for savings—and more effective priority setting—from centralization of functions.
- Provinces should commit to a phased introduction of activity-based funding to drive improvements in efficiency in the hospital and other sectors. Provinces should review comparative cost data (published by the Canadian Institute for Health Information) to ensure that provincial payment rates are set at efficient levels.
- Introduction of activity-based funding should be accompanied by measures to promote improved quality, whether through pay for performance, non-payment for poor performance, or increased surveillance and accountability.
- As part of activity-based funding implementation, provinces should consider introduction of incentives on hospitals to reduce waiting times.

# CHAPTER 7

# GETTING HOSPITALS AND ACUTE CARE RIGHT

Many authors have described hospitals as the cathedrals of the twenty-first century (e.g., Deber, 2006), and the vaulted atriums have some parallels in architectural terms. But the analogy has more to it than the architecture. In medieval times cathedrals were centres of inspiration and inerrancy, places to worship and to hope for miracles. They were centres of power and great wealth too, with the rest of life revolving around them. Miracles might appear to occur in hospitals, but unlike a century ago, these miracles are fully explicable in scientific terms.

As much as we might hope for a patient-centred health system, with services in orbit around the patient, unfortunately the cathedrals analogy hints at a pre-Copernican health system, with patients and other health services organized around the hospital. But this model is under challenge, with policy reforms in almost all countries aiming to strengthen primary care, and to rebalance the system away from an emphasis on acute care.

In an emergency, though, we all want what hospitals offer. At their best, they can marshal immense diagnostic power, quickly. The highly trained staff can initiate treatment that literally saves lives. And this happens every day, 24/7. We also need hospitals for scheduled surgical care, dealing with causes of pain so that we can go about our daily lives.

In Chapter 2 I proposed this goal for the health system: *The right person enables the right care in the right setting, on time, every time.* Unfortunately, we know that the end components of this are not really happening. Not necessarily the right care, nor the right setting, not on time, not every time. And this is what we have to address to get hospitals and acute care right.

## The quality agenda: The right care, every time

The first decade of the twenty-first century might in retrospect be seen as when the issue of patient safety came firmly onto the policy agenda in the developed world. In the United Kingdom it was in the aftermath of the tragic deaths at the Bristol Royal Infirmary (Kennedy, 2001); in the United

States the Institute of Medicine's report *To Err Is Human* (Kohn, Corrigan, & Donaldson, 2000) was the game changer. In Canada the movement was not so palpable, but nevertheless institutional structures changed with the creation of the Canadian Patient Safety Institute in 2003. Patient safety should be top of mind for every manager, policy maker, and clinician, but there is "a discrepancy between the gravity of the problem and the frailty of the solutions implemented to date" (Leistikow, Kalkman, & de Bruijn, 2011, p. 1).

"Quality" is broader than safety, the former including a boy-scout list of additional attributes: acceptability, accessibility, appropriateness, effectiveness, and efficiency.[96] Degos and Rodwin (2011) distinguish between a "care-centred approach" that focuses almost exclusively on safety (prevalent in the United States) and a "system-centred approach," focusing on the continuum of care including clinical prevention and access. The "acceptability" dimension highlights the fact that quality measurement and conceptualization from the perspective of clinicians may differ from what patients value (Duckett & Ward, 2008). Unfortunately, contemporary approaches to measurement of the patient experience are "seriously flawed" (Gill & White, 2009), highlighting the need for better conceptualization of service quality measurement in the health sector (Dagger, Sweeney, & Johnson, 2007; Zeithaml, Parasuraman, & Berry, 1990). Accessibility and efficiency will be dealt with separately in this chapter.

### Safety of health care

What do we know about the safety of health care in Canada? The major Canadian study (Baker et al., 2004) showed that about 7.5 percent of all admissions had an adverse event, with higher rates (10.3 percent) in teaching hospitals; in about 20 percent of cases, these adverse events resulted in death. The concept of preventability of adverse events, though, has limitations.[97] Physician reviewers in the Baker et al. (2004) study estimated that about one third of the adverse events were preventable (given current knowledge), and that an adverse event almost doubled the length of stay in smaller hospitals and in teaching hospitals (see Table 7.1)

So an adverse event causes extra days of care, with associated costs (Jha, Chan, Ridgway, Franz, & Bates, 2009), adding a financial imperative to the moral one to "first, do no harm" (Smith, 2005). The Canadian rates of adverse events are in line with those found in other countries, at least where a similar record-review method was used (Baker et al., 2004; de Vries, Ramrattan, Smorenburg, Gouma, & Boermeester, 2008). The key strategies to improve quality have cultural transformation as an essential element. The culture change required is of two kinds: first to create a "just and trusting culture" and second, a culture of efficient teamwork.

**TABLE 7.1**
**Length of hospital stay associated with an adverse event, by type of hospital**

| | Small hospitals | | Large hospitals | | Teaching hospitals | |
|---|---|---|---|---|---|---|
| | Patients without adverse event | Patients with adverse event | Patients without adverse event | Patients with adverse event | Patients without adverse event | Patients with adverse event |
| Mean length of stay | 7.6 | 16.2 | 7.7 | 14.0 | 7.8 | 17.7 |
| Additional days of stay identified by physician reviewers as directly related to an adverse event | | 7.7 | | 3.6 | | 6.2 |

## Creating a safety-enhancing culture

Fifty years ago, the predominant culture in health care was one of inerrancy: things rarely went wrong and, if they did, it was the fault of an errant individual. But our understanding today is different. We now accept that mistakes happen in health care. What is important is that we learn from those mistakes to reduce the likelihood that the same mistake will happen again. Individual fault is not seen as a good starting point for analyzing why things went wrong. We now understand mistakes to be a result of a "web of causation," with multiple contributing factors,[98] many of which are organizational or "systems factors" (Perrow, 1999; Reason, 1990, 2000).

If system factors are more likely to be causative than individual fault, then individuals who see or make mistakes should feel free to report them. Although health professionals often blame themselves for mistakes (Bryant, 2007; Delbanco & Bell, 2007), organizations can encourage reporting—and hence the ability to learn from mistakes—if individuals feel that they will not be blamed or punished when they come forward. This approach was originally called a "no blame" culture (Wachter & Pronovost, 2009), and it was seen as one of the key elements of an encompassing "safety culture." Recognition *inter alia* that there are blameworthy events (e.g., working while intoxicated), and that not all health professionals are, like children in Lake Wobegon, above average (Berwick, 2009), has led to the descriptor "just and trusting culture" being preferred.

Feeling free to report is not the only element of a safety-enhancing culture. What is also required is freedom to intervene. Health care organizations are extremely hierarchical (Freidson, 1970), and personnel further down the hierarchy might feel reluctant to raise safety issues involving people higher in the pecking order.

Creating a just and trusting culture is not wholly in the control of an individual health service: the media still will often sensationalize quality issues (Dentzer, 2006) and personalize the causal path when mistakes happen. Further, the risk/blame balance in politics is more oriented to blame (Hood, 2002), resulting in politicians also looking for an individual to be labelled at fault.[99]

At the broad conceptual level, describing what a safety or just and trusting culture is trying to achieve is easy. Defining and measuring it is more difficult. Definitions of a just and trusting culture and the broader concept of a "safety culture" abound (Guldenmund, 2000; Weiner, Hobgood, & Lewis, 2008), but the definitions are not consistent as different researchers emphasize different elements (Halligan & Zecevic, 2011). With no consistency in definition, there is no consistency in approaches to measurement or in what dimensions of a safety culture should be measured (Colla, Bracken, Kinney, & Weeks, 2005; Singla, Kitch, Weissman, & Campbell, 2006). Indeed, the quest for a rigorous measurement approach appears to be illusory (Ginsburg et al., 2009). Despite these difficulties, the first step in comprehensive approaches to improving patient safety is measuring the culture, however inadequately (Provonost et al., 2005; Reason, 1997), as there is a link between hospital safety culture and hospital-level safety performance (Singer, Lin, Falwell, Gaba, & Baker, 2009). The occupational health literature shows that improving safety culture leads to improved safety performance and accident prevention (S. Clarke, 2006), and the same probably holds true for patient safety. As a minimum, systematic reporting and subsequent learning cannot be effective if they are inconsistent with the organizational culture.

If measurement of culture is step one, step two will often be attempting to change the culture. This will require multiple interventions, including broad patient safety and management education programs. Unfortunately, the track record of achieving measurable change is poor (Benning, Ghaleb, et al., 2011; Parmelli et al., 2011), possibly because of a poor understanding of underlying change, motivational, and other theory (Grol, Bosch, Hulscher, Eccles, & Wensing, 2007).

### Efficient teamwork

The second cultural transformation required to improve quality is to build more effective health care teams. There is almost no health care intervention that involves only a single professional, and transitions of care from one professional (or team) to another involve an "information loss" and the potential for mistakes, for example, missed test results when moving across settings (Callen, Georgiou, & Westbrook, 2011). Communication issues are among the most commonly cited underlying causes of adverse events (Sutcliffe, Lewton, & Rosenthal, 2004), but these may be symptoms of intra-organizational conflict (Hewett, Watson, Gallois, Ward, & Leggett, 2009). Poor handover between shifts and in interhospital transfers is a symptom of poor communication, and is also a risk factor for adverse events (Cohen & Hilligoss, 2010; Ong & Coiera, 2011). Despite the importance of good communication and teamwork, Clements, Dault, and Priest (2007, p. 27) note pessimistically that effective teamwork is "so far not at the tipping point where workers or employers expect it," in contrast to patients who assume it is in place.

Improvement in the quality of health care thus relies on improving the functioning of health care teams and the environment in which they work (Greenfield, Nugus, Travaglia, & Braithwaite, 2011). Nelson, Batalden, and Godfrey (2007, p. 233) define clinical microsystems as the sharp end of care, "the place where patients, families, care teams, and information come together." Microsystems, they argue, should be the focus of improvement efforts as the quality of care a patient receives is "a function of the quality of care provided to that patient in each of the microsystems ... where he or she receives care, plus the quality of the interactions of all the microsystems providing care to that patient" (p. xxxiii).

Effective teamwork requires a combination of knowledge (what is the role of other team members) and skills (e.g., meeting management), coupled with personal traits and a motivation to make the team work (Leggat, 2007). Full 360° feedback can be used to assess team contributions; indeed, colleague and patient evaluations are now being used as part of physician performance appraisals (Campbell et al., 2008). Team effectiveness can be improved by appropriate interventions, but unfortunately, "taken as a whole, published studies do not provide clear direction on how to create or maintain high-functioning teams" (Lemieux-Charles & McGuire, 2006, p. 295); this conclusion was confirmed in a later review by Bosch et al. (2009).

In addition to improving communication, clinical teams (or micro-systems) have a key role in improving the efficiency of processes of care (to be discussed below). Teams also provide a venue to discuss how to reduce variability in clinical processes. The Plan-Do-Study-Act (PDSA) cycle is now recognized as the *sine qua non* of quality improvement processes (Deming, 1993; Langley et al., 2009). Teams can be powerful mechanisms for sharing and learning, especially if the standardization is based on evidence, and even more so if the evidence is local from a PDSA cycle.

Although the quality journey is often seen as a continuous or never-ending one, PDSA cycles should only continue until the desired aim has been achieved. The task then is to standardize the process to ensure that the measured aim is achieved in every case. PDSA cycles should thus lead to a "standardize-do-study-act" cycle, recognizing that even once a process is standardized it might still result in anomalies or have opportunities for further improvement (Nelson, Batalden, & Godfrey, 2007). Standardization can present a challenge to some clinicians who value their individual autonomy highly. But autonomy should be regarded as an intermediate goal, valued insofar as, and only insofar as, it contributes to better care outcomes.

### Patient safety interventions

There are a myriad of interventions being undertaken to improve patient safety in health care facilities across Canada and internationally (Cohen, Restuccia, et al., 2008; Wensing, Wollersheim, & Grol, 2006). Few of these are rigorously evaluated, or at least as documented in published studies (Hoff, Jameson, Hannan, & Flink, 2004), and many have no sound (or at least no clear) theoretical base for their implementation approach (Dixon-Woods, Bosk, Aveling, Goeschel, & Pronovost, 2011). Good, simple ideas for promoting safety and improving quality are advocated passionately and persuasively (e.g., Gawande, 2009a), but subsequent evaluation may produce equivocal results (Ko, Turner, & Finnigan, 2011).

There are many competing priorities for organizational investment, both patient safety and otherwise. Hoff et al. (2004), following their review of patient safety interventions, recommended that managers

1.  prioritize the kinds of medical errors and safety issues that their institutions need to address first;
2.  specify clear outcomes (i.e., dependent variables) desired for those issues and make sure timely, accurate data can be produced to assess changes in outcomes; and
3.  develop an intervention approach that not only reflects a systems approach to dealing with the error or safety problem (i.e., there are multiple factors at work) but also allows the opportunity to evaluate the relative effects and cost-benefit of one type of organizational intervention versus another. (p. 29)

Implementing safety interventions successfully is not simple: as with any system disruption, it requires good change management, supported by training and support.

The quality improvement cycle starts with detection: identifying when things have gone wrong (Dückers et al., 2009). There are multiple ways to measure and report adverse events, and these methods have different strengths and weaknesses. Despite development of a World Health Organization taxonomy for incident reporting (Runciman et al., 2009; World Alliance for Patient Safety Drafting Group et al., 2009), there is little uniformity as to how incidents are reported or analyzed, inhibiting cross-institutional learning (Noble, Panesar, & Pronovost, 2011). *The Canadian Patient Safety Institute should develop guidelines for incident-reporting systems and mechanisms to share lessons from incident reviews across Canada.*

As argued above, underpinning good detection is the existence of a "just and trusting culture" that encourages identification and reporting of adverse events and near misses. Introduction of incident reporting has been shown to increase detection (Dückers et al., 2009). Routine ("administrative") data can also be used for systematic monitoring of adverse events (Carroll, McLean, & Walsh, 2003). The United States' Agency for Healthcare Research and Quality has developed a set of "patient safety indicators" that can be extracted from the routine data for monitoring purposes (McDonald et al., 2002; Miller, Elixhauser, Zhan, & Meyer, 2001; Rivard et al., 2008). Introduction of "condition onset flags" or "date stamping" of diagnoses and procedures enhances the potential of the routine discharge data sets for monitoring purposes (Bahl, Thompson, Kau, Hu, & Campbell, 2008), as does the development of a way of summarizing and classifying reported adverse events (Jackson, Michel, Roberts, Jorm, & Wakefield, 2009).[100] *The Canadian Institute for Health Information and provinces should develop feedback strategies to provide hospitals with information on hospital-acquired diagnoses.*

Patient safety interventions have been shown to be successful in addressing a range of proximal causes including medication errors, diagnostic errors, falls (Dückers et al., 2009), and bloodstream infections (Pronovost, Marsteller, & Goeschel, 2011). High-profile broader interventions, across multiple hospitals, have not always reported the same positive impact (Benning, Dixon-Woods, et al., 2011; Benning, Ghaleb, et al., 2011), reinforcing the importance of context in implementation of quality improvement initiatives, especially local leadership (Kaplan et al., 2010). Multi-institutional quality improvement collaboratives have also been advocated but, again, the published evidence suggests with mixed results (Schouten, Hulscher, van Everdingen, Huijsman, & Grol, 2008; Strating, Nieboer, Zuiderent-Jerak, & Bal, 2011).

Conventional wisdom about quality improvement involves a number of handy hints suggesting that better performance on quality measures is associated with broader hospital involvement, more involvement of senior management, and more physician involvement. Not all of these stand up empirically (Weiner, Alexander, Baker, Shortell, & Becker, 2006; Weiner, Alexander, Shortell, et al., 2006), nor does the suggestion that greater adoption of information and communication technologies will unequivocally improve care (Perry, Wears, & Cook, 2005).

Woodward et al. (2010), however, have identified a set of recommendations that are worth pursuing (see Table 7.2).

**TABLE 7.2**
**Recommendations to improve patient safety**

| | |
|---|---|
| For policy makers | 1. Create higher-level groups to drive changes in safety. |
| | 2. Support the creation and running of reporting systems. Reporting system data and trends should be reviewed to identify possible areas of concern and best practice, to be investigated further. |
| | 3. Focus on patient safety but understand that behavioral change will be slow. |
| | 4. Apply principles of social change to the problem of medical error. |
| | 5. Support the implementation of disclosure policies. |
| For managers | 1. Recognize the value of standardization of practice and establish standard operating procedures. |
| | 2. Evaluate patient safety initiatives using patient outcomes. |
| | 3. Give visible support to patient safety initiatives. |
| | 4. Acknowledge that IT is an investment; savings will accrue in the long-term. |
| | 5. Implement disclosure policies. |
| | 6. Understand that staff buy-in to safety initiatives is essential and avoid overly didactic approaches. |
| For clinicians | 1. Reduce the individualistic approach to clinical care; seek to work effectively within teams and across divisions of care. |
| | 2. Hand hygiene is a good way to start. |
| | 3. Acknowledge IT not as a threat but as an aid. |
| | 4. Be aware of the dangers of workarounds. |
| | 5. Be open about errors. |
| For patients | 1. Confirm own identity to health care providers. |
| | 2. Carry information about allergies, medications, and existing health conditions and share them with all health care providers. |
| | 3. Request clear information about medication dose, indication, interaction, and side effects. |
| | 4. Find out how and when test results will be received, and keep copies where appropriate. |
| | 5. Play an increased role in detecting and reporting error, challenging unsafe practice, and actively taking part in standard procedures, such as checklists. |

Source: From "What Have We Learned about Interventions to Reduce Medical Errors?" by H. I. Woodward et al., 2008, *Annual Review of Public Health, 31*(1), p. 492. Copyright 2008 by Annual Reviews Inc. Reprinted with permission via Copyright Clearance Center.

## Effectiveness and the challenge of variation

Addressing quality or safety in health care is often conceptualized as chasing (and preventing) errors and mistakes. But as Brennan, Gawande, Thomas, and Studdert (2005) point out,

> The … notion of individual accidental death … oversimplifies the causal realities of iatrogenic injuries, overpromises on achievable gains, and threatens to skew

priorities in quality-improvement initiatives. Moving away from a focus on saving lives solely by preventing errors and instead emphasizing the implementation of evidence-based practices to improve the quality of care more generally will yield better long-term results. (p. 1405)

Health care faces an evidence overload, but the evidence is not implemented: Glasziou and Haynes (2005, p. 4) refer to a "practice famine amidst the evidence glut." There are many steps along the way to implementing evidence-based practice, requiring that evidence be easy to access at the bedside, that the evidence be implemented as a quality-improvement task, and that patients accept and adhere to the prescribed treatment (Dougherty & Conway, 2008; Glasziou & Haynes, 2005).

The last few years have seen an increasing interest in one aspect of evidence-based practice: addressing variation in medical care. Underpinned by a long history of research (Wennberg, 2010), the reality of significant variation in hospital admission rates was popularized by an article in *The New Yorker* magazine in June 2009 that examined the contrasting experience of two Texan towns with vastly different practice patterns (Gawande, 2009b). Most of the "variations" research has been undertaken in the United States. We know that there is variation in utilization in Canada, both between provinces and within (Duckett et al., 2012), but Canada does not have the solid *national* corpus of evidence that has been developed in the United States over the last few decades.[101] The results of the few Canadian variations studies are consistent with the United States' studies: Coyte, Wang, Hawker, and Wright (1997), for example, reported a threefold variation[102] in the rate of knee replacement between geographical areas (public health units) in Ontario after adjusting for age, sex, and disease prevalence. In a related study, Wright et al. (1999, p. 953) found that "surgeons' opinions or enthusiasm for the procedure was one of the major determinants of geographic area variation."

As Appleby (2011, p. 26) points out, "the first step in addressing unwarranted variations in health care is the systematic and routine collation, analysis and publication of data on such variations." *The Canadian Institute for Health Information should be tasked and funded to expand publication of data on variation in utilization rates across Canada.*

Wennberg's (2010) careful research has shown that higher utilization rates are not associated with improved outcomes, and this has been known for decades. However, as Evans (1990b) pointed out, "Knowing is not the same as doing. The most striking fact about the large and extensively documented variations in patterns of medical practice, throughout the developed world, is the minimal impact that this information has had on health policy" (p. 117).

Moving from analysis to action involves disentangling types of variation, as different underlying causes need to be addressed by different strategies.

Wennberg (2010) distinguishes three types of care: effective or necessary (where the critical issue is potential underuse), preference sensitive, and supply sensitive (Table 7.3).

**TABLE 7.3**
**Attributes of preference- and supply-sensitive care**

| | |
|---|---|
| Preference-sensitive care | • Uncertainty in medical opinion about treatment choices<br>• Weak influence of patient preferences in treatment choices |
| Supply-sensitive care | • Supply of health care resources (physicians, hospital beds) leads to more intense care for chronic illnesses<br>• Worse patient experience (more deaths in intensive care units, more patients with two or more physicians) |

Source: Derived from Wennberg (2010, pp. 10-11).

In contrast to the policy paralysis that Evans (1990b) lamented, Wennberg (2010, p. 5) has now identified four strategies to address variation:

1.   promoting organized systems of health care delivery;
2.   establishing informed patient choice as the ethical and legal standard for decisions surrounding elective surgeries, drugs, tests, and procedures, and care at the end of life;
3.   improving the science of health care delivery; and
4.   constraining undisciplined growth in health care capacity and spending.

Although influenced by his United States' context, these have relevance in Canada. The issue of organized systems of delivery has been discussed in Chapter 4; the other three strategies will be discussed below.

### *Promoting informed choice*

In the face of uncertainty about the evidence, clinicians can legitimately differ in their treatment recommendations. Wennberg (2010) and others have argued that the appropriate and ethical response to this uncertainty is to strengthen the hand of the consumer in the decision-making process (Falit, 2008; Moulton & King, 2010), an example of "postmodern medicine" (Gray, 1999). Different consumers will place different valuations on having surgery (vs. watchful waiting), and on the potential side effects of surgery. As a result, there can be significant differences between surgeons' opinions about whether a procedure is indicated and patient willingness to have the operation (Hawker et al., 2001).

A key way to assist patients to make informed choices is through use of "patient decision aids" that are designed to

1. provide evidence-based information about a health condition, the options, associated benefits, harms, probabilities, and scientific uncertainties;
2. help patients to recognize the values-sensitive nature of the decision and to clarify, either implicitly or explicitly, the value they place on the benefits, harms, and scientific uncertainties ... and
3. provide structured guidance in the steps of decision making and communication of their informed values with others involved in the decision e.g., clinician, family, friends. (O'Connor et al., 2009, p. 3)

Patient decision aids are now available covering a wide range of preference-sensitive conditions,[103] and it is estimated that in 2006 patient decision aids were accessed, mostly on the Internet, 9 million times (O'Connor et al., 2007).

Patient decision aids have been shown to influence patient choices, resulting in lower rates of surgery and improved patient satisfaction with the decision-making process (Leatherman & Warrick, 2008; O'Connor et al., 2009). However, patient decision aids are not yet part of routine practice, despite implementation of a range of methods to increase their uptake (Légaré et al., 2010). O'Connor et al. (2007) have suggested financial incentives and a new legal standard be used to encourage wider use of decision aids. Consent forms can incorporate material from patient decision aids, tailored to the outcomes experience of the index hospital (consistent with Etheredge's [2007] concept of a rapid learning health system). Patient decision aids can also be tailored to the characteristics of the individual patient (Decker et al., 2008). *Provinces should fund health-care-provider access to a suite of patient decision aids and should encourage hospitals to use patient decision aids as part of their routine consent procedures for preference-sensitive conditions.*

Initiatives to address variation should be evaluated so lessons can be shared nationally. *The Canadian Institutes of Health Research should be tasked and funded to establish a research program to evaluate provincial (and regional) initiatives to address variation in utilization rates.*

Patient decision aids are oriented toward the patient's decision about whether or not to have surgery (or a screening test), not where the surgery should be undertaken. There has been extensive attention, especially in the United States, to public "report cards" to stimulate quality improvement and/or to change patient flows. The evidence of the use of report cards by patients is weak (Fung, Lim, Mattke, Damberg, & Shekelle, 2008), but more important, report cards may be inconsistent with the concept of promoting a just and trusting culture.

## Improving the science of delivery

Bohmer and Sepucha (2005) identify a "zone of complexity" in health care decision making that is the mid area on both a certainty-uncertainty axis and an agreement-disagreement/variation (in terms of valuation or prefer-ences as to utilities or outcomes) axis.[104] In addition to being the zone where patient preferences can be given greater prominence, it is also the zone that cries out for knowledge creation. The current scientific paradigm sees knowledge creation occurring by comparison of current practice with the new alternative. The comparison can occur in a randomized clinical trial or through natural experiments and analysis of experience as documented in large routine data sets, leading to what Etheredge (2007) calls the "rapid learning health system."

But both models require a much more systematic approach to clinical practice and clinical innovation than is common in health care today. Rather than every patient being treated according to the preferences and styles of his or her practitioner, described as the "cottage industry" approach by an array of US health care luminaries (Swensen et al., 2010), the new paradigm requires standardization of approaches to care. Adoption of standardized pathways reduces in-hospital complications and probably reduces length of stay (Rotter et al., 2010). Although the methods to bridge the evidence-practice gap through standardization are still somewhat unclear (Evensen, Sanson-Fisher, D'Este, & Fitzgerald, 2010), standardization at least requires clinical leadership and widespread clinical involvement, and appropriate decision support to ensure easy access to clinical paths and standardized practices or order sets[105] (Blackmore, Mecklenburg, & Kaplan, 2011; Brennan, Mattick, & Ellis, 2010; Moxey et al., 2010). Nelson et al. (2007) argue that this can take place within a clinical "microsystem" or small clinical team at the facility level, and this is true. But cross-facility learning and sharing may be more powerful, allowing learning from a more heterogeneous set of experiences, and addressing the idiosyncrasies of local practice patterns (including supply effects) that impact care (de Jong, Westert, Lagoe, & Groenewegen, 2006).

One mechanism to facilitate this cross-facility learning is to create prov-incial "clinical networks." Originally developed to improve cancer care in Scotland, then adopted more widely throughout the National Health Service in the United Kingdom (Carter, Garside, & Black, 2003; Cropper, Hopper, & Spencer, 2002) and imported to Australia (Duckett, 2007, 2009) and thence Alberta, clinical networks have been defined as "linked groups of health professionals and organizations from primary, secondary and tertiary care working in a co-ordinated manner, unconstrained by existing professional and organizational boundaries to ensure equitable provision of high-quality effective services" (Edwards, 2002, p. 63).

Although the benefits of clinical networks may not always be realized (Addicott, McGivern, & Ferlie, 2006), clinical networks have the expertise to develop and the legitimacy to facilitate implementation of standard pathways, practice approaches, and methods of comparing clinical performance. Their key strength is that they are grounded in clinical practice (Addicott, McGivern, & Ferlie, 2007; Guven-Uslu, 2006), and with that focus can become a powerful quality-improvement force (Frank, Marshall, Faris, & Smith, 2011; Gooch et al., 2009).

*Provinces should create and fund clinical networks to provide leadership in sharing good practice to improve access, quality, and sustainability of health care.*

Clinical networks can contribute to ensuring good referral networks are created within and between provinces, and can endorse appropriate paths for referrals to facilitate procedures being undertaken where there is appropriate expertise (Brennan et al., 2010). The relationship between volume and outcomes is so strong that Urbach, Stukel, Croxford, and MacCallum (2005, p. 2) commented, "In our review, we were not so much struck by the observation that volume-outcome associations were so prevalent, but by the remarkable finding that it was impossible to identify a health service that had been evaluated in more than one study that did *not* have a volume-outcome association."

The volume effect is partly due to reduced complications (Allareddy, Ward, Allaready, & Konety, 2010) and is more pronounced for some procedures (Finks, Osborne, & Birkmeyer, 2011). Centralization of services involves complex trade-offs between clinical outcomes and multiple factors: travel time for patients and their visitors; local politics and employment; and the destabilizing effect on local hospitals (including potentially impacting their viability) of removing some services. When confronted with travel time versus outcome trade-offs, different patients will have different responses, and there are different patterns for different conditions (Kronebusch, 2009). The costs of centralization can, to some extent, be ameliorated by taking the service to the patient through telehealth technologies (Praxia Information Intelligence & Gartner, 2011). The overall pattern is that a high proportion of patients will prefer treatment locally if outcomes are the same; but the more outcomes are better at centralized facilities, the more patients will be prepared to travel (Chang et al., 2004; Finlayson, Birkmeyer, Tosteson, & Nease, 1999; Tracey & Zelmer, 2005). Although clinical networks can make recommendations about the benefits of service centralization, local communities should be presented with the potential outcome differences and consulted on their preferences. Espoused preferences and revealed preferences should be tracked over time with (non)-centralization decisions regularly reviewed for their appropriateness.

Finally, clinical networks can be appropriate authorizing bodies for standardized, evidence-based care paths, including reviewing the multiplicity of inconsistent guidance and care paths developed by external "authoritative bodies" (Keyhani, Kim, Mann, & Korenstein, 2011) or by commercial groups such as Map of Medicine (Brennan et al., 2010; Goldmann, 2010; Vanhaecht, Panella, Van Zelm, & Sermeus, 2009).

The *Canada Health Act* criterion about comprehensiveness imposes an obligation on provinces to cover "necessary" services, a concept that is vague and undefined (see discussion in Chapter 1). An appropriate contemporary qualifier to "necessary," or indeed an alternative, could be to limit required coverage to "effective," or better, "cost-effective" services.[106] The risk here is that provinces could establish differential standards of parsimony, masquerading as effectiveness, and so covered services might diverge across Canada, undermining the national consistency of Medicare. Two approaches could be followed to mitigate this risk:

- Any provincial process to assess effectiveness/cost-effectiveness should be transparent and independent of government (Flood & Choudhry, 2002, 2004).
- A national body (such as the Canadian Agency for Drugs and Technologies in Health) could establish a register of candidate technologies that could be deemed potentially ineffective, and provinces' autonomy would be limited to excluding technologies on the register. This would guarantee a national core of common covered services.

The two approaches are not alternatives and both could be pursued. Highlighting the importance of effectiveness as a criterion for coverage could stimulate effectiveness and cost-effectiveness research in Canada.

*The comprehensiveness criterion in the* Canada Health Act *should be amended to include an obligation on provinces to cover effective services, with a requirement that effectiveness be determined in a transparent way.*

Over time, it would be appropriate for the effectiveness criterion to be replaced by a cost-effectiveness one. This evolution should be preceded by further public debate on the issue of value for money in the Canadian health care system and the place of cost-effectiveness assessment in ensuring that.

### Addressing capacity

It is now 50 years since an analysis of the impact on the admission rate and length of stay of a significant expansion of beds in upstate New York led to Roemer's Law: that a built bed becomes a filled bed.[107] Additional supply (of beds, physicians) leads to additional use, but that additional use does not lead to improvement in health status or patient satisfaction (Léonard, Stordeur, & Roberfroid, 2009; Wennberg, 2010). Unfortunately, this reality applies across the health system. More use of nursing home beds, for example, does not necessarily lead to reduction in use of acute beds (Wennberg, 2010).

The supply effect is endemic, in both rural and urban areas, but is more an issue in some provinces than others (see Figure 7.1). There were substantial utilization rate differences between provinces in 2005–06 from a high of around 12,000 admissions per 100,000 population in Saskatchewan to around in 7,500 in Ontario. Although there was a reduction in utilization over the decade (average of around 25 percent), utilization rate patterns are surprisingly stable with a strong correlation between the provincial rates at the beginning and end of the period (r = 0.94).

**FIGURE 7.1**
**Age-standardized inpatient hospitalization rates (per 100,000 population), by province, 1995–1996 and 2005–2006**

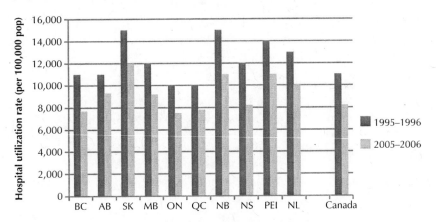

Source: Canadian Institute for Health Information (2007b, Table 2).

Players in decisions about hospital capital expansion have a range of motives, not solely related to improving health or even health care, and the relationship between local hospital management and central funders can become quite complex (Thompson & McKee, 2011). Strategies to reduce supply (and preference) sensitive utilization include developing rigorous and agreed priority-setting criteria for admissions, which should build on the work of the Western Canada Waiting List Project;[108] monitoring appropriateness of admissions and length of stay (Fontaine et al., 2011; Gertman & Restuccia, 1981; Shortt, 1998); and seeking to understand patient preferences.[109] As with centralization of services, addressing capacity issues is not easy (Sinclair, Rochon, & Leatt, 2005), and hospital closures have traditionally been a "no go" in health policy. But there is increasing recognition of the economic, staffing, and quality costs of keeping non-viable facilities open (Torjesen, 2011). Certainly, expansion proposals should now be rigorously reviewed to assess whether intrahospital flow improvement strategies or development of community-based alternatives are more cost-effective (Fisher, Bynum, & Skinner, 2009; Scott, 2010).

*Provinces should request clinical networks (when established) to review differences in intra- and interprovincial utilization rates. Networks should be invited to develop and/or update priority-setting criteria.*

### Access: Getting the right care, on time

Canadians wait too long for access to care: for primary care, to see a specialist, in an emergency, for elective procedures (see Figure 7.2). Waiting times in Canada are longer than in many other countries (Schoen et al., 2010). The data reported in Figure 7.2 are from the New York–based Commonwealth Fund, which conducts annual surveys of experiences of health care in a number of countries. Canada's own tracking of wait times is patchy and inconsistent, and "much of the wait time picture remains clouded in mystery" (Wait Time Alliance, 2010, p. 1). Patients want clearer, better information (Bruni, Laupacis, Levinson, & Martin, 2010). There is no standardization of definitions between provinces, and in some cases there is no standardization within provinces (Sanmartin & Steering Committee, 2003).[110] Public wait-time reporting is almost exclusively limited to the five "priority areas" established as part of the 2004 Accord: joint replacement (hip and knee), cataract surgery, coronary artery bypass graft, diagnostic imaging (MRI and CT), and radiation therapy. There is no evidence that these conditions are serving as indicators for whole-system performance, and a continued focus on a limited range of conditions seems inappropriate.

**FIGURE 7.2**
**Canadians' experience of waiting for care, 2010**

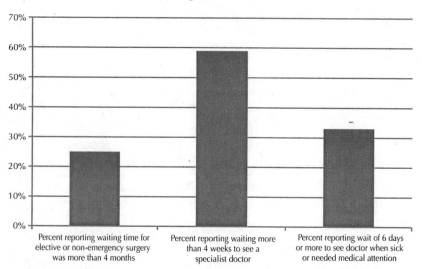

Source: Schoen et al. (2010).

In addition to interprovincial differences, waits differ by age, income, and region (Maddison, Asada, & Urquhart, 2011).

For elective procedures, from a patient's perspective, the critical wait is from when a family physician makes a referral through to when a definitive procedure occurs (if one is necessary), but this is rarely what is reported. Public reporting typically focuses on the wait from when a surgeon decides a procedure is necessary, ignoring the first wait up to the specialist consultation. For cancer care, different pathways (medical oncology, radiation oncology) have different waits (Maddison et al., 2011).

There is no magic policy or management bullet that will fix waits (Siciliani & Hurst, 2005). No single strategy, uniformly applied, will address the wait-time problem, as the causes and symptoms vary across Canada. But there are some generic approaches:

- start with measurement, as without knowing the extent of the problem, management is not possible;
- consider both demand and supply issues, for example, focus upstream (prevent where possible); and
- recognize that multifaceted strategies will be required.

## Measurement and targets

Measurement of waits is not simple. In the case of elective procedures, it requires new data collections so that the total wait from family physician referral can be calculated. Component waits (time to consultation, time to procedure) should be separately reported, which means consistency of definitions of each component: Is the second wait from the time a surgeon makes a decision that a procedure is necessary? The time the hospital is notified that an operating slot will be required? The time that a patient decides that he or she wants the procedure, considering all the options and the potential side effects (see the earlier discussion about patient decision aids)? There are technical issues as well, including whether reporting should be based on the actual experience of those who waited, or on census measures of waiting lists (Armstrong, 2009, 2010a, 2010b). Lists with long waiting times may include people whose needs have changed since originally listed, and so these lists should be reviewed both administratively and clinically before the data can be reliably used for public reporting (Stainkey, Seidl, Johnson, Tulloch, & Pain, 2010).

*Provinces should commit to adopting common definitions of waiting times for the full patient journey.*

Measurement goes beyond simple counting: as argued above, there needs to be consistent priority-setting processes to ensure more urgent cases are dealt with expeditiously.

Although measuring provides the base, measurement without active intervention is futile. Incentives on services to manage waiting lists—through targets with sanctions and rewards—are effective in bringing down long waits (Hauck & Street, 2007; Propper, Sutton, Whitnall, & Windmeijer, 2008, 2010; Siciliani & Hurst, 2005) and, although they carry a gaming risk (Kreindler, 2010), should be part of all service-funding regimes. The English waiting-time targets are much more aggressive that Canada's, covering the whole wait of a patient, in a much shorter time. Implementation has been driven aggressively and waiting times in England have dramatically improved (Appleby, 2011). Quebec has given some force to its waiting-time targets by introducing a "guarantee" that where targets are not achieved, the patient has redress through funded access to alternative provision (Prémont, 2007). A guarantee, of course, is only necessary if there is failure to achieve the announced targets: in Quebec the guarantee was a response to a Supreme Court decision. Guarantees rely on alternative providers, but creation of an alternative supply may create a different range of problems (Duckett, 2005b; Iversen, 1997).

*Federal, provincial, and territorial leaders should agree on waiting-time targets for a broad range of services. Provinces should publish consistent data on achievement of these targets at least quarterly, and the Canadian Institute for Health Information should collate and publish these data at least annually.*

The *Canada Health Act* does not specifically mention wait times as part of the accessibility principle:

> In order to satisfy the criterion respecting accessibility, the health care insurance plan of a province
>
> (a) must provide for insured health services on uniform terms and conditions and on a basis that does not impede or preclude, either directly or indirectly whether by charges made to insured persons or otherwise, reasonable access to those services by insured persons. (s. 12(1))

The only barrier specifically mentioned in the Act is extra-billing, for which there are strict penalty provisions. But long waits are a clear example of impediments to reasonable access. Additional force can be given to agreed waiting-time targets by making them the basis for additional penalty provisions. *The 2014 Accord should expand the penalty provisions in the* Canada Health Act *to incorporate penalties for consistent failure to reach agreed waiting-time targets.*

### Demand-side interventions

A key driver of health care demand is growth and aging of the population, which impacts differentially in different locations. But demographic demand is mediated by a range of other factors: population health programs to improve health; the propensity of a person with a particular set of symptoms to convert that to health-service utilization, in secondary care, as guided by a particular physician; and the availability (and convenience) of alternative treatment options. Demand-side strategies have been described as "somewhat problematic" because of the perceived relative intractability of demand (Kreindler, 2010). The lead times for these factors obviously vary, with some public health interventions taking years to have an impact. However, shorter-term impact is achievable: implementation of more informed patient decision making can have an immediate impact for preference-sensitive conditions, and improving management of chronic illnesses impacts outcomes and utilization within 12 months, at least in terms of family physician and emergency department visits (Lorig et al., 2001). Development of alternative services such as free-standing procedure centres are effective in alleviating waits for elective procedures, but these centres have longer lead times associated with construction (Lowthian et al., 2011).

## Supply-side interventions

Access issues are created when demand and supply are not in balance. Demand is best measured as a flow: how many patients arrive per hour in the emergency department, per day in primary care, and so on. Supply then should also be measured in terms of flow. The critical issues are not how many emergency department spaces there are, how many family physicians, and how many hospital beds but rather what these services do. What is the flow? Of course capacity is one factor that impacts flow, but so too is productivity. What is the length of stay in those beds? How many patients are seen per physician per day? (This will be discussed more fully in the next section about efficiency.)

Successful supply-side strategies require supportive local leadership, physician engagement, and sometimes seed funds to kick-start projects (Pomey et al., 2010). In general, more direct wait-time strategies are more successful:

> Paying for treatment activity, buying capacity locally to support increased treatment and providing strong incentives for organizations to meet wait-time targets are demonstrated strategies for reducing wait times. There is also evidence that the use of existing capacity can often be greatly improved … In contrast, indirect strategies—for instance, depending on an internal market to provide the right incentives for wait reduction, on increased private financing to generate an adequate supply of needed care, on the reporting of wait-time information to encourage patients to redistribute themselves, or on unenforced guarantees to spur changes in provider behaviour—have a poor record. (Kreindler, 2010. p. 28)

## The efficiency imperative

Total health spending is the result of the interaction of costs and volumes. The variations discussion above focused on the importance of controlling volume, but controlling costs or prices paid is equally important—more important,

White (2011) argued and, from a policy perspective, more effective. From a theoretical perspective, price regulation may be more effective than volume regulation when marginal benefits increase relatively slowly (at least relative to marginal costs), a situation that is typical in health care (Hepburn, 2006).

There is considerable variation in unit costs of care (cost per patient treated, cost per lab test, cost per physician visit) across the health system, both within and between provinces. In addition to waste in the system associated with this (technical) inefficiency, there is waste associated with social or allocative efficiency: the right care is not being provided in the right setting.

Bentley, Effros, Palar, and Keeler (2008) have developed a framework for conceptualizing waste in the health care system, distinguishing

- administrative waste (due to administrative complexity);
- operational waste (from inefficient ways of producing services); and
- clinical waste (due to "low value" outputs such as unnecessary admissions or tests).

### Administrative waste

The Canadian health system is not administratively top heavy, at least as compared to the United States (Cutler & Ly, 2011; Morra et al., 2011; Woolhandler, Campbell, & Himmelstein, 2003). The 1990s saw a wave of provincial reviews and regionalization in Canada that eliminated countless separate boards (Naylor, 1999) each with associated administrative overhead; the notable exception is Ontario, which maintains an elaborate structure (Flood & Sinclair, 2004). Of course regionalization does not guarantee elimination of administrative waste, and a 2002 survey reported lack of clarity by participants of relative roles in regionalized systems (Lewis & Kouri, 2004), predisposing to a degree of administrative waste.

Regionalization is not a panacea (Casebeer, 2004), and further administrative savings can be achieved. However, reorganization/restructuring of health service delivery agencies per se rarely realizes the postulated benefits (Braithwaite, Westbrook, & Iedema, 2005). The continued pursuit of reorganization-based strategies has been described by one English commentator as "the triumph of hope over experience" (Edwards, 2010) and ridiculed by others (Oxman, Sackett, Chalmers, & Prescott, 2005). Notwithstanding these cautions, consolidation of Alberta's nine regions and three provincial boards into Alberta Health Services led to significant reductions in the number of senior administrators, as well as savings through economies of scale from centralization of procurement decisions and other functions (Duckett, 2011).

*Provinces should review current administrative structures to identify the potential for savings—and more effective priority setting—from centralization of functions.*

## Operational waste

The last decade has seen the widespread use of systematic techniques (such as LEAN or Six-sigma) in the health sector to reengineer work flows and processes to eliminate waste (Barnas, 2011; DelliFraine, Langabeer, & Nembhard, 2010; Glasgow, Scott-Caziewell, & Kaboli, 2010; Poksinska, 2010; Toussaint, 2009). The favourite or dominant technique changes almost at fashion-frequency, being described as "pseudo-innovation" (Walshe, 2009), with a suggestion that the underlying theory behind these approaches is weak (Grol et al., 2007).

"LEAN thinking" emphasizes that there are two types of activities in organizations: value adding and waste (the latter often labelled with the Japanese word for waste, *muda*). Waste is defined broadly to include rejects (in the health sector this category would include quality issues), transport waste, and motion waste (Imai, 1997). Various tools have also been developed to identify operational waste such as those of the Institute for Healthcare Improvement (Resar, Griffin, Kabcenell, & Bones, 2011).

Fundamental to LEAN redesign is improving flow (Womack & Jones, 2003). In the health sector this should cover the entire value stream from referral to rehabilitation (Frank et al., 2011). For the operating room, flow improvement covers elective and emergency cases, and the hospital services that are upstream and downstream, such as intensive care units (Cardoen, Demeulemeester, & Beliën, 2010). Flow improvements can occur through a number of channels: creation of new clinical decision units or medical assessment units associated with emergency care (Daly, Campbell, & Cameron, 2003; Hassan, 2003); creation of "23-hour units" to focus on ensuring appropriate discharge quickly (Ryan, Davoren, Grant, & Delbridge, 2004); and flow redesign on clinical units (National Nursing Research Unit, 2010) and in outpatient settings (Rouppe van der Voort, van Merode, & Berden, 2010). These improvements can be led internally or involve external consultants (Scott et al., 2011), but are always premised on involvement of those in the affected work place (Imai, 1997). Niemeijer, Trip, Does, De Mast, and Van Den Heuvel (2011) have identified nine generic categories of improvement projects, six of which are associated with cost or waste reduction.[111] These strategies aim to reduce costs by improving productivity of personnel, utilization of equipment/facilities, purchasing processes, and safety (by reducing complications and incidents); and by reducing unnecessary use of resources and inventory.

Operations research techniques, including queuing theory, and simulation and systems dynamics techniques can also be used to guide potential areas for system improvement (Homer & Hirsch, 2006; Lane & Husemann, 2007).

Another form of operational waste is poor-quality care, which costs money in longer stays (see Table 7.1), in returns to the operating room (Birkmeyer et al., 2001; Ploeg, Lange, Lardenoye, & Breslau, 2008), in avoidable attendances at emergency departments at the end of life (Barbera, Taylor, & Dudgeon, 2010; Earle et al., 2003), and in avoidable readmissions (Halfon et al., 2006; Jack et al., 2009; van Walraven et al., 2010; van Walraven, Bennett, Jennings, Austin, & Forster, 2011). Addressing quality variation and implementing safety practices are thus potential efficiency strategies (Huerta, Thompson, & Ford, 2011; Mitton, Dionne, Peacock, & Sheps, 2006), a conclusion reinforced by Ludwig, Van Merode, and Groot (2010) who suggest that efficiency and quality "go together" as complements rather than substitutes. Reduction in adverse events is not the only way in which improved quality can lead to reduced costs; improved booking processes can, for example, reduce the "did not attend" rates in clinics (Marshall & Øvretveit, 2011). Reinforcing the efficiency benefit of improved quality, Mark, Jones, Lindley, and Ozcan (2009) found many nursing units were operating inefficiently, but that

> traditional targets for efficiency improvements, such as providing fewer hours of nursing care and reducing operating expenses, are not managerial strategies that would yield the largest efficiency gains. Our analysis suggests that it is in the reduction of medication errors and patient falls— two critical patient safety targets—where the greatest efficiency gains are likely to be seen. (p. 184)

The link between efficiency and high quality has also been found within a single health system: the United States Veterans Health System (Gao et al., 2011).

## Clinical waste

Bentley et al. (2008, p. 644) define clinical waste "as spending to produce services that provide marginal or no health benefit over less costly alternatives." They provide eight examples in the United States, accounting for at least 1.9 percent of US health spending: excessive antibiotic use for viral upper respiratory infections and otitis media; avoidable emergency department use; avoidable hospitalizations of nursing-home patients; overuse of cytology for cervical cancer screening; inappropriate hysterectomies; unnecessary hospital admissions in emergency department triage of chest-pain patients; overuse of non-invasive radiologic imaging; and inappropriate spinal-fusion surgeries. Hoffman and Pearson (2009) use the term "marginal medicine" and identify four types of examples: inadequate evidence of comparative net benefit; use beyond boundaries of established net benefit; higher cost when net benefit is comparable to other options; and relatively high cost for incremental benefit compared to other options.

Probably the most significant example of clinical waste in Canada is attributable to alternate-level-of-care patients; as pointed out in the previous chapter, failure to provide alternate care means that such patients occupy about 5,200 acute hospital beds on any given day.

Another class of patients indicative of clinical waste is patients admitted to hospital with diagnoses that could have been prevented (e.g., vaccine preventable diseases) or whose risk of admission could have been reduced with good primary health care or prevention. Termed ambulatory care sensitive conditions (Ansari, 2007; Ansari, Laditka, & Laditka, 2006), these diagnoses accounted for one in eight medical admissions in 2006–07 (Sanchez, Vellanky, Herring, Liang, & Jia, 2008) and more than one in ten hospital-bed days overall (Sanmartin, Khan, & LHAD Research Team, 2011). The age-sex standardized admission rate for ambulatory care sensitive conditions per 100,000 population per annum varies from 251 in British Columbia to 497 in Prince Edward Island. There is a sixfold difference across Canada in rates of admission at the regional level: from 157 per 100,000 population in the area served by the York regional health unit in Ontario to 1,040 in the Burntwood region in Manitoba.[112] This form of waste—excess admission rates for ambulatory care sensitive conditions—can be addressed at least in part by the chronic disease management strategies discussed in Chapter 4, and by home care investments (Lavoie, Forget, Dahl, Martens, & O'Neil, 2011).

In addition to ambulatory sensitive conditions, there are a number of conditions where intensive acute treatment can be provided in the home instead of in a hospital: programs to facilitate this are often called "hospital in the home" (Montalto, 2010; Montalto, Lui, Mullins, & Woodmason, 2010). Clinical outcomes from these programs do not appear to differ from inpatient treatment and are less expensive (Iliffe & Shepperd, 2002; MacIntyre, Ruth, & Ansari, 2002; Shepperd et al., 2008), and so failure to use these programs to the full is another example of waste.[113]

Overuse of laboratory tests and diagnostic imaging is another source of waste (Jha et al., 2009; Sistrom et al., 2009; You et al., 2007). Studies of inappropriate use of acute beds regularly find high levels of excess length of stay and inappropriate admissions (Fontaine et al., 2011; McDonagh, Smith, & Goddard, 2000), a further example of clinical waste. Inclusion of experienced physiotherapists in the orthopedic care path reduces the need for visits to a surgeon (MacKay, Davis, Mahomed, & Badley, 2009; Oldmeadow et al., 2007). Introduction of specialist nurse roles ("pivot nurse") can also achieve efficiency improvements in orthopedic clinics (Poder, Bellemare, Bédard, He, & Lemieux, 2010).

Finally, another form of clinical waste is use of treatments of low clinical value. The Croydon (London) Primary Care Trust has developed a list of such procedures including

- those where more cost-effective alternatives should be tried first (e.g., hysterectomy in cases of heavy menstrual bleeding);
- those with a close benefit-and-risk balance in mild cases (e.g., wisdom teeth extraction);
- potentially cosmetic procedures (e.g., orthodontics); and
- those considered to be relatively ineffective (e.g., tonsillectomy).

Although there may be disagreement about some of the items on the list, the United Kingdom Audit Commission (2011) has estimated that, given the current incidence of these procedures in the United Kingdom, reduction in incidence could yield savings of around C$15 per head of population.

The United States–based Good Stewardship Working Group (2011) has identified a top five list of "don'ts" for internal medicine, family practice, and pediatrics, adoption of which would also lead to reduction in clinical waste.[114]

Ensuring good end-of-life care is important in terms of patient and family experience. But given the concentration of health care costs in the last few months of life (as discussed in Chapter 2), improvements in care here may also reduce costs. There is good evidence about a range of medical interventions to improve end-of-life care (Lorenz et al., 2008). Discussing patient and family expectations and wishes about treatment options at the end of life and for older people is associated with improved satisfaction and communication (Detering, Hancock, Reade, & Silvester, 2010; Teno, Gruneir, Schwartz, Nanda, & Wetle, 2007). In this context, it becomes possible for treatment teams to address waste issues in end-of-life care, for example by discontinuing treatment that has no life-extending impact and reduces quality of end-of-life care (Saito, Landrum, Neville, Ayanian, & Earle, 2011).

Addressing waste requires a combination of strategies: measurement of inappropriate use (McDonagh et al., 2000), involvement of the clinical networks to identify potential indicators of clinical waste, involvement locally to improve flow, involvement of regional or provincial decision makers to ensure cost-effective alternatives are implemented. Stronger incentives should also be introduced to encourage local management to address efficiency variations.

## Incentives to improve efficiency

Financial incentives on providers can be used to promote a range of policy objectives, and incentive arrangements need to be matched to the contemporary policy goals (Custers, Hurley, Klazinga, & Brown, 2008). The 1990s regionalization wave in Canada was associated with introduction of a new funding system: population-based funding to regions and global funding to services. Although population-based funding (termed capitation in the United States) provides the incentives for both technical and social efficiency, the reality is that after almost 20 years of implementation, it does not appear to have achieved this. This may be due to incomplete implementation: regions rarely have responsibility for the full spectrum of health care (pharmaceuticals for ambulatory patients and physician budgets being the most notable exclusions), and political overrides may change funding allocations to vitiate incentive effects of the funding formulas.[115]

Under global budgeting there is no direct relationship between the allocated funding and the services provided, and each region tended to develop its own approach to establishing the global budget for the institutions for which it had responsibility. Comparisons of efficiency between institutions were inhibited for a range of reasons including inter-regional mistrust and differences in data systems and definitions. Inevitably, facilities diverged in their efficiency.

Over the last two decades there has been an increasing international interest in one technique for addressing efficiency variation—activity-based funding. In Canada this approach, termed "service-based funding," was recommended in the Kirby Report (Senate, 2002a).[116] The idea is simple: hospitals and other sectors should be paid on the basis of what they do (their activity). But there agreement ends. The concept has "more names than a mobster on the run" (Collier, 2008, p. 1407), and the policy permutations similarly vary, including at the most basic level whether funding to a facility should be capped or uncapped and what method should be used to describe activity (Jegers, Kesteloot, De Graeve, & Gilles, 2002).

Activity-based funding has two key elements:

- A hospital's (or other service's) revenue is directly linked to the volume and acuity of patients (clients) treated.
- The payment per patient (or client) is determined prospectively, independent of the specific hospital/service.

Health services funded under an activity-based funding system have a strong incentive to provide services up to the level of any funding/volume cap, and to ensure that what they do is done efficiently as they face the same payment rates as other services. Activity-based funding has been shown to drive management responses and significant efficiency improvements (Biorn, Hagen, Iversen, & Magnussen, 2010; Busato & von Below, 2010; Conrad & Guven Uslu, 2011; Cutler & Ly, 2011; Duckett, 1995; Moreno-Serra & Wagstaff, 2010; Vos, Wagner, et al., 2010), but carries an inherent risk of evoking inappropriate responses through adverse selection or moral hazard (Laffont & Tirole, 1993), including up-coding and cream skimming (Simborg, 1981). The perverse incentives of activity-based funding can and should be addressed in the design of the case-mix classification used, in other elements of system design, and through monitoring and surveillance systems (Duckett, Hatcher, Murphy, & Richards, 2011).

Activity-based funding is not always possible or the best policy option. Like any quasi-market strategy, it relies, for example, on good descriptors of the services being purchased (Williamson, 1975, 1986), and where there is little variation in volumes or costs, block contracts/global budgets may be preferred (Chalkley & McVicar, 2008).

There are many choices to be made in the design of activity-based funding systems (Deber, Hollander, & Jacobs, 2008; Street & Maynard, 2007a). Activity-based funding can be designed to promote a range of disparate objectives (Street & Maynard, 2007b), and so it is likely that there will be interprovincial variation in design as a result of different emphases in policy between the provinces.

Activity-based funding systems evolve: in the United States where activity-based funding for Medicare patients in hospitals (called prospective payment) has been in place for almost 30 years (Russell, 1989), there are now calls to extend the unit of measurement for payment beyond hospital walls to incorporate more elements of the patient's journey, creating a bundled episode of care payment (Averill, Goldfield, Hughes, Eisenhandler, & Vertrees, 2009; Bach, Mirkin, & Luke, 2011; Davis, 2007; Hussey, Sorbero, Mehrotra, Liu, & Damberg, 2009; Sood, Huckfeldt, Escarce, Grabowski, & Newhouse, 2011). That said, the condition precedent for this—robust descriptors of typical patterns—does not currently exist.

Implementation of activity-based funding is likely to change the power dynamic within hospitals as hospital management seeks to engage physicians in changing their behaviour to reduce the number of services ordered (laboratory tests, diagnostic imaging) and length of stay to complement traditional strategies to reduce unit costs of services ordered (Saltman & Young, 1981; Young & Saltman, 1985). Not all hospital departments are equally efficient (Ludwig et al., 2010), and that may also generate intrafacility conflict.

Implementation of activity-based funding in Canada should not occur overnight (Sutherland, 2011; Sutherland, Barer, Evans, & Crump, 2011). Hospitals should be given time to prepare, and should be supported with the necessary management infrastructure. Activity-based funding may drive increased demand for hospital substitutes (such as home care), and further investments may be needed there too.

*Provinces should commit to a phased introduction of activity-based funding to drive improvements in efficiency in the hospital and other sectors.*

Because of the provincial basis of the Canadian health care system, and the further decentralization of funding policies associated with regionalization, there is substantial variation in cost per patient treated across Canada (after taking severity into account). As each province develops its own activity-based funding approach, care needs to be taken that these provincial variations are not inappropriately incorporated into the design of the funding system. *Provinces should review comparative cost data (published by the Canadian Institute for Health Information) to ensure that provincial payment rates are set at efficient levels.*

## Pay for performance

Among the blizzard of funding reform proposals in the United States[117] are many that link service funding to other aspects of performance such as quality. Pay for performance is being considered or introduced in a number of countries with publicly funded health care (Annemans et al., 2009; OECD, 2010e; van Herck et al., 2010) with different mixtures of the key design elements: which measures to reward, what is the basis for the reward, and how much reward.

A move away from global funding facilitates the incorporation of incentives for a broad range of policy goals, including incentives to reduce waiting times (Duckett, 2008). Almost all contemporary implementations of funding reform involve a blend of efficiency and pay-for-performance (P4P) aspects (McClellan, 2011; Schneider, Hussey, & Schnyer, 2011). Yet the evidence to support such enthusiasm is weak (Christianson et al., 2008; Tanenbaum, 2009; Van Herck et al., 2010). Further, it has been argued that the preconditions for pay for performance to provide the desired incentive effects are not present (Nicholson et al., 2008), or that such incentives misconstrue the importance of a balance between reputational and financial rewards among health professionals (Frølich, Talavera, Broadhead, & Dudley, 2007). Pay for performance also has the potential to exacerbate the prevalent inequality in access in the United States (Blustein, Borden, & Valentine, 2010), although the quality and outcomes framework in the United Kingdom appears to be equity-enhancing (Doran, Fullwood, Kontopantelis, & Reeves, 2008).

So there is legitimate skepticism about pay for performance among Canadian policy leaders (Coutts & Thornhill, 2009; Lewis, 2009). Pay for (quality) performance relies on good measurement (Nicholson et al., 2008). Although routine data sets and clinical registries perform similarly in predicting risk of hospital death (Aylin, Bottle, & Majeed, 2007), measurement of quality of hospital care using readily available data is still challenging (OECD 2010d, 2010e; Pronovost & Lilford, 2011)—at least to the standard necessary to be of use in making comparative judgments. An analysis of commercially available methods of predicting in-hospital deaths using a Massachusetts data set showed little agreement between calculated in-hospital mortality rates and individual mortality-risk probabilities (Shahian, Wolf, Iezzoni, Kirle, & Normand, 2010). There is also little agreement between rankings of hospitals using different data sets (Stausberg, Halim, & Faerber, 2011), with data exhibiting random variation that may preclude "rankability" (van Dishoeck, Lingsma, Mackenbach, & Steyerberg, 2011; van Dishoeck, Looman, van der Wilden-van Lier, Mackenbach, & Steyerberg, 2011). Hospitals that perform well on a composite measure may not even be in the top quintile on most individual measures (Shwartz et al., 2011). There is a degree of underlying instability in some of the measures used in pay-for-performance (and public) reporting: hospitals with zero mortality in prior years appear no different (or worse) than other hospitals in subsequent years (Dimick & Welch, 2008), with low stability also reported for measures of organization performance in health maintenance (Swaminathan, Chernew, & Scanlon, 2008). In order to mitigate these risks, the OECD (2010d) has developed principles to take into account when using and developing quality indicators, including addressing the risk of gaming.

A negative form of pay for performance is not to pay for non-performance, or identified safety issues. Averill, Hughes, and Goldfield (2011) distinguish this from pay for performance by referring to it as pay for outcomes. Incentives can be structured as bonuses or penalties, with different effects (Balch, 1980); a long stream of behavioural research in this area suggests that avoidance of penalties is a very strong motivator. In addition to any monetary effect of a penalty, penalties for quality-related infringements (or poorer performance) carry stigma or reputational-risk costs. Incentive structures for hospitals should thus balance positive and negative reinforcement strategies.

The routine hospital data sets used for activity-based funding distinguish pre-existing comorbidities present on admission and hospital-acquired complications. The United States' Medicare payment system has recently been modified to exclude a limited list of hospital-acquired conditions from being used in assigning cases in the case-mix classification and thus from impacting activity-based payment (Averill, Vertrees, McCullough, Hughes, & Goldfield, 2006; Hoff & Soerensen, 2011; McNair, Luft, & Bindman, 2009; Rosenthal, 2007). Proposals have also been advanced and implemented to absorb costs of any readmissions in the index admission (de Brantes, Rastogi, & Painter, 2010; Mechanic & Altman, 2009; Rosenthal, 2008).

*Introduction of activity-based funding should be accompanied by measures to promote improved quality, whether through pay for performance, non-payment for poor performance, or increased surveillance and accountability.*

Pay-for-performance incentives may more reliably be introduced for other policy goals such as access: incentives could be introduced that link additional activity targets, for example, to reduction in waiting times (Street & Duckett, 1996). *As part of activity-based funding implementation, provinces should consider introduction of incentives on hospitals to reduce waiting times.*

## The next steps

Hospitals are expensive and highly visible parts of the health system. Getting hospitals and acute care right has both symbolic benefits and the potential for significant efficiency improvements. What has been shown in this chapter is that there are challenges, and the potential to improve, on all three critical system goals of access, quality, and sustainability. As shown, there are interactions between these goals: quality improvements, for example, can improve efficiency (sustainability).

The provinces have a central role in improving hospitals and acute care, and more than half the proposals made in this chapter are strategies for improvement at the provincial level. Federal agencies can facilitate provincial improvement actions, and several proposals are directed accordingly.

# Word cloud: Ensuring the right skill set is available

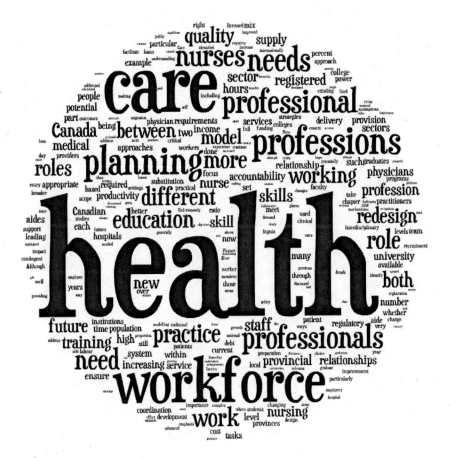

In this chapter I propose the following policy initiatives:

- Health services delivery organizations should implement or continue systematic programs for care model redesign to facilitate all professionals' working to their top scope of practice. The Canadian Institutes of Health Research should be tasked and funded to establish a funding stream to evaluate implementation of care model redesign and associated role redesign.
- Health Canada should convene a conference of provincial health ministries and regulatory bodies to share leading practice in regulation of basic and advanced nursing roles.
- Provinces should model workforce planning requirements for the larger health professions at least every five years. Health Canada should support the provinces in a national approach to modelling workforce planning requirements for the smaller health professions. Planning for Canada and the larger provinces should aim for net self-sufficiency.
- The Canadian Institutes of Health Research should be tasked and funded to create research training initiatives in professions where there is a shortage of faculty.
- The federal government should explore with the provinces interest in developing a national income-contingent loan program for health professions, coupled with loan forgiveness programs for employment in hard-to-recruit areas.
- Provinces should examine non-traditional sources for recruitment of entry-level workers, including providing on-the-job training opportunities.
- Provinces should establish formal mechanisms for planning and cooperation between universities and colleges and the major health providers. Health providers should consider mechanisms at the local level for the same purpose.
- Federal, provincial, and territorial leaders should review current health professional regulatory structures to facilitate further interprovincial migration and provision of health care across provincial borders.

# CHAPTER 8

# ENSURING THE RIGHT SKILL SET IS AVAILABLE

With the exception of the health professional acting as a passerby Good Samaritan at an accident scene, there is almost no health care encounter today that does not involve other professionals or support staff. In order to emphasize this involvement of others, the health system goal articulated in Chapter 2 might more appropriately be phrased as *The right member of the health care team enables the right care in the right setting, on time, every time.* But with this phrasing we need a caveat that family members and other caregivers would also have to be regarded as members of the health care team.

Ensuring the availability of an appropriate team is critical to delivering good quality care, efficiently. But the right team is not always available, or at least, used.

Imbalances in the health workforce have multiple antecedents and are impacted by factors within the health system (stakeholders, regulatory frameworks, payment design, market power) and outside the health system, including broad economic conditions (Zurn, Dal Poz, Stilwell, & Adams, 2004).

Although the health workforce challenge is often expressed as "Will we have enough [*insert profession of your choice*] to meet health care needs into the future?," this mono-disciplinary focus is the wrong place to start and will inevitably lead to workforce planning mistakes. We first should identify the health care needs to be met in the future, the work to be done to meet those needs, then who should do the work—and only then how many might be required (Buchan & O'May, 2000).

The missing first steps in the typical approach are based on an implicit assumption that the existing division of labour is ideal and cannot or should not be changed. As discussed in the previous chapter, health care supply and utilization vary significantly across regions, and there is scant evidence that additional supply leads to better health outcomes. A policy focus on extrapolating current provision ratios and identifying a "shortage" or a "workforce crisis" is the wrong diagnosis and almost certainly leads to the wrong prescription (Goodman & Fisher, 2008).

In parallel with thinking about the demand side of the health workforce equation (what needs are to be met, what work is to be done, what skills are needed, how many people will be needed to do this), and the supply side (where the people to do the work will come from), workforce planning needs to take into account the context or environment within which the work is done, and how work is to be organized—especially the role of teams (Simoens, Villeneuve, & Hurst, 2005). Other contextual factors include regulatory factors and payment approaches (as discussed in Chapter 4).

## The demand side

As argued above, workforce planning should start with health needs: what is required to keep a population healthy, respond to acute needs, and provide care to the chronically ill. The skills of health care providers are critically important inputs into those processes, but the objective of workforce policy is to ensure there is an adequate workforce to meet identified needs. As obvious as that sounds, this is not necessarily the way workforce planning is done today. Productivity measures used in monitoring the health workforce often focus on how many patients are seen by a professional, rather than considering what is done by the professional and how that contributes to meeting needs: a health professional can work very efficiently providing unnecessary care.

### *Cost, quality, and workforce planning*

In the past much workforce planning was simplistic and fixed-ratio based: planning was based on a target ratio of health professionals per capita, so that a target number of visits or procedures per annum could be undertaken. Workforce planning now is much more clearly linked to the service agenda, including the quality and access agendas. This quality-improvement context provides an important foil to the old, profession-based planning approaches. The quality improvement and waste discussions in the previous chapter highlighted the importance of process reform in improving both quality and efficiency. It was also pointed out in that chapter that quality initiatives can be cost saving.

The relationship between cost and quality is complex: for some conditions high cost is associated with better quality, but for others the reverse is true (Chen et al., 2010; Glance, Dick, Osler, Meredith, & Mukamel, 2010; Lagu et al., 2011). Similarly some hospitals perform well on both cost (efficiency) and quality, while others perform poorly on both metrics (McKay & Deily, 2005). Low-performing hospitals tended to have more staff per patient than other hospitals, while high-performing hospitals have fewer staff than other hospitals (McKay & Deily, 2005). This suggests fixed-ratio planning approaches, which assume that more staff is inevitably better, are inappropriate bases for workforce planning. Similarly, rigid regulatory approaches that specify particular staff ratios and/or maintain obsolete assumptions and workplace hierarchies may also militate against flexible response to emerging health care needs and hinder implementation of local quality-improvement strategies.

But obviously, health care provision will always rely on an appropriate mix of qualified staff. The knowledge, skills, and attitudes of the health workforce are critical to the quality of care received by a patient or consumer and, in a very real sense, health workers define the very nature of health care services. Skill is to be interpreted broadly, not just as technical skill, but the full skill set including the ability to communicate, work in teams, and so on. The Royal College of Physicians and Surgeons of Canada has articulated this broader concept well in its CanMEDS framework,[118] identifying the roles of competent physicians as medical expert (the central role), communicator, collaborator, health advocate, manager, scholar, and professional, each elaborated with defined competencies. This list can be mapped to those of other health professions (Verma, Paterson, & Medves, 2006).

## Practice change

The nature of health professional practice is changing, and must continue to evolve. In previous chapters, I've argued the need to change the current balance of service provision: more emphasis on supporting self-management and expanding assisted living, to give two examples. The shift in emphasis from treating acute disease to managing chronic illnesses requires a different mindset for the system, and different skill sets too. The skills of a physician or a registered nurse will always be required. But the emphasis is changing.

The image of the omniscient and omnipotent physician as portrayed by Norman Rockwell or on television shows of the 1950s is no longer apposite (Dranove, 2008). Multiple professions bring different skills to bear in working with and for their patients. All this has real consequences for the way work is organized in health care settings. Health care delivery is now more of a partnership, with each profession contributing its mite. The skill sets of each profession are expanding: what was done yesterday only by physicians is now part of the skill set of a number of professionals. The two-year hospital-based training for registered nurses, preparing them for a particular role at a particular time, has been replaced by a four-year university degree. Licensed practical nurses now fill the two-year training slot in a number of provinces.

The de facto scope of practice (as determined by employers or as reflected in funding system design) and, to a lesser extent, the de jure scope of practice determined in legislation or by regulatory bodies, have not kept pace with the competencies that many health professionals have acquired through university or college preparation, experience, and continuing education. Writing of the United States' situation, the Pew Health Professions Commission observed:

> The varying objectives and levels of specificity found in different professions' scopes of practice are more than frustrating; they have encouraged a system that treats practice acts as rewards for the professions rather than as rational mechanisms for cost-effective, high quality and accessible service delivery by competent practitioners.... Scope of practice battles have come to resemble contests for more patients, more status and power, more independence, and more money. (Finocchio et al., 1995, p. 10)

The situation in Canada today is no different.

There is nothing immutable about the current division of roles. As Mintzberg (1979) describes the choice:

> Every organized human activity—from the making of pots to placing man on the moon—gives rise to two fundamental and opposing requirements: the division of labour into various tasks to be performed, and the coordination of these tasks to accomplish the activity. The structure of an organization can be defined simply as the sum total of the ways in which it divides labour into distinct tasks and then achieves coordination among them. (p. 2)

Different organizations will make different decisions about how roles are to be divided and how coordination is to be achieved. The central point here is that local coordination mechanisms need to be purposively developed lest functions fall between roles or there is a lack of clarity about when one profession's role starts and another's finishes.

Health professionals are bright people and, having gone through a challenging preparation, it is no surprise they want to use their skills to the full, to work at the top of their regulated scope of practice. But very often the rules and routines of health care provision (especially in the larger settings such as hospitals) are ossified in old role delineations and mindsets of what is seen as appropriate. Traditionally the health sector has responded to new needs by creating new roles, increasing coordination problems in service delivery. Although this is still occurring, "role expansion" of existing professions is now occurring with increasing frequency.

Remuneration of health professionals is influenced by the length of their training (Frogner, 2010). System design that leaves a gap between what a professional has the skills to do and what he or she actually does is a form of waste. This becomes more of a problem when the higher-level skills are in short supply.

Both the Kirby (Senate, 2002a) and Romanow (Commission on the Future of Health Care, 2002) reports identified the need for role redesign as part of addressing workforce challenges. The health system has no choice if it is to meet workforce needs of the future but to use the available staff to their maximum potential. This requires redesign of care models, clarifying who currently does what, whether it needs to be done at all, and who should do what into the future. This is the fundamental and most critical task to ensure a health workforce that is sustainable into the future.

Care model redesign can draw on extensive experience of different approaches internationally, although the difficulty of importing international experience needs to be recognized (Marmor et al., 2005; Dubois & McKee, 2006).

*Health services delivery organizations should implement or continue systematic programs for care model redesign to facilitate all professionals' working to their top scope of practice. The Canadian Institutes of Health Research should be tasked and funded to establish a funding stream to evaluate implementation of care model redesign and associated role redesign.*

Working to top scope of practice will require changes for all professionals: nurses will take on roles previously the preserve of physicians, licensed practical nurses will take on roles previously the preserve of registered nurses, and health care aides will take on some of the duties of nurses. Workforce redesign will not only be about moving skills up or down a mono-disciplinary hierarchy (NHS Modernisation Agency, 2003). Other types of redesign should also be contemplated:

- expanding the breadth of a job (for example, rehabilitation practitioners working across traditionally determined boundaries, nurse practitioners in remote areas, pharmacists providing immunizations)
- increasing the depth of a job (for example, nurse practitioners in critical care)
- creating new roles formed by combining tasks in a new way, such as nurses performing endoscopies

## Collaborative practice

The twentieth century was one of increasing specialization in health care, starting with the Flexner reforms of medical education, which led to an emphasis on research and university affiliations. But the Flexner-driven cleanup of medical education created a sad legacy:

> The rigorous education envisioned by Flexner had an unintended consequence, i.e., the development and approval of policies that fostered—and continue to foster—a balkanized guild structure, which in turn has imposed occupational control. New health professions that emerged in the 20th century have also embraced this guild structure. Policies created to achieve Flexner's ... goals [of] university affiliation and full-time faculty ... have played out in a manner that isolates professions. Each guild lives within its own compound, e.g., professional associations, learned journals; subscribes to its own belief system, e.g., codes of ethics, scopes of practice; and erects intellectual fences, e.g., entry to practice requirements. (Gilbert, 2008, p. S12)

This balkanization of the medical and other health professionals may have initially been quality-enhancing as individual professionals developed deeper skills across a narrower range of areas. By the end of the century, though, there was a recognition that this increasing specialization has a downside in increased coordination costs, leading to inefficiency and problems of continuity of care.

Care model redesign in chronic care and rehabilitation will involve new forms of working for all professions. There is already a set of skills common to many professions: communication, assessment, program planning, implementation, and monitoring (Marriott, Reid, Jones, de Villiers, & Kennedy, 2005), although the language and underlying frameworks of the different professions are different. Each profession also brings its own unique skill set, for example, nurses with wound management and infection control; physiotherapists with expertise in mobility; occupational therapists with environmental adaptations; speech therapists with swallowing; social workers with family support.

The foundations of collaborative practice or interdisciplinary working need to be laid in the initial preparation of health professionals through interdisciplinary subjects incorporated in the curriculum—and not just foundation subjects such as physiology, where students are educated alongside one another, but subjects where they work on issues common to their respective professions. Yet good interdisciplinary education will be otiose if it is not reinforced by the practice that new graduates see and undertake (Gilbert, 2008).

In a collaborative-practice model, each professional is taught by the other professionals and teaches some of his or her skills to the others (Marriott et al., 2005, provides an example of this approach). Collaborative practice improves understanding of the skill set of the other team members (reducing communication and hand-over issues) and allows better integration of services to clients. This can potentially reduce the number of separate professionals involved in a client's care, improving continuity of care and client satisfaction. The specialist expertise of each professional would continue to be available where needed on a consultancy basis, as part of the assessment and monitoring process, and for the design of care plans that can be implemented by team members.

## Role substitution and supplementation

In addition to introducing interdisciplinary ways of working, care model redesign can involve reassigning tasks or roles from one type of health worker to another (role substitution) or providing additional services to enhance quality (role supplementation). There are many examples of potential substitutions: pharmacists or nurses for physicians being the most common (Dennis et al., 2009). A recent study showed that registered nurses' perception of their workload was not correlated with the actual nursing hours per patient day but with the adequacy of assistive personnel (Kalisch, Friese, Choi, & Rochman, 2011), suggesting that nurses are well aware of the potential productivity-enhancing benefits of task-substitution strategies.

There is a vast literature evaluating role revisions, in both primary care and hospital settings. In their meta-synthesis, Laurant et al. (2009) identified 18 systematic reviews of this literature! Evaluations of task substitution are generally favourable in terms of maintaining outcomes/quality and potentially showing improvements. On costs, Laurant et al.'s conclusion is more cautious: "The effect on overall health care costs is mixed, with savings dependent on the context of care and specific nature of role revision" (p. 82S).

Care model redesign could be undertaken for a variety of reasons, not only cost reduction. In an environment of potential shortages of some professions, cost-neutral role substitution that maintains quality but reduces use of professionals in short supply would still be beneficial.

Since nursing is the largest health profession, the potential for role revision affecting nurses—both development of advanced roles and delegation—has been a particular focus in a number of countries. Although Canada was an early adopter of nurse practitioners (Delamaire & Lafortune, 2010), there are still barriers to effective working of nurse practitioners such as ability to discharge patients (Donald et al., 2011). Consideration of the potential for nurses to work in advanced roles does not appear to be a routine part of health workforce planning (DiCenso, Martin-Misener, et al., 2011).

*Health Canada (or the Conference of Deputy Ministers) should convene a conference of provincial health ministries and regulatory bodies to share leading practice in regulation of basic and advanced nursing roles.*

## Challenges to care model redesign

Changing roles will mean confronting existing professional hierarchies and challenging the status quo. This will not be easy. Development of almost all professions has involved struggles over turf (Abbott, 1988), and the next generation of changes can be expected to lead to further public debates (Durier-Copp & Wranik, 2005). Balkanization of the professions has created multiple self-regulating professions, each with their own fiefdoms and roles to protect. Although the purpose of professional regulation is to protect the public, (regulatory) colleges often seek to promote their profession in public debates and as part of demarcation disputes generated by care model redesign.[119]

Bloor and Maynard (2003) lamented the lack of consideration of skill-mix change in workforce planning:

> This continued behaviour may be a product both of unthinking habits and the desire of the medical profession to resist changes in skill mix. That such

behaviour is tolerated by regulatory authorities in all countries is a reflection of the political sensitivity of unrest amongst medical practitioners. Conflicts of this type can seriously damage governments, both directly by threats of withdrawing services, and indirectly by failing to collaborate in the pursuit of policy objectives.... Internationally the medical profession has used its market power to maintain high relative levels of remuneration, high rates of return to investment in medical education over the life cycle, and substantial professional autonomy. (pp. 24-25)

Bloor and Maynard's comments focus on the medical profession: other health professions do not have the same power as physicians (in either public debate or internal organizational politics), but are still able to stymie change.

However, many health professionals recognize the weaknesses of the current situation, with unsystematic and unplanned role overlap and consequent role confusion. White et al. (2008) found that "insufficient role differentiation among nurses and between nurses and other healthcare professionals leaves some nurses feeling devalued and not respected for their contribution to healthcare delivery" (p. 45).

Nevertheless, role revision within nursing (moving tasks/roles within a nursing/health care aide hierarchy) is still controversial, particularly in hospital settings. There have been a large number of cross-sectional studies that demonstrate an association between a richer nursing staff mix, in the sense of a greater proportion of registered nurses, and better care outcomes in hospitals and long-term settings (Buchan & Dal Poz, 2002; Buerhaus & Needleman, 2000; Clarke & Donaldson, 2008; Kane, Shamliyan, Mueller, Duval, & Wilt, 2007; Lang, Hodge, Olson, Romano, & Kravitz, 2004; Lankshear, Sheldon, & Maynard, 2005). There are significant methodological issues in this stream of research (Lang et al., 2004; Mark, 2006), and the evidence from longitudinal studies is weaker than that from cross-sectional studies (Mark, Harless, McCue, & Xu, 2004).

Cross-sectional studies cannot demonstrate causation, although that language is sometimes used to describe the results. Meta-analysis (Kane et al., 2007) shows a dose-response relationship for staffing variables (patients to registered nurses per shift, registered nurse hours per patient day), so as there are more registered hours per day, for example, there is an increased likelihood of improved quality outcomes being demonstrated. But the relationship appears to be curvilinear (Lankshear et al., 2005), and so whether the relationship exists in a particular setting depends on the starting ratio.

The impact of staff shortages was not assessed in these studies. If the desirable registered nurse staffing is x for a given nursing unit, and a registered nurse cannot be recruited, what is the marginal impact of replacing the registered nurse with a licensed practical nurse or a health care aide? What is the marginal impact of decreasing the number of patients to be treated in the nursing unit and extending waiting times?

## The importance of productivity

The number of person hours required is clearly influenced by the productivity of each worker (Dubois & Singh, 2009), which in turn "depends on a variety of factors including the intensity of work (proportion of paid hours given to patient care), how work is organised, technological inputs, and inputs of other types of professionals" (Birch et al., 2008, p. S7). Birch et al. (2008) illustrated the importance of improving productivity in an analysis of the relative impact of different strategies to achieve a balance in nursing workforce requirements in Atlantic Canada. In their simulation study, compared to a baseline scenario where intakes into nursing programs would need to be increased by 2,975 places per annum to avoid future shortages, if a productivity improvement of 0.5 percent per annum was achieved, the required intake would drop to 825 places.

Evans, Schneider, and Barer (2010) highlighted the importance of improved productivity but also cautioned about the difficulties in measuring productivity, in particular the need to focus not only on inputs per output (e.g., health worker hours per patient treated) but beyond that on the relationship between inputs and health benefits. These findings link to the issue of the marginal return to health of increasing health care and the issue of supply-sensitive care discussed in the previous chapter.

Related to productivity is the conversion rate of a graduate to full-time paid hours. This is affected by whether graduates work full- or part-time in their first few years, and more particularly by whether they work in their chosen profession at all. New graduates can feel marginalized (Boychuk Duchscher & Cowin, 2004) and, as a result, leave their profession after a short period. Some professions, including nursing, are particularly exposed to high attrition in early years of practice. Strategies such as "graduate year" programs and mentorship can reduce these attrition rates (Block, Claffey, Korow, & McCaffrey, 2005).

## How many staff of which kind?

Once the care model redesign has been completed, the next stage is to project demand for the desired skill mix. Unfortunately, workforce planning has a poor track record (Walker & Maynard, 2003).[120] Bloor and Maynard's (2003) indictment of physician workforce planning applies to all professions: "The basis of current physician workforce planning is incomplete and mechanistic, using fixed ratio relationships that have no empirical validity" (p. 24). New technology has meant that "fixed ratio" and other mechanistic approaches can now be easily replaced by modelling that allows testing different assumptions about staffing patterns and the sensitivity of the assumptions involved in model development.

For this reason, leading practice workforce planning typically incorporates a range of scenarios, modelling different options (Barber &

Lopez-Valcarcel, 2010; Lavieri & Puterman, 2009; Masnick & McDonnell, 2010). Starting workforce planning with care model redesign helps to base workforce needs in a new reality; modelling approaches also allow testing the effect of different productivity, skill-mix, and working-hour assumptions. These approaches thus help address the weaknesses of traditional workforce planning highlighted by Bloor and Maynard (2003).

The Canadian population is growing, according to the medium projections from Statistics Canada, 11 percent over the next decade and 10 percent in the decade after that.[121] The older population is growing faster, and so the question is not whether there needs to be more health workers but how many. Because of the importance of linking care model reform to workforce requirements, workforce planning should be led by those with delivery responsibilities, rather than by universities/colleges or professional associations. Those stakeholders should be involved through consultation rather than leading the planning exercise. For the smaller health professions where training is not offered in every province and interprovincial flows are therefore high, workforce planning cannot effectively be undertaken by a single province.

Canada as a whole and most provinces rely on internationally educated health professionals: in 2005, internationally educated nurses made up 6.5 percent of the nursing workforce, and internationally educated physicians made up 22 percent of the physician workforce (Canadian Institute for Health Information, 2007a). Although some countries appear to pursue an explicit strategy of overproduction of health professionals for export, the ethics and appropriateness of relying on international recruitment is under challenge (Runnels, Labonte, & Packer, 2011). Migration (both internal and international) of health professionals is inevitable: for further training, family reasons, and travel. However, planning for a wealthy country such as Canada should at least be on a "net self-sufficiency" basis, with inflows and outflows in balance.

*Provinces should model workforce planning requirements for the larger health professions at least every five years.*[122] *Health Canada should support the provinces in a national approach to modelling workforce planning requirements for the smaller health professions. Planning for Canada and the larger provinces should aim for net self-sufficiency.*

### The supply side

Supply of health professionals in Canada has been growing steadily over the last decade, with annual rates of growth above 1 percent per annum for nurses, and physician growth increasing in recent years (Figure 8.1).

Workforce planning recommendations traditionally focused on increasing university/college intakes and graduations as the main strategy to address future supply. Contemporary workforce planning is more comprehensive. First, it increasingly starts with a "skill set requirement" approach, informed by role substitution potential—for example, planning for "care hours" that could be met by registered nurses, licensed practical nurses, or health care aides—rather than planning for a single profession. Second, it recognizes the manifold sources for increasing supply: increasing workforce participation being the most obvious (Antonazzo, Scott, Skatun, & Elliott, 2003; O'Brien-Pallas et al., 2003; Vujicic & Evans, 2005; Vujicic, Onate, Laporte, & Deber, 2011). Take physicians, for example: the trend over the last 20 years has been for decreasing hours of work for male physicians, with no noticeable age-cohort effect (Crossley, Hurley, & Jeon, 2009). Increasing hours of work of existing professionals can occur by changing incentives for part-time hours, making it easier for women with children to participate in the workforce, and making it easier for people to stay in the workforce at older ages.

**FIGURE 8.1**
**Average percentage growth in physician and nursing workforce, Canada, 2000–2009 (physicians), 2005–2009 (nurses)**

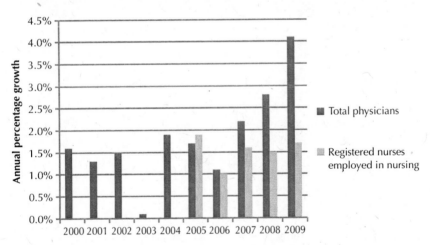

Data source: Canadian Institute for Health Information (2010d), *Supply, Distribution and Migration of Canadian Physicians in Canada, 2009*; and (2010c), *Regulated Nurses: Canadian Trends, 2005 to 2009.*

### Expanding university and college places

The traditional workforce supply solution of expanding university-college places faces challenges over the next decade. First, medium population projections suggest a decline in the 15–19 and 20–24 cohorts, the typical university and college entrant population, between now and 2021.[123] This means that the health professions will need to increase their proportion of school leavers and graduates choosing to enter the health professions relative to other professions. Second, there are continuing difficulties in recruiting qualified faculty for most health professions, other than medicine (Aiken, Cheung, & Olds, 2009; Berlin & Sechrist, 2002; Patry & Eiland, 2007). Strategies to address the faculty shortage include academic innovation, partnering between institutions to facilitate faculty development, and special funding to develop faculty (Allan & Aldebron, 2008).

*The Canadian Institutes of Health Research should be tasked and funded to create research training initiatives in professions where there is a shortage of faculty.*

### Increasing diversity in university and college populations

Students who are entering health professional education do not have the same profile in terms of wealth, ethnicity, or rurality as the people they will serve on graduation (Dhalla et al., 2002; Etowa, Foster, Vukic, Wittstock, & Youden, 2005). In addition to creating issues of cultural acceptability in service delivery and rural access, drawing on a narrow recruitment base will be less viable in the future with the reduction in the university and college entrant population.

### Increasing access to health professional education

Health professional education is not free to students, and graduates face a significant debt upon graduation (Finnie, 2002). Higher debt appears to affect the social composition of medical schools: Quebec, a province with lower medical school fees (and consequentially where students have lower debt on graduation) has more students enrolled who grew up in low-income neighbourhoods and had lower parental income than other provinces (Merani et al., 2010). Finnie (2002) has proposed revising the Canada Student Loan Program to incorporate income-contingent loans. Australia has more than 20 years' experience with income-contingent loans, which appear to have an impact on increasing equity, albeit moderate (Chapman & Ryan, 2005).

The evidence about whether students from lower-income backgrounds are (student) debt averse is somewhat mixed (Callender & Jackson, 2005; Eckel, Johnson, Montmarquette, & Rojas, 2007), but debt aversion appears to affect subject choice (Callender & Jackson, 2008), and high debt tends to encourage graduates to take high-income jobs (Rothstein & Rouse, 2011). This suggests that a combination of strategies is needed to improve student-body diversity. One such approach would be to couple income-contingent loans with upfront loan forgiveness for working in hard-to-recruit geographic areas or specialties. This would build on existing provincial programs expanding on the scheme announced in the 2011 federal budget to provide loan forgiveness for physicians and nurses in rural and remote locations.

Income-contingent loans at the provincial level (where loans are recouped via taxation) may have the perverse effect of encouraging labour mobility, hence federal leadership would be required in this area.

*The federal government should explore with the provinces interest in developing a national income-contingent loan program for health professions, coupled with loan forgiveness programs for employment in hard-to-recruit areas.*

### Expanding recruitment of health care aides

Care model redesign and the need to expand seniors' care will require an increase in the number of health care aides and other support staff. The OECD estimates that the long-term care workforce will need to grow from around 1 percent of the Canadian working population in 2008 to 1.6 percent in 2050 (Colombo et al., 2011). Again, strategies need to be developed to recruit from non-traditional sources.

Meeting the care needs of the future will rely on care model redesign discussed above and, in the case of seniors' care, an expansion of both home care and assisted living facilities. In both cases, a mix of professional staff and health care aides will be required. The largest growth in care-worker demand will be for health care aide positions. Expanding the proportion of health care aides in the workforce could be challenging; R. I. Stone (2004) goes so far as to describe it as "the third rail of home care policy." But health care aides already have a valuable role in health and seniors' care (Thornley, 2003) and, with appropriate training, they can reliably identify need for professional intervention and support (Boockvar, Brodie, & Lachs, 2000).

Health care aide positions are entry level to the health sector and can be entry level to the workforce (Stone & Wiener, 2001). In the past, many health care aide roles have been conceptualized as requiring limited (if any) training. The Alberta approach, in contrast, was to move to certification of health care aides, with the equivalent of about three months' training.[124] Training both allows health care aides to undertake a broader range of tasks safely, and gives nurses and other supervisors more assurance in delegating tasks (Mackey & Nancarrow, 2005). Training for health care aides also helps to increase their attachment to the health sector, which is particularly important in volatile economies.

Health care aide training can be seen as a way of transitioning people into the workforce, the health workforce in particular (Deshong & Henderson, 2010). One strategy explored in Alberta Health Services was to create health care aide-in-training positions as entry level into the workforce, particularly for older/middle-aged people. Trainees could recoup training costs from the employer, thus making training accessible to low-income people. In addition to tapping into a new recruitment pool, moving people from unemployment to employment has broader health improvement benefits.

Career-laddering strategies should also be used to encourage health workers to upgrade their skills—health care aides to licensed practical nurses, and practical nurses to registered nurse qualifications. These opportunities are available by distance education, and so staff do not have to move from their current homes. Employers should support distance education courses as part of regular staff development options.

*Provinces should examine non-traditional sources for recruitment of entry-level workers, including providing on-the-job training opportunities.*

## The interaction between the health and education sectors

Health workforce planning will fail unless there is a close and productive relationship between the suppliers (education institutions) and the demanders (the health sector). A recent international review of preparation of health professions had this to say about the consequences of weak relationships: "Professional education has not kept pace with ... [contemporary health service] challenges, largely because of fragmented, outdated and static curricula that produce ill-equipped graduates" (Commission on Education of Health Professionals, 2010). The health and education sectors therefore need to be closely linked. This is already the case in some, but not all, health professions.

The education sector is responsible for preparing most professions, but it relies on the health sector for clinical placements, leading to a complex set of flows between the two sectors (Duckett, 2009). The health sector has significant (and underutilized) power in this relationship that could potentially be used to influence curricula to ensure a better fit between health sector needs of the future and the type of graduates being produced.[125] An example might be an expectation of stronger team-working skills. But the health sector's power comes with a quid pro quo—that clinical placements of the right kind will be available to meet the negotiated intake levels and curriculum design. Universities and colleges are key players in shaping the workforce of the future, and so collaboration and partnership between the two sectors is going to be mutually productive.

Work readiness of new graduates is also perennially questioned (Wolff, Regan, Pesut, & Black, 2010), with the health sector responding with "graduate nurse year" programs. Universities and colleges guard their historical autonomy, but that autonomy leads to development of curricula that differ across institutions, creating problems for students and future employers alike: inhibiting student transfers, and potentially leading to differences in work readiness that employers need to address.

Unfortunately, the two sectors may be worlds apart. The time frames of health service providers are often expressed in days and months, while educational providers take years to revise curricula and introduce new courses. Leaders in the two sectors need to understand the differences between the two cultures—the different funding incentives, constraints, and aspirations. Closer working relationships will not occur without both will and action.

Improving working relationships between the health and education sectors requires three critical steps. First, there needs to be a recognition that the old ways are not working and we need to do things differently. Second, each sector needs a better understanding of the other (Regan, Thorne, & Mildon, 2009). This may come from closer cooperation but certainly requires action at both provincial and local levels. Local educational institutions need to work very closely with relevant health services to identify the extent to which service needs are changing. Third, health services also need very close working relationships with the educational institutions that supply new entrants to their workforce. Health and education institutions need to work together to ensure appropriate clinical placements are available to meet agreed levels of intakes into universities and colleges.

Flexibility is going to be required on both sides to ensure appropriate responses to changing health service needs. Educational institutions will need to develop new products (shorter courses, retraining, modular provision), and the health sector will need to be more flexible as to how it provides clinical education and clearer about articulating its needs.

Currently, the formal relationships between the education and health sectors are mostly indirect, mediated through relevant provincial ministries that have variable knowledge of day-to-day issues or longer-term requirements. Direct relationships are generally informal, often based on historical agreements. Coincidence of interest may be accidental, rather than planned. Improved understanding in both sectors and the closer working relationships described above may identify the joint requirements and ensure appropriate responses. But if funding arrangements and incentives are not aligned and do not reinforce the need for responsiveness (on both sides), then all the understanding and goodwill in the world may be to no avail. New formal arrangements at local, provincial, and/or national levels thus may be necessary to facilitate joint planning and better outcomes in terms of matching the supply of health professionals to the needs of the populations they serve.

*Provinces should establish formal mechanisms for planning and cooperation between universities and colleges and the major health providers. Health providers should consider mechanisms at the local level for the same purpose.*

## The context of health roles

Health professionals work within a complex web of accountability arrangements, involving upward, downward, and sideways accountability of varying degrees of formality.

The individual clinical professional clearly has accountability to the patient or consumer, but increasingly health providers are being held to account by a broader group of potential consumers through the publication of comparative performance measures, such as comparative case fatality rates.

Health care employees experience a vertical (upward) accountability, and, for physicians working within hospitals, there may be employer-like accountabilities as well. This relationship to the employer is quite a complex one as the managerial hierarchy may often not be seen as having legitimacy, competence, or power to control professional practice (Pollitt, 1993). Employment accountability is thus typically supplemented by horizontal accountability of the clinician to professional peers through organized specialty or unit meetings in a hospital, for example. The clinician is also accountable to a broader peer population through specialist societies and to the relevant professional registration body. In addition, clinicians have obligations and some form of accountability to multidisciplinary colleagues.

The accountability relationships described here are often implicit rather than explicit. Generally, the less formalized the relationships, the weaker the accountability. The most formalized relationships are the upward to employer and sideways to professional registration bodies. Both of these can ensure that the downward accountability to the consumer is working effectively.

In an environment of high interprovincial migration, there needs to be close and effective relationships between provincial registration boards. The Canadian Agreement on Internal Trade[126] (and regional supplements such as the western Canada Trade, Investment and Labour Mobility Agreement) is supposed to lead to improved labour mobility. Unfortunately, this has been slow to be realized. Cross-border provision by health professionals is still generally regulated by both relevant provinces, hindering efficient provision of services. There are a variety of ways to deal with cross-border provision and interprovincial migration: national registration as pursued in Australia is one option, but the "driver's licence model," where there is immediate and unbureaucratic recognition interprovincially, is a potential easy step (Carlton, 2006).

*Federal, provincial, and territorial leaders should review current health professional regulatory structures to facilitate further interprovincial migration and provision of health care across provincial borders.*

## Conclusion

One aspect of sustainability of the health system is whether there will be an appropriate workforce to meet future needs (Ricketts, 2011). What is argued here is that there can be, provided that the health and education systems, and the health professions, are not locked into the straitjackets of the past. Health services need to embrace new ways of working, to ensure that all health workers can work to their top scope of practice. It will require careful work redesign to ensure that the staff have the skills to perform the new roles, and understand the new coordination issues. With these changes, highly skilled professionals will be liberated to fulfill the functions they are prepared for and, at the same time, our health care system will be able to meet future needs.

# Word cloud: What others have said: Diagnoses and prescriptions for health care in Canada

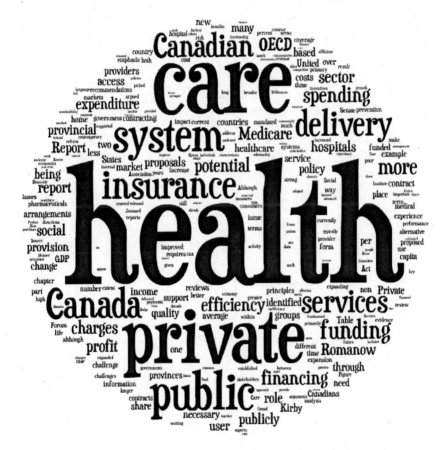

In this chapter I propose the following policy initiatives:

- The public administration criterion in the *Canada Health Act* should be rephrased as being about public governance and public insurance.
- Canadian health care is best served by a continuation of tax financing. Expansion of private insurance into core areas should not be pursued.
- Provinces should continue to contract with the private sector for service delivery. Contracts for private delivery should incorporate marginal pricing and robust measures of quality.

# CHAPTER 9

# WHAT OTHERS HAVE SAID: DIAGNOSES AND PRESCRIPTIONS FOR HEALTH CARE IN CANADA

The health policy landscape in Canada is awash with policy proposals. Over the last decade Canada has seen two major health system reviews (Kirby and Romanow) that built on an earlier Prime Ministerial National Forum on Health; health stakeholders are preparing for the 2014 Accord renewal and weighing in with their proposals; and there are regular reports from "think tanks" peddling alternative nostrums. The lens adopted by the various commentators to some extent shapes their proposed policy directions. Is the Canadian health system in crisis? If so, is the private prescription the one to swallow?

## Provincial reviews

This contemporary policy activity is nothing new: practically every province conducted some form of review into its health system in the 1980s or 1990s. Cost-sharing had been abolished as the basis for federal-provincial health financing arrangements in 1977, a "bad bargain" for the provinces as the economy slowed but health costs did not (Davidson, 2004). A flurry of provincial reviews took place as provinces grappled to respond to contemporary challenges (Crichton, Hsu, & Tsang, 1994; Mhatre & Deber, 1992). There was a remarkable similarity in the rhetoric of the reports and their recommendations: an emphasis on prevention, home care, strengthening the hand of consumers vis-à-vis providers, and workforce reform. Desirable directions for care reform have been stable for over 30 years. What has been missing is action to transform the rhetoric into reality. The one exception to this inertia is organizational: most of the provincial reports recommended better linking of hospitals to other aspects of the health system, leading to establishment of regional administrative structures in most provinces.

In addition to provincial reviews, some provinces (led by Alberta and Ontario) shifted the fiscal challenge by demand-side or revenue measures: increasing (in the case of hospital care) or allowing (in the case of medical care) user charges and copayments. This in turn led to pressure for a federal response to address the problems of access so created, and the 1984 *Canada Health Act* provisions that eliminated any benefit to the provinces by allowing extra-billing.

## National Forum on Health

The National Forum on Health, established and chaired by Prime Minister Chrétien, aimed "to involve and inform Canadians and to advise the federal government on innovative ways to improve our health system and the health of Canada's people." The Forum released a number of issue or background papers that informed its work (http://www.hc-sc.gc.ca/hcs-sss/pubs/renewal-renouv/1997-nfoh-fnss-v2/index-eng.php). Its final report, released in 1997, concluded that the Canadian health care system is fundamentally sound, that enough money was already spent on health care, but there was room to improve.

Again, the directions for reform were similar to those identified in the provincial commissions:

> If we were building a health care system today from scratch, it would be structured much differently from the one we now have and might be less expensive. The system would rely less on hospitals and doctors and would provide a broader range of community-based services, delivered by multidisciplinary teams with a much stronger emphasis on prevention. (National Forum on Health, 1997, "Straight Talk")

The Forum recognized the broader determinants of health and the critical role of public sector financing, arguing that "increasing the scope of public expenditure may be the key to reducing total cost." The Forum's report identified and made recommendations about key gaps in the contemporary funding and delivery arrangements: home care, pharmaceutical coverage, and reforming primary care. This same list is identified in the Kirby and Romanow reports.

An important concept that does not appear to have been picked up in the subsequent reports is that of balance: between the health sector and the rest of the economy (How much of gross domestic product should be spent on health care?); within the health sector (balance of funding on hospitals, home care, etc.); and in terms of public and private roles. The subgroup of the Forum that dealt with balance argued for improved accountability and transparency including collection and dissemination of improved information about health and health system performance on a range of dimensions.

## Kirby and colleagues

The Kirby Report was released in October 2002 following a two-year review by the Senate Standing Committee on Social Affairs, Science and Technology (Senate, 2002a). Chaired by Liberal senator Michael Kirby, the committee was multiparty, and the report was unanimously supported by the seven Liberals, three Progressive Conservatives, and one Independent who comprised the committee.

The final report was informed by principles that had been articulated in the committee's fifth interim report, released six months earlier in April 2002. The principles were said to be based on recognition of "three fundamental realities":

1. Canada's publicly funded health care system is not fiscally sustainable given current funding levels;
2. Canadians want a strong role for the federal government in facilitating health care restructuring and renewal; and
3. There is a need to introduce incentives for all participants in the publicly funded hospital and doctor system—providers, institutions, governments and patients—to deliver, manage and use health care more efficiently. (Senate, 2002b, p. 5)

If the principles articulated in the fifth volume were adopted, the Canadian health system would be reshaped to establish and split the functions of purchaser, provider, and independent evaluator of health care, and to create an "internal market" in health care. Splitting the functions of purchaser and provider was the contemporary policy fashion internationally in the mid-to-late 1990s, and was seen as a way of reducing provider power, and ensuring both social and technical efficiency (Chernichovsky, 1995; Jérôme-Forget, White, & Wiener, 1995; Preker & Harding, 2003; Saltman & von Otter, 1995).[127] Splitting the roles requires changing the basis for funding flows to providers to introduce the potential for contestability or "internal markets" within a publicly funded health system, in turn allowing for introduction or expansion of private delivery of publicly funded health services. Under internal market reforms, purchasers would procure services based on desired activity, replacing global or historical budgets with activity-based funding.

The final report of the committee deemphasized the rhetoric of the internal market and purchaser/provider split, but adopted the principles articulated in the interim report as the basis for its policy prescriptions.

Consistent with a position that Medicare in its current form was unsustainable, the Kirby Report included a number of recommendations to promote efficiency: core to the report was a move toward activity-based funding (termed "service-based funding"). The report explicitly endorsed the concept of private provision of health care, although it anticipated that the "overwhelming majority" of institutional providers would remain as either public or non-profit.

The Kirby Report emphasized the importance of maintaining a single (public) funder of Medicare:

> The Committee is keenly aware that shifting more of the cost to individual patients and their families via private payments, the facile "solution" recommended by many, is really nothing more than an expensive way of relieving or, at the least, diminishing governments' problem. Regardless of how it is expressed (as a share of GDP, share of government spending, etc.), there is only one source of funding for health care—the Canadian public—and it has been shown conclusively that the most cost-effective way of funding health care is by using a single (in our case, publicly administered or governmental) insurer/payer model. (Senate, 2002a, p. 9)

The Kirby Report proposed expanding public responsibility and funding into new areas of health care, such as home care and pharmaceuticals. It also proposed a Health Care Guarantee:

> For each type of major procedure or treatment, a maximum needs-based waiting time be established and made public. When this maximum time is reached, the insurer (government) pay for the patient to seek the procedure or treatment immediately in another jurisdiction, including, if necessary, another country (e.g., the United States). (Senate, 2002a, p. 117)

## Romanow recommendations

Released a few weeks after the Kirby Report, the Romanow Report (Commission on the Future of Health Care, 2002) was bold and expansionary. The mandate Romanow was given set the context for his review: it referred to an endorsement of the principles of the *Canada Health Act* and the "strong attachment" Canadians have to the health system. The title of the report was *Building on Values*, and Romanow emphasized the value-base of Medicare throughout his report. To Romanow, health care was not just some other commodity but an embodiment of what it means to be a Canadian, of the commitments Canadians have to each other, part of the glue that binds Canadians together in a "compassionate society."

Referring to the 40th anniversary of Medicare (which had passed shortly before he completed his report), Romanow argued that "the next big step for Canada may be more focused, but it will be no less bold. That next step is to build on this proud legacy and transform Medicare into a system that is more responsive, comprehensive and accountable to all Canadians" (Commission on the Future of Health Care, 2002, p. xxi). And he went on to make this challenge:

Getting there requires leadership. It requires us to change our attitudes on how we govern ourselves as a nation. It requires an adequate, stable and predictable commitment to funding and co-operation from governments. It requires health practitioners to challenge the traditional way they have worked in the system. It requires all of us to realize that our health and wellness is not simply a responsibility of the state but something we must work toward as individuals, families and communities, and as a nation. The national system I speak about is clearly within our grasp. Medicare is a worthy national achievement, a defining aspect of our citizenship and an expression of social cohesion. Let's unite to keep it so. (p. xxi)

Some aspects of his challenge have clearly been accepted and addressed: the 2004 Health Accord, for example, delivered a "stable and predictable commitment to funding"—an important, tangible outcome. Whether others were picked up may lie in the eye of the beholder: Is funding ever adequate? The tenor of the previous chapter (and to some extent Chapter 4) is that the health employers and professions have not picked up the Romanow challenge of new ways of working.

Romanow's recommendations covered the full gamut of health care: proposing expansions in home care, improvements in access, and introduction of electronic health records. Some of his recommendations were adopted in more or less the form he advised (the Health Council of Canada, Canada Health Transfer), and others were picked up in a modified form (it could be argued that Romanow's proposed Diagnostic Services Fund has been incorporated in a broader waiting-times initiative). But in other areas his recommendations led nowhere (catastrophic drug provision), despite some positive rhetoric (home care).

On the contentious issue of the private role, Romanow distinguished between direct care (no private for-profit role) and ancillary support such as food preparation, cleaning, and laundry, where he found a private role acceptable. Romanow had two arguments to support private provision of ancillary services: quality was measurable, and contestable (outside health care) markets existed (p. 6). Both echo Williamson's (1975, 1986) theoretical arguments for conditions when purchasing from markets would be preferred to provision from within the firm, but there may be some debate about whether aspects of direct health care can be adequately described, with robust measures of quality.

## The views of health stakeholders

The health sector in Canada is a large employer nationally, provincially, and locally, and employee and professional groups have a critical stake in the future of the health system.

The Canadian Medical Association (2010) has advanced its prescription for "health care transformation." Although the CMA endorsed the current five *Canada Health Act* principles, they proposed two additions: patient-centred care and sustainability. In terms of specifics, the CMA proposed

- a patient charter,
- changed incentives to enhance timely access and to support quality care,
- a new pharmaceutical scheme,
- enhanced access to continuing care,
- more effective workforce planning,
- more effective adoption of health information technologies, and
- better system accountability.

The Canadian Nurses Association, in contrast, has established an "expert commission" to formulate its position, although it has established policies that indicate preferred directions. In its first contribution, the Canadian Federation of Nurses Unions has emphasized the contribution of nurses to the health system and nursing-specific issues (Coutts, 2010).

The institutional provider organization, the Canadian Healthcare Association (2010), has also published proposals and identified six priority areas for reform: funding; health human resources; Pharmacare; wellness (health promotion/disease prevention); continuing care (home, long-term, respite); and leadership.

Table 9.1 summarizes key stakeholder proposals published at time of writing. Despite some differences in emphasis and language, there are many similarities in the directions proposed. First is a general orientation toward coverage or service enhancement, suggesting health stakeholders are aware of the limitations of the current framework and provision. Second, although two groups identify funding and system efficiencies as priorities, there is no call from any group to expand private funding. Third, there is an emphasis on the need to invest "upstream" or in non-institutional services: prevention, primary care, or home care. Fourth, there is common recognition (three of the four groups) of the need to improve access to pharmaceuticals and to address waiting times for care. In terms of system enablers, three of the four groups identified the importance of addressing issues relating to the health workforce and the need for system leadership.

### The alternative nostrums

A number of self-identified "think tanks" and other non-health groups or "policy shops" have advanced proposals for health system change. In contrast to the service-expansion orientation of the health stakeholders,

**TABLE 9.1**
**Prescriptions for change, key health stakeholder groups, May 2011**

| Issue | Canadian Healthcare Association | Canadian Medical Association | Canadian Nurses Association | Canadian Federation of Nurses Unions |
|---|---|---|---|---|
| Prevention and promotion | ✓ | | ✓ | |
| Primary health care reform | | | | ✓ |
| Home care/continuing care | ✓ | ✓ | | |
| Access to pharmaceuticals | ✓ | ✓ | ✓ | |
| Access/wait times | | ✓ | ✓ | ✓ |
| Patient safety/quality of care/patient-centred care | ✓ | | | |
| Health workforce issues | ✓ | ✓ | ✓ | |
| Interdisciplinary care issues | | | ✓ | |
| System efficiencies | | | | ✓ |
| Funding | ✓ | | | ✓ |
| Information and communication technologies | | ✓ | | |
| Accountability | | ✓ | | |
| Leadership | ✓ | | ✓ | ✓ |

Note: ✓ indicates that the stakeholder group has covered this aspect of change in its proposal.
Source: Derived from an analysis by Pamela Fralick (2011), which was based on available information at the time and included a broader range of organizations.

these non-health bodies place a much greater emphasis on financial issues. Similarly, the discourse of these bodies tends to be replete with "crisis" and unsustainability language, setting the scene for potential solutions that may be unpalatable to the average Canadian.

## C.D. Howe Institute

The topic of the C.D. Howe's Benefactors' Lecture in 2010 was health care, entitled "Critical Condition: A Historian's Prognosis on Canada's Aging Healthcare System" (Bliss, 2010). Historian emeritus professor Michael Bliss reviewed trends over the previous 150 years and formulated "lessons" to guide policy. He was pessimistic about the potential to moderate future health expenditure, describing "the record of attempts to curb the growth of healthcare spending in Canada (as sometimes seeming) like a chapter in the biography of King Canute" (p. 18). His lessons included revisiting universality and expanding the role of the market in provision and/or insurance.

In 2011 the C.D. Howe Institute again entered the fray with a paper co-authored by former governor of the Bank of Canada David Dodge and colleague Richard Dion on health with the main title "Chronic Healthcare Spending Disease" (Dodge & Dion, 2011). Dodge and Dion do not make any specific proposals for change but rather leave us on the horns of a dilemma, denying the possibility of an alternative, more palatable, future:

> Even if we in Canada are incredibly successful in improving the productivity, efficiency and effectiveness of the healthcare system—our optimistic case—we face difficult but necessary choices as to how we finance the rising costs of healthcare and manage the rising share of additional income devoted to it.... Some combination of the following actions will be necessary to manage the "spending disease":
>
> 1.  a sharp reduction in public services, other than healthcare, provided by governments, especially provincial governments;
> 2.  increased taxes to finance the public share of healthcare spending;
> 3.  increased spending by individuals on healthcare services that are currently insured by provinces, through some form of co-payment or through delisting of services that are currently publicly financed;
> 4.  a major degradation of publicly insured healthcare standards—longer queues, services of poorer quality—and the development of a privately funded system to provide better-quality care for those willing to pay for it. (p. 11)

### Fraser Institute

The Fraser Institute's contribution (Skinner & Rovere, 2011) also questions sustainability, particularly focusing on the share of provincial government expenditure allocated to health care. Skinner and Rovere suggest that the main provincial strategies to address spending growth have essentially been rationing, as demonstrated by waiting times for many health services and limitations on publicly supported access to new pharmaceuticals.

According to Skinner and Rovere (2011), the *Canada Health Act* principles constrain provincial responses to the issues identified. They propose that "the Federal government should temporarily suspend enforcement of the *Canada Health Act* for a five-year trial period to allow the provinces to experiment with new ways of financing medical goods and services" (p. 3). This new-found freedom would allow provinces to implement Skinner and Rovere's other prescriptions that include

- allowing reintroduction of user charges over and above current government payments to providers;
- introducing private insurance for services currently covered by Medicare; and
- expanding the role of for-profit providers in service delivery.

## TD Economics

In its 2010 report on health care in Ontario, TD Economics (Drummond & Burleton, 2010, p. 10) also highlighted sustainability challenges, colourfully referring to health care as "the Pac Man of provincial budgets." In contrast to other non-health groups, the report did not support an expanded role of private funding for currently publicly funded services, noting that this simply shifted costs, and was probably not politically achievable in any event. However, the TD Economics report supported a form of social insurance ("pre-funding") for pharmaceuticals and an expanded role for private sector provision, together with a set of broader proposals such as promoting healthy lifestyles. The report included a number of efficiency-enhancing initiatives (changing the way doctors are compensated; changing hospital funding from global budgets to activity-based funding; increasing bulk purchases of drugs) and new revenue sources (health care benefit tax).

## Social insurance

A number of writers have proposed social insurance as a way of financing expansion of Medicare into currently uncovered areas such as pharmaceuticals (Morgan, 2008) and long-term care (Hébert, 2011). Social insurance was the subject of a two-day conference sponsored by the Ontario Ministry of Health and Long-Term Care in 2006 (Flood, Stabile, & Tuohy, 2008b). The Wildrose Alliance in Alberta has also quoted with approval European models of health care based on social insurance principles.[128]

Social insurance is the Bismarckian alternative to the tax-financed Beveridge approach to universal health systems. Social insurance may mandate coverage by an insurer but allows consumers to elect the insurer from which they will obtain coverage. It has the potential to create a competitive purchasing market. Compared to voluntary insurance, mandated social insurance is more equitable in ensuring redistribution of risk over the life cycle (Glied, 2008a).

## The perspective(s) of the OECD

The Organisation for Economic Co-operation and Development (OECD) undertakes and publishes biennial "country surveys" about member nations; the most recent Canadian one was released in 2010 (OECD, 2010a). In addition to a review of the economy of the country, the surveys typically have a chapter focusing on a special issue: in 2010 that issue for Canada was health care. The survey lauded some aspects of Canadian health care, referring to "top-notch" care for Medicare services, but qualified this by identifying problems relating to non-covered services, cost pressures, and waiting lists.

The OECD report used strong language to ring alarm bells based on its perceptions of the impact of health policy for the whole economy:

In the longer run the soundness of Canada's public finances will likely be largely determined by the decisions taken regarding the health-care system.... With health already accounting for around half of total primary provincial spending, meeting the fiscal and demographic challenges will require that the growth of public health spending be reduced from an annual rate of about 8 percent seen over the last decade toward the trend rate of growth of nominal income in coming years (estimated to be less than 4 percent per year), the only alternative being to squeeze other public spending or to raise taxes or user charges. (2010a, p. 17)

Although the survey recommended expansion of the scope of services covered by "the core public package" (home care being the most notable example), it coupled this with recommending expansion of private funding, both through private insurance and increased use of copayments.

The OECD has a long track record of publishing analyses of comparative performance of health systems. In recent years it has published a series of reports that use a statistical technique known as data envelopment analysis to identify possibility "frontiers" from different combinations of policies and experiences. Using this multivariate technique, one can measure how far any country is from the technically feasible frontier so that it is possible to identify both output inefficiency (how much outputs could be improved or expanded if the country functioned at the optimal level of efficiency) and input inefficiency (whether inputs could be reduced to achieve the same outputs; Worthington, 2004).

The OECD report identified potential for Canada on both dimensions, but did not highlight the implications of these findings (OECDa, p. 143).

Most OECD countries have the potential to learn from each other in terms of improving life expectancy—one of the key output measures adopted in the OECD analyses (Joumard, André, Nicq, & Chatal, 2008; Joumard, André, et al., 2010; Joumard, Hoeller, et al., 2010). Although Canada performs relatively well on life expectancy, and hence has relatively less potential to improve than the average OECD country, pursuing a different mix of policies (such as expanding vaccinations, in Canada's case for example, for diphtheria) would allow Canadians to expect to live just over two years longer (see Figure 9.1).

The OECD researchers also addressed the potential for efficiency improvement, examining per capita health expenditure. Per capita health expenditure and health expenditure as a share of gross domestic product has been increasing across OECD countries, and Canada is no exception. Over the decade 1997–2007, Canadian per capita health expenditure increased 45 percent, approximately at the OECD average of 48 percent (see Figure 9.2). With unchanged policies, and projecting forward the impact of growth and aging of the population, Canada should expect a similar pattern for the 2007–2017 decade.

## FIGURE 9.1
## Estimated potential additional years of life expectancy at birth if "output inefficiency" were eliminated, selected countries

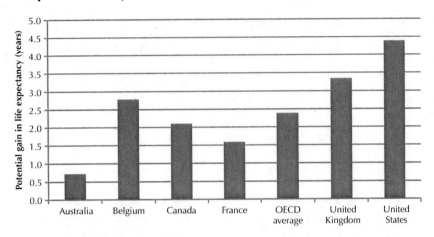

Source: Joumard, Hoeller, et al. (2010).

## FIGURE 9.2
## Increase in per capita spending 1997–2007 and estimated increase in per capita spending 2007–2017 if "input inefficiency" were eliminated, together with potential savings in health share of GDP, selected countries

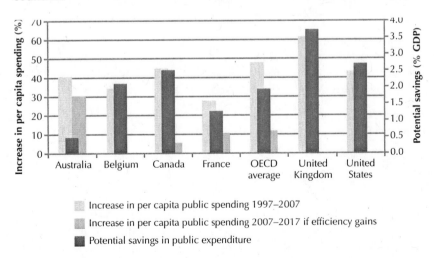

Increase in per capita public spending 1997–2007

Increase in per capita public spending 2007–2017 if efficiency gains

Potential savings in public expenditure

Source: Joumard, Hoeller, et al. (2010).

But as with life expectancy potential, again the OECD estimated the impact of changed policy settings and practice patterns: Canada, for example, has a longer average length of stay for hospitalizations for cancer than the OECD average. With different policy settings—for example, stronger primary care gatekeeping, less reliance on fee-for-service remuneration of physicians—Canada could achieve better value for money in its spending and meet projected demand with a smaller than otherwise per capita increase in spending. The OECD papers estimated that a 5 percent increase would be required over the 2007–2017 decade to potentially save around 2.5 percent against the otherwise projected health share of gross domestic product.

## Some common themes

There are a number of common themes running through most (but not all) of these commentaries and reviews. First is the sustainability challenge. This was an issue addressed in Chapter 2 where I argued that, to the extent aging is an issue, it will occur gradually and thus the health system will be able to adapt to its impact. Other challenges are the result of conscious policy decisions to enhance health care (more technology, funding a new range of services). These decisions can and should be accompanied by strategies for sustainable funding, which brings us to the pursuit of social efficiency discussed in Chapter 5 and technical efficiency in several chapters.

The second theme of many of these reviews and commentaries is the pessimism about the potential to address future expenditure needs through improved efficiency. Efficiency agendas can be pursued successfully. In the late 1990s, for example, Ontario established a Health Services Restructuring Commission. Despite legal challenges and local adverse community reaction, change did occur. Key participants observed,

> Perhaps the most important [achievement] is that, for the time being at least, [the Commission] broke the mould of the *status quo ante*. By exercising its power, [the Commission] demonstrated that it is possible to make changes to health care—or at least restructure hospitals. (Sinclair et al., 2005, p. 213)

More recently, the creation of Alberta Health Services led to significant reductions in administrative layers and saved hundreds of millions of dollars through centralization (Duckett, 2011).

### The public/private challenge

The third common theme relates to the role of the private sector: other than health stakeholder proposals, all the other reviews and proposals canvassed this issue, with the Romanow Report (Commission on the Future of Health Care, 2002) being the solitary standout in not recommending or foreshadowing the potential for greater private roles.

The Kirby Report (Senate, 2002a) drew attention to what it described as the "misunderstanding" of the fifth *Canada Health Act* principle, public administration. The phrasing of the principle is about the administration of provincial "insurance" arrangements; it is not about service delivery arrangements. It could be argued that private delivery is part of Medicare's fundamentals as the vast majority of physicians are not public health sector employees; most medical practices are incorporated and function as independent private services.

The reality is that the Canadian health system currently involves a mix of private financing and private delivery (see Table 9.2). In terms of universal coverage, public financing covers the core Medicare services: hospitals and medical services. There are other publicly funded services for some age groups in some or all provinces (veterans, seniors' drug coverage). Hospital services are primarily publicly provided, although there are many not-for-profit hospitals (primarily of religious foundation), and some private services acting under contract to the public sector.

**TABLE 9.2**
**Examples of public and private financing and delivery in Canadian health care**

| | | Financing | |
|---|---|---|---|
| | | Public | Private |
| Delivery | *Public* | Hospitals | Emergency medical services |
| | *Private* | Medical services | Out-of-hospital pharmaceuticals<br>Dental care |

Emergency medical services are primarily (with some provincial variation) delivered by the public sector, but again not entirely, relying on private funding either through direct user trip charges or through provincial insurance arrangements. Pharmaceuticals have the same funding sources but delivery is almost entirely private, at least for community-based provision.

So, it is only one cell of the two-by-two matrix that is about health care publicly delivered and publicly financed, albeit an important sector—hospital care, one which shapes images of health care.

One approach to clarifying the contemporary misunderstanding of the legitimate role of private delivery is to update the language of the *Canada Health Act* to focus on governance, which has a stronger connotation of oversight (Flood & Choudhry, 2002, 2004), while maintaining the emphasis on public insurance. *The public administration criterion in the Canada*

*Health Act should be rephrased as being about public governance and public insurance.*

The reviews and commentaries take different positions on expansion of the private sector in delivery and/or financing (see Table 9.3).

**TABLE 9.3**
**Positions on the future for public and private financing and delivery in Canadian health care**

|  |  | Private financing | |
|---|---|---|---|
|  |  | *Maintain status quo* | *Expand* |
| **Private delivery** | *Maintain status quo* | Romanow Report<br>Health stakeholders |  |
|  | *Expand* | Kirby Report<br>TD Economics | C.D. Howe<br>Fraser Institute |

## Private financing

A number of arguments are advanced for expanding private financing, not all of which are consistent (Tinghőg, Carlsson, & Lyttkens, 2010). One line of argument, for example, proposes increases in user charges, arguing that price signals will provide strong incentives on consumers to moderate (unnecessary) use of health services and hence moderate escalation in provision. Alongside this argument are proposals to expand the role of health insurance, which, of course, would dampen (or eliminate) any direct price signal effect on consumers.

### User charges

User charges or copayments attract vigorous debate (Weale & Clark, 2010). There is a robust literature on the effect of user charges (Baicker & Goldman, 2011; Carrin & Hanvoravongchai, 2003; Stoddart, Barer, & Evans, 1993) supported by a significant empirical study in the United States, the RAND health insurance experiment (Newhouse & Health Insurance Experiment Group, 1993). Essentially, the RAND study can be summarized as follows:

- user charges change utilization patterns;
- user charges impact more on the poor than the wealthy; and
- people whose behaviour changes as a result of user charges reduce both "necessary" and "unnecessary" care ("necessary" as judged by professionals).

All of this is consistent with what could be expected. User charges are typically flat fees per visit and, coupled with the average poorer health of lower-income groups, the cumulative impact on a poor person's (or family's) disposable income can be expected to be greater than on a wealthy person (or family). The result is that user charges, on average, exacerbate inequity.

The findings that user charges reduce both "necessary" and "unnecessary" care also have a logical explanation. The extent of health literacy varies in the community and consumers are not always good judges of what signs or symptoms are indicative of serious underlying problems. As a result, user charges may lead to deferral of necessary care and increased costs with later presentation.[129]

Universal health care is introduced to ensure a more equitable distribution of costs from the sick to the healthy, and from the poor to the wealthy. User charges are antithetical to that underlying premise, and expanding the role of user charges has not been supported by the Canadian public or politicians. Evans, Barer, Stoddart, and Bhatia (1994) colourfully describe the persistence of user-charging proposals: "Like zombies in the night, these ideas may be intellectually dead but are never buried. They may lie dormant for a time … but when stresses build up either in the health care system or in the wider public economy, they rise up and stalk the land" (p. 1).

Voluntary user charges, allowing people to pay privately for services covered by Medicare, are also "zombies." Often couched as allowing "freedom of choice" for the wealthy, this option would formalize a two-track (or two-tier) system of Medicare where ability to pay would explicitly be designed to affect access (Marchildon, 2005). If long waiting times are caused by shortages of health personnel, creation of a private track could exacerbate the problem as personnel in short supply shift their time to the more lucrative private market (Duckett, 2005b).

Two-track systems have the potential to weaken social support for the health system. Medicare is designed to ensure that all Canadians have equal access to publicly financed care. This in turn means that all Canadians have a stake in ensuring that the public system functions effectively; Medicare thus contributes to social cohesion and social solidarity. The more Medicare is relegated to being a system for the "poor," and the more middle-class or wealthy individuals seek to opt out of a public system to rely on private insurance and private services for their care, the more social solidarity will be weakened and government expenditure on Medicare and the public system will be questioned by those groups who do not see themselves benefiting from that expenditure.

### Insurance

The alternative to out-of-pocket costs and user charges as a way of increasing "private" contributions is through insurance, either voluntary or mandated. Voluntary insurance tends to be used by high-income groups, leads to differential access, and may impact adversely on public provision (Colombo & Tapay, 2004; Cuff, Hurley, Mestelman, Muller, & Nuscheler, in press; Duckett, 2005a, 2005b; Glied, 2008b; Stabile, 2008). The Australian experience with parallel systems of public and private insurance suggests that, if introduced into Canada, it

> would redistribute income (in general, from sick, low-income individuals to healthy, high income individuals, and from members of society more generally to health care providers and insurers), increase inequality in access to health care, and increase choice for those who can afford private insurance. (Hurley, Vaithianathan, Crossley, & Cobb-Clark, 2001, p. 29)

Wider uptake of private health insurance is seen as a necessary precondition for development of private markets in health care (to ensure a greater proportion of the population has access to private services). But, for a host of reasons, private markets do not exist or work in health care, at least in those aspects of health care that are regarded as necessary for health (rather than beauty). As Evans (1997) concludes, "There is in health care no 'private, competitive market' of the form described in the economics textbooks, anywhere in the world. There never has been, and inherent characteristics of health and health care make it impossible that there ever could be" (p. 428).

Tax-funded Medicare and other forms of mandated insurance involve two types of redistribution: in terms of income, so access by poorer people is subsidized by wealthier people, and for an individual, over his or her life cycle (Barr, 2001). This latter function means that all Canadians benefit directly from Medicare and have a stake in its success. If upper- and middle-income Canadians could address this life-cycle redistribution need outside Medicare, through private insurance arrangements, the political support for Medicare could be undermined (Casamatta, Cremer, & Pestieau, 2000).

Health insurance markets, both voluntary and mandated, require complex regulatory regimes (Colombo & Tapay, 2004; Dror & Preker, 2002; Laffont & Tirole, 1993; Saltman, Busse, & Mossialos, 2002,) that may be beyond the regulatory capacity of many countries where these regimes have been introduced (Wagstaff, 2010). Mandated insurance requires complex risk adjustment as well, but the technology to do this is still underdeveloped. The leading researcher in this area, Dutch health economist Van de Ven (2011), describes the "quality of the risk equalization system in many countries ... as poor to moderate" (p. 149).

One form of mandated insurance is "social insurance," the predominant health-financing model in those European countries that have followed the Bismarckian tradition (most of northern continental Europe). Under these models, social insurance contributions are mandated, typically as part of employment arrangements.

Recent social insurance reforms in The Netherlands broke the nexus with employment and allowed greater choice of insurance fund, although insurance was still mandated. These changes were designed to strengthen competitive forces in social insurance but appear to have resulted in little consumer take-up of the new-found freedoms, in part because of inadequate information about switching insurers (Boonen & Schut, 2011; Reitsma-van Rooijen, de Jong, & Rijken, 2011). A feature of social insurance is choice of plans (in contrast to Beveridge-type arrangements), which raises an equity risk that "those with a lower income would opt for less-expensive plans and a lower standard of care in some dimensions than those with higher incomes" (Blomqvist, 2008, p. 36).

The allure of social insurance is still great, but the performance is weak. As Evans (2009) summarizes, social insurance "costs more, yields no better average health outcomes, reduces participation in the formal labour force and, in developing countries, typically falls far short of universality" (p. 23). World Bank economist Adam Wagstaff in his latest review of the experience with social insurance concluded that it "is thus far from the panacea it is often portrayed to be" (2010, p. 515).

Does private spending really substitute for public spending?

An expanded role for private funding is often couched as "taking pressure off public spending," the implicit assumption being that public and private spending on health care are substitutes. Cross-national comparisons do not support that hypothesis (Figure 9.3).

**FIGURE 9.3**
**Public and private health expenditure as share of gross domestic product by per capita GDP, selected OECD countries, 2008**

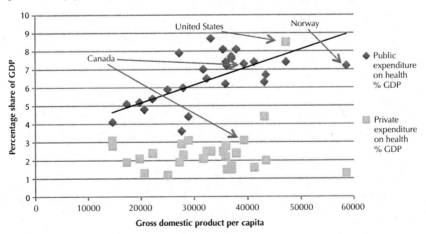

Source: Author's analysis of OECD data.

Total health expenditure as a percentage of gross domestic product (GDP) increases with GDP, primarily driven by an increase in public spending. The anomalous experience of the United States affects the strength of the relationships: public spending is strongly correlated with per capita GDP (r = 0.67 for all countries, 0.72 excluding the US and Norway), but private spending only exhibits a weak correlation for all country data (0.21) or no correlation excluding the two outliers (0.09).

A visual inspection of the data shows the slope of the relationship between private expenditure and GDP per capita is flat, in contrast to the public expenditure–GDP relationship, further emphasizing the lack of relationship between public and private expenditure. An examination of the United States' experience is sobering: US public spending on health care is close to expectations given the size of its GDP. The excess US expenditure on health care appears to be driven entirely by its excess private expenditure. All this suggests that the international comparative experience provides no evidence to support a hypothesis that increasing private expenditure on health would substitute for public spending or make health care more affordable.

Although advocates of expanded private financing often couch their proposals as being able to respond to challenges facing the public sector as a result of pressure on public funding, what has been shown here is that private financing is a risky path to tread: it may not deliver the promised benefits and will almost certainly challenge the equitable underpinnings of Canadian health care. As White (2001) argued in a somewhat similar context, the greatest threat to Canadian Medicare may be from the campaign to "save" it. In summary, an expanded private financing share is "more likely to harm than help" (Tuohy, Flood, & Stabile, 2004, p. 393).

*Canadian health care is best served by a continuation of tax financing. Expansion of private insurance into core areas should not be pursued.*

### Private delivery

Private delivery is an inherent part of Canadian Medicare and other parts of Canadian health care (see Table 9.2). Private delivery and private financing of care are two separate and not necessarily linked concepts: indeed, private delivery within a publicly financed system already occurs in Canada in primary care, long-term care and, to a lesser extent, in acute care.

However, expansion of private delivery into some areas where it has not been traditional is still contentious. As shown in Table 9.2, most medical services are already provided as private sector operations; private provision of laboratory medicine and diagnostic imaging are logical outgrowths of private medical provision and appear less publicly contentious than private surgical facilities. However, contracts for private diagnostic services still need to be negotiated to ensure efficiency dividends accrue to the public payer and appropriate quality controls are in place.

For obvious reasons (lack of data elements), there is no Canadian evidence on the relative merits of private delivery of acute services and, as discussed in Chapter 6, only weak evidence about private delivery of long-term care.

There are a number of arguments advanced for private delivery, some stronger than others. For example, private delivery does not obviate payment for capital, despite claims sometimes made to the contrary. Private delivery only shifts the incidence of capital costs from upfront payment to service charges paid on a periodic basis.

Private delivery is often claimed to facilitate innovation and to be more efficient than public delivery and, in theory, that will be true when the assumptions of a competitive market hold true: that there are no externalities in production or consumption, that the product is not a public good, that the market is not monopolistic in structure, and that information costs are low (Megginson & Netter, 2001, p. 329). In practice these assumptions are often violated in the health sector; for example, hospitals may typically be local monopolies, and information costs are high. Competitive markets in the United States are not associated with improved quality of care (Scanlon, Swaminathan, Lee, & Chernew, 2008). Arguments for private delivery and privatization are thus often made on ideological grounds (Braithwaite, Travaglia, & Corbett, 2011; Palley, Pomey, & Forest, 2011), with the evidence or relative performance of public versus private being irrelevant (Currie, Donaldson, & Lu, 2003).

The evidence about the benefits of private delivery is mixed. Hollingsworth (2008) reviewed 317 studies and found not-for-profit hospitals were, on average, more efficient than for-profit, although he cautioned that the strength of the difference might be setting-dependent and influenced by study methods. Different model specifications, for example, shift US for-profit hospitals from being more efficient than not-for-profits to being no different (Rosko & Mutter, 2008). Results are also sensitive to the concept of "efficiency" being studied: although German private and non-profit hospitals are less (technically) efficient than public hospitals (Herr, 2008), if "profit efficiency" (driven by both cost efficiency and revenue generation) is the measure, the ranking changes as private hospitals earn higher surpluses/profits than public hospitals (Herr, Schmitz, & Augurzky, 2011). Shukla, Pestian, and Clement (1997) found no difference in traditional efficiency and productivity indicators between for-profit and not-for-profit hospitals, but differences in emphasis on revenue strategies; the higher surpluses/profits in for-profit hospitals were attributable to revenue strategies rather than cost and efficiency management.

The *ceteris paribus* assumption endemic to economics studies is important in interpreting these findings too. Not all economic analyses standardize for quality differences in their measures of efficiency, and this can materially influence efficiency rankings (Mutter, Rosko, & Wong, 2008). A systematic review by Devereaux et al. (2002) showed that for-profit facilities performed worse than not-for-profit in terms of mortality outcomes.

## Contracting

If private delivery is to occur within a public framework, then well-specified contracts need to be developed. The *sine qua non* of a contract is specification of the service to be contracted. This is a non-trivial task, but developments in case-mix research over the last few decades have improved the ability to describe health care services. Provider contracts, of course, also need to describe quality of services, and this is still somewhat more difficult.

Service description is not the only complexity in contracting. Indeed, Oliver Williamson shared the 2009 Nobel Prize in economics for his work on identifying when internal production or market procurement was to be preferred (the "make or buy decision"). Health care contracts might also involve "asset specificity," another issue identified by Williamson (1975, 1986): if an asset brought into use as part of a contract has no alternative use, this creates "bilateral dependency" in the contract. Williamson (2002) argues that this leads to a "fundamental transformation" of the contracting process: no longer are there many buyers and many sellers—the assumption underpinning market economics—and continuity of the relationship becomes critical. In public sector contracting, this exposes the transaction to political interference risks. The risks of asset specificity can be mitigated by longer-term contracts and by financing arrangements that allow leasing of premises and equipment.

Structuring of pricing arrangements in contracts involves policy choices, for example, whether to have fixed "administrative pricing" or to have "competitive pricing" derived from a bidding process. The different pricing arrangements require different information and different skills to administer, and evoke different political responses from providers (Coulam, Feldman, & Dowd, 2011). Poorly designed contracts can result in the public purchaser's overpaying private providers (Dranove, Capps, & Dafny, 2009; Pollock & Kirkwood, 2009). Any efficiency benefits from private delivery may then accrue solely to the private provider, making moot a potential reason for contracting. Good practice in contracting should also incorporate marginal pricing rather than paying for all contracted service delivery at full average cost (Laffont & Tirole, 1993), and provide for sharing of productivity gains. This does not appear to be the uniform current practice in Canada.[130]

Where there is a market there should be risk, as profit is in part a payment for risk taking. Risk involves the potential for contract failure through default or bankruptcy. Although the financial costs of default will fall primarily on investors (and possibly on employees), consumers may also suffer because of short-term withdrawal of capacity in the health system. Again, contract negotiations need to include safeguards in the event of default.

Most contracting health authorities have limited experience in contracting with commercial operators, but more experience in contracting with not-for-profit providers. For-profit providers and health authority contract negotiators may not share culture assumptions, influencing preferred models for contract specification (Mackintosh, 2000). In the context of limited contracting experience, different cultural norms, and occasional poor ability to specify what is being purchased, it is not surprising that weak contracts are written and that the public sector does not achieve the putative benefits of private sector provision.

Private delivery has potential in Canada but carries risks, especially with poorly specified contracts, inappropriate incentives, and potential overpayments. And because of asset specificity, private providers have strong incentives to seek contract negotiations outside business processes. Nevertheless, private delivery may stimulate innovation and improved efficiency. *Provinces should continue to contract with the private sector for service delivery. Contracts for private delivery should incorporate marginal pricing and robust measures of quality.*

### So how good is the Canadian health care system? And how much change is necessary?

The reviews and commentaries canvassed in this chapter are all predicated on the premise that the Canadian health care system needs to change. Previous chapters of this book have also advanced proposals for change. Does the combination of all of this mean that "fundamental change" is necessary, or does the system need to be rebuilt, to use the Commonwealth Fund survey language (Schoen et al., 2010)?

At the most fundamental, the phrase "Canadian health care system" embodies the problem: there is no single Canadian system. Rather, Canada has a provincialized approach to management and policy direction (Di Matteo, 2009), and "no province, nor Canada as a whole, has a ... [health care system], if we take the word system to mean an organization in which the many different and diverse parts function together" (Sinclair et al., 2005, p. 23).

Ham (2010) has identified ten characteristics of high-performing health systems. Table 9.4 shows my assessment of Canada's performance against these criteria drawing on the evidence and arguments in the previous chapters.

In my assessment, Canada does not have a high-performing health system. This is not to say it is not better than many other systems. Access is better for the poor, and the system overall is more efficient than the United States' system, for example. There are pockets of excellence in the United States, and so too in Canada. However, the issue, returning to the goal articulated earlier in this book, is whether we have a system where *the right person enables the right care in the right setting, on time, every time.* Regrettably, the answer is no.

The next chapter outlines how we might get there from here.

**TABLE 9.4**
**Ten characteristics of high-performing health systems**

| Characteristic | Canadian performance (author assessment) |
|---|---|
| Universal coverage | Exists for access to hospital and medical care |
| Care is free at the point of use | Exists for access to hospital and medical care |
| The delivery system focuses on the prevention of ill health | Questionable: to some extent the "prevention" system is separated from the service delivery system. Hospitals have very little involvement in prevention |
| Priority is given to patients to self-manage their conditions with support from caregivers and families | Self-management support unevenly developed across Canada |
| Priority is given to primary health care | Not in place |
| Population management is emphasized | Not in place, despite regionalization in many provinces |
| Care is integrated to enable primary health care teams to access specialist advice and support when needed | Referral arrangements generally ad hoc. Few systems for referral in place |
| The potential benefits of information technology are exploited to improve chronic care | Not in place |
| Care is effectively coordinated | Not in place |
| These nine characteristics are linked into a coherent whole as part of a strategic approach | Not in place |

Source: Author's analysis using characteristics from Ham (2010).

**Word cloud: How to get there from here: How the efficiency agenda (broadly defined) is at the heart of protecting health care access and quality in Canada**

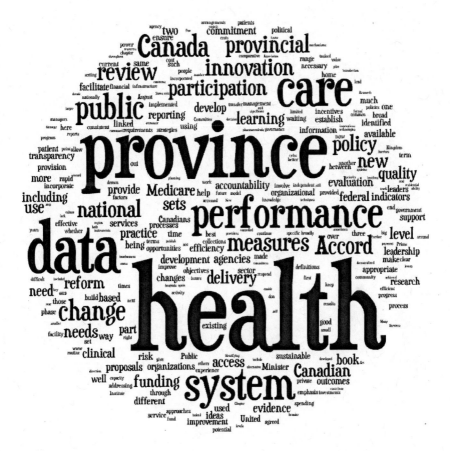

In this chapter I propose the following policy initiatives:

- The 2014 Accord should be for a ten-year period, and should guarantee funding increases to the provinces of 6 percent per annum.
- The new Accord should reaffirm the principles of the *Canada Health Act*, modifying the comprehensiveness criterion to focus on effective care determined in a transparent way and the public administration criterion to focus on public insurance.
- The 2014 Accord should provide that, if and when a national pharmaceutical program is introduced, federal funding to the provinces should be reduced to offset any provincial savings that accrue due to substitution of new federal spending for past provincial spending.
- Federal, provincial, and territorial leaders should agree on a (limited) set of performance measures to be published annually.
- The Canadian Institute for Health Information should be tasked to develop a national health data dictionary that would incorporate the data elements necessary for derivation of the agreed performance measures.
- The 2014 Accord should make any transfer payments to a province conditional on the province's contributing to a national data set the data necessary to derive the agreed performance measures using the nationally mandated data definitions.
- Provinces should leverage the power of existing data collections through linked data sets that are available for use in research and system evaluation.
- Federal, provincial, and territorial leaders should commit to achieving access to national linked data by 2020. The Canadian Health Services Research Foundation should be tasked to develop a road map for the most effective and efficient way to develop national access.
- Provinces should fund the infrastructure to establish pilot sites for facility-level rapid-learning health system evaluation. The Canadian Institutes of Health Research should be tasked and funded to establish a funding stream for rapid-learning health system evaluation.
- The 2014 Accord should incorporate a commitment to conduct mid-term and end-of-term independent reviews of health care in Canada to inform the 2024 renegotiations.
- Federal and provincial governments should develop governance structures to facilitate broadly based, whole-of-government approaches to address factors influencing health.
- Provinces should build on the nationally agreed performance measures to develop clear performance measures for health and health care in the province and for every separately incorporated health-delivery agency in the province.
- Provinces should develop strategies for public reporting of performance of delivery agencies, and processes to build accountability for performance of agencies.
- The 2014 Accord should make provision for a broadly based Federal/Provincial/Territorial Advisory Committee, consisting of people able to represent consumer views as well as people drawn from the health sector. The committee should be tasked with identifying issues and making recommendations to deputy ministers or ministers. The functioning and worth of the committee should be reviewed two years after its first meeting.
- Delivery agencies should review their current approaches to public participation to assess whether they are addressing contemporary needs. Provinces should establish guidelines for minimum standards of public participation. Health Canada should convene a conference every three years to share delivery agencies' experiences with public participation.

CHAPTER 10

# HOW TO GET THERE FROM HERE: HOW THE EFFICIENCY AGENDA (BROADLY DEFINED) IS AT THE HEART OF PROTECTING HEALTH CARE ACCESS AND QUALITY IN CANADA

This book is about directions, about "Where to from here?" I argued in Chapter 2 that health care in Canada is sustainable and indeed the subtitle of this book is *Keeping Medicare Sustainable*, emphasizing the tasks that need to be taken. So the book is very much about what we have to do now and into the future to keep Medicare sustainable.

There are certain themes that flow through the book, guided by the orientations articulated in Chapter 2:

- a concern for disadvantaged populations and addressing unmet needs
- an emphasis on the least restrictive alternative
- the three perspectives on value: patient, clinician, and economic
- the use of economic incentives
- the potential of different provider forms

The key to ensuring the health system responds to the needs of a growing and aging population in a sustainable way is to make sure existing resources are used to their best. The efficiency agenda is not simply about cost cutting, or spending less. It is about using limited resources wisely: it is about ensuring that every service that needs to be provided is provided in the most efficient way, and that the services that are provided do indeed need to be provided and are the best investments to improve outcomes. This is what is meant by efficiency "broadly defined."

I have made around 60 proposals for change in this book, many directed at provinces, calling for change in priorities, approaches, and management. There are some big things, most notably looking to coverage of pharmaceuticals, but most are small and incremental changes. This is for two reasons. First, the fundamentals of health care in Canada are right. Canada does not need "big bang" reform and, in any event, the track record of big bang proposals is not good (Hutchison et al., 2001). Second, I have an eye to implementability. The small changes I have proposed are all achievable and can be implemented incrementally.

But just because they are small changes, it does not mean that their cumulative effect could not be profound. With these changes—better investments, more efficient services—there is no doubt that Medicare will continue to be sustainable.

## The levers for change

There are three broad levers, instruments or factors that shape health system direction and change: financial levers and incentives; laws, regulations, and governance arrangements; and values, norms, culture, and collegial workings. The evolution of the Canadian health system, and how it has responded to challenges over time, has demonstrated the strength of the latter factor (Tuohy, 1999). In this book a mix of instruments is used, including financial incentives and collegial insights, to reshape care.

Former United Kingdom prime minister Blair's strategy unit identified four sets of forces that were being used to reshape public services there (Prime Minister's Strategy Unit, 2006). Two related to incentives and governance, the latter called "top-down performance management" in their parlance, and included target setting and performance assessment. A third was pressure from users "shaping services from below," and included funding following user choices: activity-based funding can facilitate that. The fourth pressure was termed "capability and capacity" and included leadership, workforce development and skills reform, and organizational development. Workforce issues were canvassed in Chapter 8. This chapter will address governance, leadership, and public participation—the components of cultural change.

## The importance of governance and stewardship

The importance of the governance context cannot be underestimated. As Romanow identified before the 2004 Accord (Commission on the Future of Health Care, 2002), stable and secure funding is an essential prerequisite for any change. But it is also important that the ground rules are agreed upfront. The 2004 Accord gave health care in Canada unparalleled stability. Provinces knew a decade in advance what funds would flow from the federal government, and what criteria would be used to judge the legitimacy of their actions.

The 2014 Accord should give the same certainty. The federal government has announced that it will maintain 6 percent indexation only through to 2016–17, with indexation in line with economic growth thereafter. Health spending increases faster than the economy so this represents a significant tightening, barely keeping pace with the impact of population growth and aging. Although I have argued there is room to improve the efficiency of health care in Canada, there is no reason to believe that the public wants to constrain health spending in line with economic growth. Surveys have shown time and again that the public would prioritize health spending over other potential spending priorities. Further, linking funding to economic growth does not provide the health sector with the necessary funding certainty. *The 2014 Accord should be for a ten-year period, and should guarantee funding increases to the provinces of 6 percent per annum.*

The next Accord should continue to give assurance about the broad parameters within which provinces can manage Medicare. The five principles defined in the *Canada Health Act*—public administration, comprehensiveness, universality, portability, and accessibility—provide a good and well-accepted framework but may need to be marginally revised if the scope of Medicare expands (such as to cover home care and pharmaceuticals).

The language of the *comprehensiveness* and *public administration* criteria may need to be updated too. As discussed in Chapter 1, the comprehensiveness criterion rests on the ambiguous notion of "necessary services." A more contemporary approach would be to focus public funding on effective services. Australia introduced a cost-effectiveness criterion for listing of pharmaceuticals on its national Pharmaceutical Benefits Scheme 20 years ago, and for new items on its Medicare schedule in 1998 (Duckett & Willcox, 2011). As argued in Chapter 7, effectiveness decisions need to be made in a fair and transparent way. Subject to that caveat, the comprehensiveness criterion should be revised to base coverage on effective services.

The requirements of the public administration criterion are confused in public discourse about the *Canada Health Act*. As was discussed in Chapter 9, most physician services in Canada are privately provided, and there is no prohibition in the Act against private provision of covered services. What the Act does proscribe, and what should be maintained, is private administration of provincial insurance arrangements. Perhaps the criterion could be reframed and reworded as a "public insurance" criterion to describe its purpose better.

*The new Accord should reaffirm the principles of the* Canada Health Act, *modifying the comprehensiveness criterion to focus on effective care determined in a transparent way and the public administration criterion to focus on public insurance.*

In previous chapters I have advanced a number of proposals for change in the federal role, some of which require increases in federal spending. Many of the proposals are inexpensive and should be able to be absorbed as part of the routine business of government priority-setting. The standout exception relates to the development of a national pharmaceuticals program, which can be cost saving but will involve a redistribution of who spends what. Chapter 5 does not make a definitive recommendation, proposing instead a process that could lead to a realignment of funding responsibilities between the federal and provincial governments. This needs to be recognized. *The 2014 Accord should provide that, if and when a national pharmaceutical program is introduced, federal funding to the provinces should be reduced to offset any provincial savings that accrue due to substitution of new federal spending for past provincial spending.*

## Accountability and transparency

Just as the health service delivery arm has embraced the concept of continuous improvement, so too should the policy arm. This requires a culture change in the current modus operandi and has a number of implications. First is a renewed emphasis on transparency in terms of performance of health care both nationally and provincially. The OECD described the current situation thus:

> Efforts to evaluate policies are hampered by an insufficiency of publicly available provincial performance data (e.g. on unit costs, volumes and quality), as well as of clinical data covering treatment outcomes. This is partly technical, as a lag exists, relative to both other sectors and countries, in adopting information and communication technologies in health care. Ministries of health, responsible for nearly half of overall provincial spending, may lack the commensurate analytical capacity. But there are transparency issues as well: provincial health ministries may not be terribly keen to expose their systems' weaknesses, and doctors may not like being subject to scrutiny, unless pushed by effective checks and balances. (2010a, p. 107)

At present, provinces use different definitions for key performance indicators, and may not contribute data to national data holdings. Despite progress over the last decade, there are still significant gaps in the data necessary to answer key questions about health system performance in Canada (Canadian Institute for Health Information, 2009b). The range of publicly available data in Canada is significantly less than in Australia,[131] and there should be wider availability of public use data sets drawn from complete national data collections (El Emam, Paton, Dankar, & Koru, 2011). This lack of access hinders transparency, inhibits accountability, and slows transfer of lessons from one part of the country to another—all to the detriment of Canadians as citizens, as potential patients, and as taxpayers.

The 2004 Accord espoused a commitment to accountability and transparency, and indeed, performance reports have been produced (see Health Canada, 2008b), but these have been criticized as inadequate for accountability purposes. The Auditor General of Canada, in her December 2008 report, concluded:

Health Canada met the specific health indicator reporting obligations that the agreements required of it—including identifying common indicators for reporting with its provincial and territorial counterparts. It has produced a health indicators report every two years.

The *Healthy Canadians* reports do not fulfill the broader intent of the agreements—to provide the information Canadians need on the progress of health care renewal. The reports provide indicators, such as wait times for diagnostic services, without providing sufficient information to help readers interpret them. There is no discussion of what the indicators say about progress in health renewal. Without interpretation, their ability to inform Canadians is limited. (Office of the Auditor General of Canada, 2008)

The federal Health Minister in an August 2011 speech to the Canadian Medical Association emphasized that the 2014 Accord would (again) include "a clear emphasis on accountability. This way, Canadians will be able to know that we are achieving *real results* in improving the system" (Aglukkaq, 2011; emphasis in original). If this commitment is to go beyond mere rhetoric, there needs to be a much higher profile given to reporting—an expectation that Health Canada, or another designated agency, will produce meaningful, consistent data with accompanying interpretation, in a form that allows assessment as to whether "real results" have been achieved.

The prerequisites for accountability and transparency are common data definitions sufficient to allow calculation of performance measures across a range of dimensions including outputs (volumes provided), outcomes (quality measures), and processes (e.g., access measures). *Federal, provincial, and territorial leaders should agree on a (limited) set of performance measures to be published annually. The Canadian Institute for Health Information should be tasked to develop a national health data dictionary that would incorporate the data elements necessary for derivation of the agreed performance measures. The 2014 Accord should make any transfer payments to a province conditional on the province's contributing to a national data set the data necessary to derive the agreed performance measures using the nationally mandated data definitions.*

Selecting performance indicators for reporting is not a technocratic or value-neutral process. It involves choices on what will be measured, prioritizing some aspects of the health system over others. Nienaber and Wildavsky's (1973) eloquent description of the problem of choosing objectives applies equally to choosing performance indicators:

Of objectives it can be said that they invariably may be distinguished by three outstanding qualities: they are multiple, conflicting and vague.... The assumption that objectives are known, clear, and consistent is at variance with all experience. Objectives are not just out there, like ripe fruit waiting to be plucked; they are man-made [*sic*], artificial, imposed on a recalcitrant world. Inevitably, they do violence to reality by emphasising certain activities (and hence organisational elements) over others. Thus the very process of defining objectives may be considered a hostile act. It they are too vague, no evaluation can be done. If they are too specific, they never encompass all the indefinable qualities that their adherents insist they have. If they are too broad, any activity may be said to contribute to them. If they are too narrow, they may favour one segment of the organisation against another. (p. 10)

The performance measures to be incorporated in the 2014 Accord requirements should be broad in scope (Smith, Mossialos, Papanicolas, & Leatherman, 2009), recognize the multidimensional nature of health and health care objectives (Hauck & Street, 2006), and respond to the concerns that Canadians have about system performance (e.g., waiting times). There should be an evidence-base to support the measures, with credible benchmarks where appropriate (Watson, Barer, Matkovich, & Gagnon, 2007) that take into account the different incentive effects inherent in different formulations of definitions (Hussey, de Vries, et al., 2009).

Performance indicators have a distribution, and attributes of that distribution should generally be reported. In some cases the distributional attributes reported should be statistical (e.g., it is now common to report the $90^{th}$ percentile for waiting times as well as the mean). More important, many aspects of health care provision vary by location, race, and socioeconomic status. So reporting of key performance indicators should enable tracking of equity of provision: Are waiting-time distributions the same for people who live in poorer areas as wealthier? The same question arises for health outcome measures.

Recommended performance measures should not be limited by existing data collections, but should take into account the cost of new data collections. A road map should be developed that provides for phasing-in of new performance measures as data become available. New measures that might be considered include patient-reported outcome measures (Fitzpatrick, 2009; Maynard & Bloor, 2010), which allow tracking of outcomes from a patient perspective, as well as derivation of true measures of productivity change (Castelli, Laudicella, Street, & Ward, 2011; Smith & Street, 2007; Sharpe, Messinger, & Bradley, 2007).

## Linked data sets

Considerable investments have been made in hospitals and other facilities in collecting data, and some provinces have made investments to use these data to shine a light on system performance. Manitoba's Centre for Health Policy[132] led the world in data linkage and leveraging the power of data to give insight into system performance and desirable directions (Marchessault, 2011; Roos, Menec, & Currie, 2004; Roos & Roos, 2011). Other provinces have followed suit: Ontario's Institute for Clinical Evaluative Sciences provides an alternate but also successful model.[133] Not all provinces have moved as speedily and as far. There are barriers to development of the linked data sets that characterized these models, not the least being to assure people that these approaches do not violate reasonable privacy concerns (Flood & Thomas, 2011). But the potential benefits from harnessing the power of information are so great (Lewis, 2011) that establishing linked data sets has moved from a "nice to have" element of research infrastructure to an essential component of system learning.

Although there should be no option about the "whether," the "how" might vary provincially. *Provinces should leverage the power of existing data collections through linked data sets that are available for use in research and system evaluation.* Larger provinces should establish their own linked data sets and make them available for use by independent researchers. Smaller provinces should either follow suit or participate as data providers to another province's data set.

These provincial moves should be accompanied by strategies to facilitate access to national linked data. This may be best effected by provincial data sets being transmitted to a national data set. Alternatively, coordinated access arrangements could be developed to provide a single point of national access that could draw on distributed data holdings. *Federal, provincial, and territorial leaders should commit to achieving access to national linked data by 2020. The Canadian Health Services Research Foundation should be tasked to develop a road map for the most effective and efficient way to develop national access.*

National strategies for data linkage should also involve linking national data, such as national population health surveys and Canadian community health surveys, to the provincial utilization data.

### Toward a rapid-learning health system

Etheredge (2007) advanced the concept of a "rapid-learning health system" that draws on the power of health data sets to facilitate innovation and quality improvement. The Institute of Medicine in the United States has convened a series of workshops to identify how these ideas might be advanced in practice,[134] recognizing that "because of their potential to enable the development of new knowledge and to guide the development of best practices from the growing sum of individual clinical experiences, clinical data represent the resource most central to healthcare progress" (Grossman, Goolsby, Olsen, & McGinnis, 2010, p. 1).

The work of the Manitoba Centre for Health Policy has demonstrated the worth of using data to evaluate policy and practice at a provincial level. The rapid-learning health system advances this in two ways: creating a new model for clinical effectiveness research (Olsen & McGinnis, 2010) and advancing facility-specific analyses.

A new paradigm for clinical effectiveness research would involve drawing on vast data sets to analyze the actual experience of newly implemented treatments to assess outcomes and cost in real practice situations, as opposed to conducting initial evaluations using randomized controlled trials with selected patients (Normand, 2010; Schneeweiss & Avorn, 2005). Retrospectively determined cohorts of matched patients can be created quickly to respond to specific concerns about patterns of complications or as part of routine post-innovation review.

Local-level data use is already part of quality improvement and Plan-Do-Study-Act cycles, although accessing timely data from the routine data sets is sometimes a challenge. Transforming access to local data sets (with comparative data drawn from provincial or national holdings) would allow a quite different approach to practice. Patients could be told about the outcomes of other patients (with matched characteristics) treated at that facility or even by that clinician in the previous year (or other valid comparative period), and these outcomes could be compared to the average in other facilities in the province. Local-level data sets can also be used to estimate the diagnostic yield from ordering investigations, against the actual patient profile seen at that facility as opposed to national averages or in academic health sciences centres. These estimates of "prior probabilities" can be used to improve test-ordering behaviour in the next generation of professionals (Davidoff, Goodspeed, & Clive, 1989). Finally, local-level data can and should be used for performance monitoring and executive decision making, despite the difficulties of gathering the right information in a timely and understandable way (Glover, Rivers, Asch, Piper, & Murph, 2010).

*Provinces should fund the infrastructure to establish pilot sites for facility-level rapid-learning health system evaluation. The Canadian Institutes of Health Research should be tasked and funded to establish a funding stream for rapid-learning health system evaluation.*

### System evaluation

Openness to innovation and a commitment to transparency and accountability should apply at all levels of the system: it should not simply be for the policy makers to impose on operational folk. Policies should be up for review, evaluation, and critique. This should start at the national level with mid-term and end-of-cycle evaluation of the Accords.

The 2004 Accord was preceded by a Senate review that led to the Kirby Report (Senate, 2002a) and by an independent commission conducted by former premier Romanow (Commission on the Future of Health Care, 2002). There has been no end-of-Accord review for the 2004–2014 Accord announced to date that could serve as a platform to consider improvements for the 2014 Accord. Time is running out for such a review.

The 2014 Accord could provide a model with an upfront commitment to review health care, in say 2022, in time for the lead up to a 2024 renegotiation. A smaller mid-term review, say in 2019, might also be warranted, especially if it is oriented to identifying what additional research might need to be commissioned in preparation for the end-of-term review. These reviews should be independent of federal and provincial governments. *The 2014 Accord should incorporate a commitment to conduct mid-term and end-of-term independent reviews of health care in Canada to inform the 2024 renegotiations.*

## Addressing the governance deficits

The World Health Organization has identified "stewardship" as an important component of the health care system and its environment (Saltman & Ferroussier-Davis, 2000). The stewardship function provides the oversight and overall governance of the health system as a whole. Stewardship is about designing the regulatory framework for the system and ensuring compliance, establishing the roles of the agencies and authorities, and adjusting the system on the basis of monitoring and feedback systems.

The Canadian health care system has a governance and stewardship deficit. As discussed earlier in this chapter, there are weaknesses in accountability. Incomplete information, collected on non-comparable bases, vitiates attempts to benchmark and compare performance of provinces. A weak federal role hinders national learning. The privileging of physician and hospital services under Medicare distorts focus away from needed investments in lower technology, community-based services.

New governance structures, to facilitate whole-of-government consideration of strategies to promote health beyond the health portfolio, are required at national and provincial levels (WHO Europe, 2011a). These are not just committees, but structures that incorporate processes to garner citizen input and that commit to change strategies. *Federal and provincial governments should develop governance structures to facilitate broadly based, whole-of-government approaches to address factors influencing health.*

But it is not only whole-of-government consideration of the health agenda that is weakened by the governance deficit. System reform is made more difficult. Outside voices cannot be heard, and the voices of interest groups that benefit from the existing structure and distribution of resources are heard loudest. I've suggested above a strategy to open up the policy process with an external advisory committee; Brandeis's (1914) disinfecting sunlight through better information has also been a theme.

At the local level, there is a governance deficit in terms of oversight of patient safety and quality:

> Canadian healthcare boards need to develop greater expertise in quality and patient safety. They need better information on organizational performance in these areas, along with improved skills in helping to create and monitor the strategic quality and patient safety plans of their organizations. (Baker, Denis, Pomey, & Macintosh-Murray, 2010, p. 4)

Addressing the governance deficit thus requires action at all levels of the health system, and it requires innovative leadership, another theme discussed above. The governance and stewardship function is about direction setting; it is about being clear about how the health system needs to evolve and ensuring the structures and processes for decision making are in place to support that.

As noted in Chapter 1, some authors have argued there is no Canadian health care system, rather a "collection of plans administered by the ten provinces and three territories" (Detsky & Naylor, 2003, p. 804) or "set of centralized provincial systems" (Di Matteo, 2009, p. 32). Although an advantage of such decentralization can be that provincial health systems are more locally responsive, to date it has come at the expense of sound, comparable information that allows honest benchmarking of differences in system performance. In the absence of such benchmarking, it is difficult to see how local populations can make sound judgments about system adequacy, or how policy makers can set priorities based on relative gaps in performance. Addressing the information lacuna is essential to improve system performance nationally, provincially, and locally. Without improved information to underpin stronger accountability, the Canadian health system will languish as a below-median performer.

## The need for leadership and innovation

The "capability and capacity" dimension in the United Kingdom's public service reform (Prime Minister's Strategy Unit, 2006) is relevant to health system reform in Canada too. A host of changes are needed to respond better to emerging needs and to keep Medicare sustainable into the future. New ideas have to be embraced. But unfortunately, innovation in health care in Canada is mostly evidenced in clinical innovation: administrative, policy, and service innovation is occurring more in pockets than as part of a systematic approach to learning and innovation throughout the whole country.

There are lots of reasons for this. Managers have big jobs and the day-to-day can squeeze out the long term. We do not really know how to help managers use evidence in their work (Perrier, Mrklas, Lavis, & Straus, 2011), and evidence-based management is a concept still in its infancy with lack of clarity about what it is and how to do it (Briner, Denyer, & Rousseau, 2009; Reay, Berta, & Kohn, 2009). The same holds true for "evidence-based policy" (Black, 2001). Risk taking is not rewarded in the public sector, rather the reverse (Hood, 2002), which leads to extreme caution in trying out new ideas. Unlike private industry, where there is seen to be a measurable risk-reward trade-off, "few health managers saw scope for any beneficial trade-off between risk and return. Instead, risk was something that had to be avoided, and if it could not be avoided then it should be minimised and controlled" (Shiell, Hawe, Perry, & Matthias, 2009, p. 80).

In times of extreme resource constraint, creating the organizational slack to provide start-up funds for innovation and meet other organizational objectives may be difficult (Greenhalgh, Robert, MacFarlane, Bate, & Kyriakidou, 2004; Zinn & Flood, 2009). Further, much of the research on organizational learning is drawn from studies of private sector organizations, yet context is a critical factor in promoting organizational learning—so again, there is a knowledge gap (Rashman, Withers, & Hartley, 2009). Parallel sources of authority (clinical and managerial) can also lead to a disconnect between willingness to initiate change and the ability to implement it (Lockett, Currie, Waring, Finn, & Martin, in press). At the broader level, the decentralized nature of health care in Canada leads to multiple players feeling they can exercise veto powers, further inhibiting change (Hacker, 2004). System inertia is in part a result of the complexity of the system (Coiera, 2011), and so each successful step in streamlining work processes and addressing waste may make the next one easier.

In traditional markets, organizations live and die (Kaufman, 1975, 1991), with innovation partly driving the change (Christensen, 1997). Public sector organizations do not have the same life cycle as occurs in the private sector (Kaufman, 1976). Even in the United States where market forces have a much more significant role, organizational innovation is not optimal. Cutler (2010) has attributed this to poor measurement of quality (which attenuates important market signals) and payment policies focusing on "volume not value." The proposals advanced above to enhance national transparency and accountability might mitigate the effect of these factors in Canada in future, but strategies to enhance provincial and local accountability are also required.

The first step in a new process involves alignment of performance measures. *Provinces should build on the nationally agreed performance measures to develop clear performance measures for health and health care in the province and for every separately incorporated health-delivery agency in the province.*

The next step is to hold delivery agencies to account for their performance through appropriate management control systems (McKillop, 2002, 2004). This should involve both some form of public reporting (e.g., for waiting-time performance, comparative efficiency) and formal performance review meetings between provincial leaders (e.g., Minister of Health) and boards of delivery agencies. Performance reviews should focus on the results achieved rather than, except to the extent that lessons can be transferred, specifying the way in which an agency achieved its results. *Provinces should develop strategies for public reporting of performance of delivery agencies, and processes to build accountability for performance of agencies.* Agencies should not be effectively rewarded for poor performance by end-of-year bailouts (Bordignon & Turati, 2009).

Encouraging risk taking and innovation is harder, but "baby steps" might help. As more organizations pursue contemporary, continuous quality-improvement approaches and undertake Plan-Do-Study-Act cycles, managers and leaders may be prepared to build on those cycles to pursue larger innovations. But continuous quality improvement is typically focused on incremental change to existing services using existing technologies, the most conservative cell of the two-by-two innovation matrix. More radical, disruptive, non-linear change (to use just some of the language in this literature; Omachonu & Einspruch, 2010) needs to be encouraged and rewarded: health care organizations need to review their processes that might foster risk aversion and inhibit innovation, and develop processes to encourage it (Nembhard, Alexander, Hoff, & Ramanujam, 2009). Building diversity among leadership teams may be one way of bringing new ideas into the mix, stimulating and rewarding right-brain approaches another (Pink, 2006). Disseminating information about what works, and the experience of others (Greenhalgh et al., 2004), also fosters innovation.

Risk aversion can lead to policy paralysis: from the perspective of the risk-averse decision maker, fear of any failure (or political opprobrium) outweighs the benefits that may accrue. Benchmarking and analysis of comparative performance may help here: accountability for the "might have beens," or opportunities foregone, should weigh equally in evaluations.

Policy-innovation risk is reduced by phrasing interventions as "pilots," but this too carries a risk. National and provincial funding of pilot projects is often easy to negotiate with ministries of finance because ongoing commitments are limited, and political credit is gained for taking action. Governments can address any risk of failure by claiming that the innovation was always to be evaluated. The predisposition to this type of policy innovation has created a situation where the health sector has more pilots than Air Canada. But when time-limited funding comes to an end, even promising projects might be discontinued, causing frustration among participants and an unwillingness to participate in innovative reforms in the future. The language probably needs to change: from pilots to demonstration projects, from summative evaluation to formative evaluation. The evaluation model needs to change, too, to recognize that "common sense" reforms have a place,[135] and that local adaptation and responsiveness is important. Evaluation will therefore involve natural experiments and action research.

The Canadian health care system is not alone in requiring reinvigoration and innovation. Part of the Obama health care reforms in the United States involves the creation of an "Innovation Center" within the Center for Medicare and Medicaid Services. Gold, Helms, and Guterman (2011) have identified three critical requirements for the new centre to be effective:

- focusing on change that matters
- documenting innovation to support effective learning and spread
- generating the evidence needed to support broad-based policy change

These same requirements provide appropriate guidance for innovation in Canada. One of the weaknesses of the highly decentralized (at least to the provincial level) structure of Canadian health care is that interprovincial learning is inhibited and sometimes discouraged: "not invented here" as a barrier is alive and well. Successful change in one province or even region can help to overcome the skeptics, but only if the successes in region/province A are known and valued in region/province B. Valuing the innovations is an attribute of the leaders, whether they are risk-takers or risk-averse, comfortable with the status quo or change-oriented. But transfer of knowledge about innovations can, is, and should be facilitated by a range of intermediaries: the Health Council of Canada, professional organizations, and the Canadian Health Services Research Foundation to name a few. The federal government could exercise more leadership here by convening conferences and using other media to facilitate knowledge transfer. New structures might also help. *The 2014 Accord should make provision for a broadly based Federal/ Provincial/Territorial Advisory Committee, consisting of people able to represent consumer views as well as people drawn from the health sector. The committee should be tasked with identifying issues and making recommendations to deputy ministers or ministers. The functioning and worth of the committee should be reviewed two years after its first meeting.* The purpose here is to open up the health system to more ideas and to facilitate innovation. Unfortunately, advisory committees that do not face the same budgetary and political constraints of those inside bureaucracies or in the political system may offer unaffordable, unimplementable, utopian solutions. But well-functioning committees can facilitate exchange of ideas and help drive needed innovation in the health system.

## The crucial role of provincial leadership

Because of the decentralized nature of Canadian health care governance, much of the burden of health care reform, the challenge of responding to emerging needs, and the benefit in terms of improved efficiency, will fall on the provinces. About half of the proposals for change in this book are directed at provinces to implement (see Table 10.1).

The implementation task is great, but the track record for successful reform is a sorry one (Contandriopoulos & Brouselle, 2010; Fotaki, 2010). Recognizing this, the OECD has established a "making reform happen" project. Hurst (2010) identified four factors that might help or hinder reform:

- the availability of information, evidence, and analysis
- the use of incentives (and disincentives)
- political leadership and political possibilities
- the availability of resources

The first two of these factors have been canvassed in this book, the third is certainly recognized and, depending on commitment, the financial aspect of the fourth can be addressed through political will.

## TABLE 10.1
## Recommendations to provinces

- Each province should publish its own goals and targets, consistent with the national goals and targets.
- Provinces and regional health authorities should publish regular reports on disparities in health outcomes.
- Provinces should develop (or continue) programs to support quality improvement initiatives in primary care—including family practices—aimed at addressing access.
- Provinces should review home care provision to ensure optimal use is being made of remote monitoring and other technologies that can enable and support community dwelling for at-risk people, including those with chronic diseases; where indicated provinces should invest in the infrastructure to implement new remote-monitoring models.
- Provinces should review the structure of their payment arrangements for family physicians to ensure that these arrangements incorporate the right set of incentives for care of patients with chronic illnesses including the ability to support self-management, community-level interventions, and the optimal division of labour.
- Provinces should consider shifting responsibility for physician services budgets to regional health authorities.
- Provinces should review their primary care funding arrangements to ensure that funding streams are adequate to allow collaborative team practice.
- Provinces should give consideration to pilot programs of primary care budget holding and to the alternative policy direction, development of integrated care organizations.
- Provinces should incorporate self-managed care as an integral part of their home care systems.
- Provinces should review their home care provision to ensure that the full benefit of strong home care provision is available throughout the province.
- Provinces should explore introduction of public reporting of quality of nursing home care.
- Provinces should review their regulatory frameworks for seniors' care to ensure that they incorporate a best-practice mix of instruments.
- Provinces should encourage and facilitate development of a broader range of accommodation options for seniors including an intermediate residential care option, assisted living.
- Provinces should ensure efficiency of residential care provision, and equity between providers, through the introduction of activity-based funding for residential care.
- Provinces should fund health-care-provider access to a suite of patient decision aids and should encourage hospitals to use patient decision aids as part of their routine consent procedures for preference-sensitive conditions.
- Provinces should create and fund clinical networks to provide leadership in sharing good practice to improve access, quality, and sustainability of health care.

*... continued*

- Provinces should request clinical networks (when established) to review differences in intra- and interprovincial utilization rates. Networks should be invited to develop and/or update priority-setting criteria.
- Provinces should commit to adopting common definitions of waiting times for the full patient journey.
- Provinces should publish consistent data on achievement of waiting-time targets at least quarterly.
- Provinces should review current administrative structures to identify the potential for savings—and more effective priority setting—from centralization of functions.
- Provinces should commit to a phased introduction of activity-based funding to drive improvements in efficiency in the hospital and other sectors. Provinces should review comparative cost data (published by the Canadian Institute for Health Information) to ensure that provincial payment rates are set at efficient levels.
- Provinces should model workforce planning requirements for the larger health professions at least every five years. Health Canada should support the provinces in a national approach to modelling workforce planning requirements for the smaller health professions. Planning for Canada and the larger provinces should aim for net self-sufficiency.
- Provinces should examine non-traditional sources for recruitment of entry-level workers, including providing on-the-job training opportunities.
- Provinces should establish formalized mechanisms for planning and cooperation between universities and colleges and the major health providers.
- Provinces should continue to contract with the private sector for service delivery. Contracts for private delivery should incorporate marginal pricing and robust measures of quality.
- Provinces should leverage the power of existing data collections through linked data sets that are available for use in research and system evaluation.
- Provinces should fund the infrastructure to establish pilot sites for facility-level rapid-learning health system evaluation.
- Provinces should build on the nationally agreed performance measures to develop clear performance measures for health and health care in the province and for every separately incorporated health-delivery agency in the province.
- Provinces should develop strategies for public reporting of performance of delivery agencies and processes to build accountability for performance of agencies.
- Provinces should establish guidelines for minimum standards of public participation.
- Provincial governments should develop governance structures to facilitate broadly based, whole-of-government approaches to address factors influencing health.

Political leadership and commitment is crucial. It can be built by stakeholders and supported by managers. Although evidence-based policy is the new vogue, the analytical capacity to support it is often absent in government organizations (Howlett, 2009). However, the experience of the impact on policy of health technology assessment (see Chapter 5) suggests that there may be lessons from that field more broadly (Whicher, Chalkidou, Dhalla, Levin, & Tunis, 2009). Lomas and Brown (2009) have also identified a range of strategies to promote the use of evidence in health policy processes. But evidence-informed policies are not enough: a review of the fate of commissions of inquiry in Quebec showed that political factors can overwhelm good evidence (Contandropoulos & Brouselle, 2010). As Fox and Markel (2010, p. 1750) point out, "the plural of anecdote is policy." Those of us committed to policy reform need to be prepared for that.

The list of proposals and provincial actions in Table 10.1 might at first seem daunting, but each one is severable, often requiring work with different players or groups of stakeholders. In this sense a provincial action plan for system transformation could start at any point, with any proposal, with the starting point determined by a "readiness assessment." As mentioned above, change can start with baby steps.

But large-scale system transformation should not be completely off the agenda; after all, the proposals in this book are linked and have common themes. Best et al. (2010) have identified characteristics of successful large-scale transformation, starting with leadership: "Large system transformation in health care systems requires both top-down leadership that is passionately committed to change, as well as distributed leadership and engagement of personnel at all levels of the system" (p. 4). Other requirements for successful change noted by Best et al. (2010) include measurement, recognition of the historical context, and engagement with professionals (especially physicians) and consumers.

## Public participation and involvement

The fourth lever used in United Kingdom public sector reform was "users shaping services from below" (Prime Minister's Strategy Unit, 2006). Patients' rights have been an increasingly dominant theme of health policy over the last decade (Toth, 2010), and were identified by Best et al. (2010) as one of the five preconditions for successful system change.

Most recently, the Canadian Medical Association (2010) has proposed a Charter of Patients Rights as part of its reform proposals, and so too has a Minister's Advisory Committee on Health (2010) in Alberta. Academic papers on public participation address a range of issues:

1. *Why* is public participation in health policy of interest?
2. *Who* constitutes "the public"?

3. *What* health policy issues are canvassed in exercises of public participation?
4. *Which* techniques of public participation are studied?
5. *Where to from here* in public participation practice and research? (Tenbensel, 2010)

Many health delivery agencies have developed formal mechanisms for user or public involvement, although there is sometimes a lack of clarity about "the why" and "the who": whether the involvement opportunities are for "lay experts" who contribute based on their experience with health care, or for ordinary citizens (Martin, 2008). Public participation is not a unidimensional construct, and "the what" can include participation in all stages of program design and delivery from assessing needs to evaluating programs. Robust methods for evaluating the extent of public participation are now available (Draper, Hewitt, & Rifkin, 2010).

The International Association of Public Participation identifies five points on a public participation spectrum—inform, consult, involve, collaborate, empower—each point representing a different goal and involving a different implicit commitment to participants.[136] Different techniques are appropriate at different points of the spectrum (Creighton, 2005).

Patient empowerment, which is further up the spectrum than simple participation, has shown to be effective in improving health (Wallerstein, 2006). Despite this, there is no consensus in the academic literature on when public participation is appropriate (Mitton, Smith, Peacock, Evoy, & Abelson, 2009), possibly because the extent of participation (and the consequent appropriate techniques) is still perceived as largely a value choice. Public expectations, though, are for increasing opportunities to participate.

Public participation can occur at all levels of an organization, from formal organization-wide advisory committees to enhancement initiatives in individual services. *Delivery agencies should review their current approaches to public participation to assess whether they are addressing contemporary needs. Provinces should establish guidelines for minimum standards of public participation. Health Canada should convene a conference every three years to share delivery agencies' experiences with public participation.*

## Conclusion

This book has attempted to walk a fine line about how much change is necessary in health care in Canada. My view is that the overall policy settings are sound. The broad institutional framework is appropriate. Medicare is sustainable.

Change is necessary though. Population needs are changing over time and the health system must respond. This requires dozens of small adjustments at every level of the system: in clinical practice, by service delivery agencies such as hospitals, by provinces, by the federal government.

Those changes should build on the current strengths of the system, including the commitment and skills of people who work in the system and the huge reservoir of good will toward Medicare and health care in general in the community. But policy leaders and the general public need to recognize that the Canadian health system is not perfect. It is expensive in international terms. There are significant disparities. There are opportunities to do better in terms of life expectancies.

Change will be uncomfortable and there will be vocal critics protecting their status quo. Part of the change process will thus require being clear about who wins and who loses from any change so the views of the vocal can be assessed in context.

Tommy Douglas, the father of Medicare, reflected on the continuing need for health system reform at a conference in Ottawa in 1979. He noted that those involved in the original development of what became Medicare saw health system reform as a two-phase process with removing financial barriers being the first phase.

> Phase number two would be the much more difficult one. That was to alter our delivery system, so as to reduce costs, so as to place the emphasis on preventive medicine.… What we have to apply ourselves to now is that we have not yet grappled seriously with the second phase. We must now move increasingly to group practice … to make possible the practice of preventive medicine. Only in that way are we going to be able to keep the costs from becoming so excessive that the public will decide that Medicare is not in the best interests of the people of this country. (Douglas, 1979)

This book is about the second phase. It is about addressing needs that go beyond removing financial barriers. The second phase is necessary to keep health costs from being excessive. As Douglas pointed out, this phase will be difficult.

Throughout this book I've identified opportunities for improvement: some to improve efficiency, some access, some quality. Many of these are similar to recommendations made by others in the past: good ideas that have never been implemented. As Sullivan and Baranek (2002, p. 92) point out, "Most health care analysts and decision makers know what needs to be done and the best ways of achieving it." But implementation gets stymied from the "strife of interests"[137] that characterizes the health sector.

Implementation of new ideas is a hard slog, requiring vision, perseverance, and occasionally funding to facilitate the transition from the old to the new. But in my view it is the obligation of leaders to pursue these incremental changes, rather than throwing up their hands, saying it is all too difficult, and pretending there is no other choice but to adopt radical solutions such as privatized funding.

Given the track record of previous proposals, I know that not all of my proposals will be implemented. But the point of this contribution is to demonstrate that there are feasible changes that together will lead to a Canadian health system that is better positioned to meet current and future needs. A system that is consistent with the values that Canadians hold dear and have endorsed time and time again.

## Postscript (January 2012)

As this book was in the final stage of production, the federal government announced its 2014 Accord decision: 6 percent indexation through to 2016–17, with indexation in line with economic growth thereafter. The proposal was non-negotiable and to come with no strings attached. At the time of writing it is unclear whether there will be any written Accord or other statement signed with the provinces to document this, or whether there will be any joint commitment to pursue health care reform. The recommendations throughout this book about the content of the next Accord may thus be off the formal agenda. However, most of the recommendations in this book are not couched in that way and are still relevant. Even the ones focused on the 2014 Accord have continuing relevance as they address real contemporary issues, issues that will not go away with the federal announcement.

The new indexation provisions will place further pressure on provinces to contain costs. The recommendations in this book to the provinces listed in Table 10.1 thus have increased importance: they provide a way, consistent with the values held by Canadians, for provinces to address the additional challenges the new funding formula brings.

# APPENDIX

# FULL LIST OF POLICY RECOMMENDATIONS CONTAINED IN THIS BOOK

### On improving the public's health

- Consistent with the language of the 2004 First Ministers' statement, a pan-Canadian set of goals and targets for improving the health status of *all* Canadians should be developed by governments to cover the period of the next Accord. Once developed, each province should publish its own goals and targets, consistent with the national goals and targets, and report progress against those targets. Regional health authorities and other organizations should also consider the development of goals and targets consistent with the national goals and targets.

- Provinces and regional health authorities should publish regular reports on disparities in health outcomes.

- The Canadian Health Services Research Foundation should be tasked to review the evidence on the use of tax incentives to promote public health objectives, including the case for a targeted tax on sugar-sweetened beverages.

- Federal, provincial, and territorial leaders should commission an evaluation of the existing Canadian Strategy for Cancer Control and recommend how it might be enhanced to reduce smoking prevalence further.

- The Public Health Agency of Canada should commission a comprehensive economic evaluation of potential policies to improve health status (and its distribution) in Canada and ensure that the evaluation is updated every five years.

- The *Canada Health Act* should be amended to require "cost-effective preventive interventions" as part of insured services.

## On building the primary care foundation

- Health Canada jointly with the Conference of Deputy Ministers should convene a regular conference of provincial telephone advisory services to facilitate exchange of information about new services being implemented by telehealth providers across the country.
- Provinces should develop (or continue) programs to support quality-improvement initiatives in primary care—including family practices—aimed at addressing access.
- Provinces should review home care provision to ensure optimal use is being made of remote monitoring and other technologies that can enable and support community dwelling for at-risk people, including those with chronic diseases; where indicated provinces should invest in the infrastructure to implement new remote-monitoring models.
- The federal government should make available a personal health record platform for all Canadians; all provinces should work with Health Canada to facilitate populating the personal health record with provincially held data.
- The federal government, as part of the next Accord, should provide support to the provinces to enable the transformation of primary care. Provinces should consider integration of home care and other community services with new (transformed) multidisciplinary primary care practices.
- Provinces should review their primary care funding arrangements to ensure that funding streams are adequate to allow collaborative team practice.
- Provinces should review the structure of their payment arrangements for family physicians to ensure that these arrangements incorporate the right set of incentives for care of patients with chronic illnesses including the ability to support self-management, community-level interventions, and the optimal division of labour.
- Provinces should consider shifting responsibility for physician services budgets to regional health authorities.
- Provinces should give consideration to pilot programs of primary care budget holding and the alternative policy direction, development of integrated care organizations.

## On ensuring access to (the right) drugs, technologies, and innovations

- Prescription pharmaceuticals should be an insured service under Medicare. Federal, provincial, and territorial leaders should, as soon as possible, commission an independent study of the most practicable way of introducing prescription pharmaceuticals as an insured service under Medicare, and consider that report as part of the negotiations of the 2014 Accord renewal.

- The Canadian Institutes of Health Research should assess on a regular basis the impact of funded health research.
- Each academic health sciences centre should identify its relative strengths and publish its research priorities, level of research investment, and outcomes of research at least every three years.
- Academic health sciences centres should review their teaching practices to identify the extent to which they reflect and encourage inefficient practice. Academic health sciences centres should document, and publicize to their students, how the centres' research leads to improvements in efficiency in the delivery of care.
- Academic health sciences centres should plan to become the centres of rapid-learning health care systems.
- Federal, provincial, and territorial leaders should task and fund the Canadian Agency for Drugs and Technologies in Health to establish the capacity (and advisory processes) to undertake a rolling program of reviews of potentially obsolescent health technologies. Provincial health technology assessment agencies should develop complementary programs to evaluate disinvestment opportunities.

## On supporting seniors' care needs

- Provinces should incorporate self-managed care as an integral part of their home care systems.
- Seniors' health care, whether provided in the home or in a residential aged-care facility, should become an insured service under the *Canada Health Act*.
- Provinces should review their home care provision to ensure that the full benefit of strong home care provision is available throughout the province.
- Provinces should explore introduction of public reporting of quality of nursing home care.
- Provinces should review their regulatory frameworks for seniors' care to ensure that they incorporate a best-practice mix of instruments. As part of this, the Canadian Health Services Research Foundation should be tasked and funded to support a review of current practice in Canada and experience internationally.
- Provinces should encourage and facilitate development of a broader range of accommodation options for seniors including an intermediate residential care option, assisted living.

- Provinces should ensure efficiency of residential care provision, and equity among providers, through the introduction of activity-based funding for residential care.

## On getting hospitals and acute care right

- The Canadian Patient Safety Institute should develop guidelines for incident reporting systems and mechanisms to share lessons from incident reviews across Canada.
- The Canadian Institute for Health Information and provinces should develop feedback strategies to provide hospitals with information on hospital-acquired diagnoses.
- The Canadian Institute for Health Information should be tasked and funded to expand publication of data on variation in utilization rates across Canada.
- Provinces should fund health-care-provider access to a suite of patient decision aids and should encourage hospitals to use patient decision aids as part of their routine consent procedures for preference-sensitive conditions.
- Provinces should create and fund clinical networks to provide leadership in sharing good practice to improve access, quality, and sustainability of health care.
- The comprehensiveness criterion in the *Canada Health Act* should be amended to include an obligation on provinces to cover effective services, with a requirement that effectiveness be determined in a transparent way.
- Provinces should request clinical networks (when established) to review differences in intra- and interprovincial utilization rates. Networks should be invited to develop and/or update priority-setting criteria.
- The Canadian Institutes of Health Research should be tasked and funded to establish a research program to evaluate provincial (and regional) initiatives to address variation in utilization rates.
- Provinces should commit to adopting common definitions of waiting times for the full patient journey.
- Federal, provincial, and territorial leaders should agree on waiting-time targets for a broad range of services. Provinces should publish consistent data on achievement of these targets at least quarterly, and the Canadian Institute for Health Information should collate and publish these data at least annually.
- The 2014 Accord should expand the penalty provisions in the *Canada Health Act* to incorporate penalties for consistent failure to reach agreed waiting-time targets.

- Provinces should review current administrative structures to identify the potential for savings—and more effective priority setting—from centralization of functions.
- Provinces should commit to a phased introduction of activity-based funding to drive improvements in efficiency in the hospital and other sectors. Provinces should review comparative cost data (published by the Canadian Institute for Health Information) to ensure that provincial payment rates are set at efficient levels.
- Introduction of activity-based funding should be accompanied by measures to promote improved quality, whether through pay for performance, non-payment for poor performance, or increased surveillance and accountability.
- As part of activity-based funding implementation, provinces should consider introduction of incentives on hospitals to reduce waiting times.

## On ensuring the right skill set is available

- Health services delivery organizations should implement or continue systematic programs for care model redesign to facilitate all professionals' working to their top scope of practice. The Canadian Institutes of Health Research should be tasked and funded to establish a funding stream to evaluate implementation of care model redesign and associated role redesign.
- Health Canada (or the Conference of Deputy Ministers) should convene a conference of provincial health ministries and regulatory bodies to share leading practice in regulation of basic and advanced nursing roles.
- Provinces should model workforce planning requirements for the larger health professions at least every five years. Health Canada should support the provinces in a national approach to modelling workforce planning requirements for the smaller health professions. Planning for Canada and the larger provinces should aim for net self-sufficiency.
- The Canadian Institutes of Health Research should be tasked and funded to create research training initiatives in professions where there is a shortage of faculty.
- The federal government should explore with the provinces interest in developing a national income-contingent loan program for health professions, coupled with loan forgiveness programs for employment in hard-to-recruit areas.
- Provinces should examine non-traditional sources for recruitment of entry-level workers, including providing on-the-job training opportunities.

- Provinces should establish formal mechanisms for planning and cooperation between universities and colleges and the major health providers. Health providers should consider mechanisms at the local level for the same purpose.
- Federal, provincial, and territorial leaders should review current health professional regulatory structures to facilitate further interprovincial migration and provision of health care across provincial borders.

## On getting there from here

- The public administration criterion in the *Canada Health Act* should be rephrased as being about public governance and public insurance.
- Canadian health care is best served by a continuation of tax financing. Expansion of private insurance into core areas should not be pursued.
- Provinces should continue to contract with the private sector for service delivery. Contracts for private delivery should incorporate marginal pricing and robust measures of quality.
- The 2014 Accord should be for a ten-year period, and should guarantee funding increases to the provinces of 6 percent per annum.
- The new Accord should reaffirm the principles of the *Canada Health Act*, modifying the comprehensiveness criterion to focus on effective care determined in a transparent way and the public administration criterion to focus on public insurance.
- The 2014 Accord should provide that, if and when a national pharmaceutical program is introduced, federal funding to the provinces should be reduced to offset any provincial savings that accrue due to substitution of new federal spending for past provincial spending.
- Federal, provincial, and territorial leaders should agree on a (limited) set of performance measures to be published annually.
- The Canadian Institute for Health Information should be tasked to develop a national health data dictionary that would incorporate the data elements necessary for derivation of the agreed performance measures.
- The 2014 Accord should make any transfer payments to a province conditional on the province's contributing to a national data set the data necessary to derive the agreed performance measures using the nationally mandated data definitions.
- Provinces should leverage the power of existing data collections through linked data sets that are available for use in research and system evaluation.
- Federal, provincial, and territorial leaders should commit to achieving access to national linked data by 2020. The Canadian Health Services Research Foundation should be tasked to develop a road map for the most effective and efficient way to develop national access.

- Provinces should fund the infrastructure to establish pilot sites for facility-level rapid-learning health system evaluation. The Canadian Institutes of Health Research should be tasked and funded to establish a funding stream for rapid-learning health system evaluation.
- The 2014 Accord should incorporate a commitment to conduct mid-term and end-of-term independent reviews of health care in Canada to inform the 2024 renegotiations.
- Federal and provincial governments should develop governance structures to facilitate broadly based, whole-of-government approaches to address factors influencing health.
- Provinces should build on the nationally agreed performance measures to develop clear performance measures for health and health care in the province and for every separately incorporated health-delivery agency in the province.
- Provinces should develop strategies for public reporting of performance of delivery agencies, and processes to build accountability for performance of agencies.
- The 2014 Accord should make provision for a broadly based Federal/Provincial/Territorial Advisory Committee, consisting of people able to represent consumer views as well as people drawn from the health sector. The committee should be tasked with identifying issues and making recommendations to deputy ministers or ministers. The functioning and worth of the committee should be reviewed two years after its first meeting.
- Delivery agencies should review their current approaches to public participation to assess whether they are addressing contemporary needs. Provinces should establish guidelines for minimum standards of public participation. Health Canada should convene a conference every three years to share delivery agencies' experiences with public participation.

# NOTES

[1] Alberta Health Services, for example, is the largest employer in Alberta and the largest employer in practically every town or city in the province. It is also the fourth- or fifth-largest employer in Canada.

[2] Discussed further in Chapter 4.

[3] In Alberta, for example, we aimed to reduce the number of beds in acute hospitals occupied by patients who had completed their acute episode but could not get accommodation in a residential care facility. We opened additional nursing home beds, which are cheaper to run and involve a more home-like environment for the people affected—an example of efficiency and quality going hand in hand. To the extent some of the beds were kept open, access to acute care improved as well.

[4] Although primarily designed to educate the public, Healthydebate.ca, a project of the Keenan Research Centre, Li Ka Shing Knowledge Institute of St. Michael's Hospital, is an important and useful resource for the media.

[5] Boychuk (2008a, p. 193) is more skeptical about the extent to which these values are embedded: "The belief that the Canadian system of health care is firmly rooted in some innate, distinctively Canadian set of values does not fit with the historical development of public health insurance in Canada. The degree to which public support of public health insurance has been politically constructed is marked.... Public support can be politically deconstructed or reconstructed."

[6] Although residents of most provinces do not pay an insurance premium, and coverage is mandatory and universal, Canadian Medicare is still legislatively described as an "insurance" scheme, hence the use of the term in this chapter.

[7] As mentioned above, the first four of these five criteria are based on criteria in the *Medical Care Act*.

[8] "Private practice, public payment" in Naylor's (1986) terms.

[9] Dental coverage is limited to certain types of dental surgery.

[10] For hospitals, the phrasing is "if the services are medically necessary for the purpose of maintaining health, preventing disease or diagnosing or treating an injury, illness or disability"; for physician services, "any medically required services."

[11] Although negotiations with physicians result in a fee schedule of individual items, each of which is supposed to be reasonable in terms of the service provided, in effect the negotiations are about the quantum of funds to flow to the medical profession, to be divided up among physicians, so the negotiations are essentially about physician income (Barer, Evans, & Labelle, 1988). Physician average remuneration increased with the introduction of universal coverage and is significantly above the average income of other Canadians (Duffin, 2011).

[12] Although even here many surgeons who do cosmetic surgery may also practice as plastic surgeons providing insured services (burns, hand surgery).

[13] A second type of imbalance is "vertical fiscal imbalance" caused by the different levels of government (federal vs. provincial) having either a different capacity to raise tax revenue or, at least, a different capacity relative to their responsibilities. "One's view of what constitutes an appropriate vertical fiscal gap for Canada will depend on what one perceives to be the appropriate role of the state in general and that of the federal government in particular" (Lazar, St-Hilaire, & Tremblay, 2004, p. 157).

[14] The sample frame varies from year to year: every third year it is a random sample of the over 18 population; in other years samples are drawn from people with chronic illness or from providers; see Duckett and Kempton (2012).

[15] "Avalanche" is Barer, Evans, and Hertzman's (1995) term; "tsunami" seems to be the contemporary preference (e.g., Maioni, 2010).

[16] In Canada, over the period 1921 to 2001, an increase of 1 percent in life expectancy led to an increase of 9.3 percent in GDP and 6.7 percent in GDP per capita.

[17] Aghion, Howitt, and Murtin (2010), however, suggest that the relationship is quite complex: it is the change in life expectancy before age 40 that drives improvement in GDP per capita. Change in life expectancy at age 80 has no statistically significant impact on GDP per capita (which in turn belies the apocalyptic fears), but during the intermediate years change in life expectancy may reduce GDP per capita.

[18] It may also be the case that older people are not treated as intensively as younger people (Moïse & Jacobzone, 2003).

[19] Seshamani and Gray (2004) show that the effect can be seen up to ten years before death.

[20] The work of Thorpe and his colleagues (Thorpe, 2005; Thorpe, Florence, Howard, & Joski, 2005; Thorpe, Florence, & Joski, 2004) suggests that treated prevalence is the more important factor, accounting for about 67 percent of expenditure growth. This conclusion has been challenged by Roehrig and Rousseau (2011) who argue that cost per case dominates, accounting for 75 percent of expenditure growth.

[21] Increased obesity is a significant issue worldwide (Finucane et al., 2011).

[22] In the case of people over 65, this depends on the extent to which retirement or health care use and income support is paid through social insurance (or other prepayment mechanisms such as retirement funds) or on a public funding "pay as you go" basis.

[23] This list is adapted from one initially developed in Alberta Health Services. I acknowledge the comments and improvements made by former colleagues to my original phrasing. The current wording is mine, not that of Alberta Health Services.

[24] International comparative data in this section are extracted from OECD (2010b) Health Data.

[25] Although a reduction in death rate in one disease will lead to changes in others (Olshansky, 1988), the assumption here, for simplicity, is that the causes are all independent and a reduction in one does not lead to an increase in the other.

[26] Note that PYLL75 will always be greater than PYLL70.

[27] This is roughly the same result as from the international analysis, which used a different set of selected causes and so is not directly comparable.

[28] CANSIM Table 101-0121.

[29] There has been academic dispute about this; see Subramanian and Kawachi (2004) and Macinko, Shi, Starfield, & Wulu (2003).

[30] Retrieved 15 August 2001 from http://www.phac-aspc.gc.ca/hgc-osc/pdf/goals-e.pdf

[31] See Terris (1984, p. 327) who enthusiastically described the report as "one of the great achievements of the modern public health movement ... the first official government statement of policy that recognized the beginning of a new era in public health, the era of the second epidemiologic revolution which, just as the first epidemiologic revolution conquered infectious diseases, will, during the next few decades, achieve the conquest of some of the most important non-infectious diseases." Glouberman and Millar (2003, p. 388) were more temperate, merely saying that the report "marked the first stage of health promotion in Canada."

[32] The first and most famous, held in Ottawa in 1986, issued the Ottawa Charter, but subsequent conferences have also issued statements; see the World Health Organization's "Global Conferences on Health Promotion" retrieved from http://www.who.int/healthpromotion/conferences/en/

[33] See, for example, *CDC Healthy Disparities and Inequalities Report – United States, 2011*, retrieved 23 August 2011 from http://www.cdc.gov/mmwr/pdf/other/su6001.pdf

[34] Unfortunately, when I attempted to use this to open up debate about disparities in Edmonton, the media response was to narrow the issue to one of more "urgent care," albeit in a needy neighbourhood; see Simons (2010).

[35] I use the term "sugar-sweetened" rather than "nutritively sweetened" for ease of public explanation and debate, even though the source of increased energy in drinks is essentially irrelevant. Any legislation should focus on the broader sweeteners.

[36] This issue is discussed further in Chapter 5.

[37] See the Cost-Effectiveness Analysis Registry website, retrieved 15 August 2011 from https://research.tufts-nemc.org/cear4/default.aspx

[38] For the purposes of these comparisons, A$1 is approximately the same as CDN$1. The Australian population is about two thirds of Canada's—22 million versus 34 million.

[39] Preventive interventions delivered by physicians are, of course, currently within the scope of the Act.

[40] Data from Statistics Canada, CANSIM Table 105-0502. These data include all physician visits.

[41] Data from the Canadian Institute for Health Information, Quickstats, retrieved 15 August 2011 from http://www.cihi.ca/CIHI-ext-portal/internet/en/ApplicationFull/types+of+care/hospital+care/CIHI021682

[42] The results, though, are vulnerable to the level of aggregation (Wright & Ricketts, 2011).

[43] In addition, hospital emergency departments are not able to provide continuity of care, probably contributing to this increase in use because of re-presentations.

[44] A point recognized by Tommy Douglas; see Tommy Douglas – 1979 S.O.S. Medicare Conference, retrieved 11 August 2011 from http://www.youtube.com/watch?v=V1A0vrz36Sc [Video file].

[45] See the case studies collated by the Health Council of Canada (2009a).

[46] Barrett, Kuzawa, McDade, and Armelagos (1998) suggest that the third epoch is about the re-emergence of infectious diseases; Susser and Susser (1996) identify three eras in epidemiology (and associated preventive approaches): sanitary statistics (first half of the nineteenth century), infectious disease epidemiology (up to the mid-twentieth century), and chronic disease epidemiology (from then).

[47] Resources and documentation of the Wagner approach are available on the Improving Chronic Illness Care website, retrieved 15 August 2011 from http://www.improvingchroniccare.org

[48] Evaluations of self-management strategies also show some positive impacts but are more equivocal (see Chodosh et al., 2005; Foster, Taylor, Eldridge, Ramsay, & Griffiths, 2007). My support for self-management is informed by the Wagner, systematic approach.

[49] In addition to not being consistent with the current gender profile of family practice!

[50] For a menu of community-based services for which there is good evidence of impact, see these documents produced for the National Health Service, retrieved 12 August 2011 from http://www.dh.gov.uk/en/Publicationsandstatistics/Publications/PublicationsPolicyAndGuidance/DH_124178

[51] A common metric used in quality improvement initiatives is the "third next available appointment."

[52] These services are, of course, relevant for the whole population, not just those with chronic diseases. The Canadian Radio-television and Telecommunications Commission has allocated the number 811 for these services, and this number is now used in British Columbia, Nova Scotia, and Quebec. Other provinces use idiosyncratic numbers.

[53] For example, for studies on heart failure see Clark et al. (2007); Clarke, Shah, and Sharma (2011); and Polisena et al. (2010); for stroke, see Johansson and Wild (2010, 2011). For studies on remote monitoring more generally see Barlow, Singh, Bayer, and Curry (2007); Bensink, Hailey, and Wootton (2006, 2007); DelliFraine and Dansky (2008); Ekeland, Bowes, and Flottorp (2010); Gaikwad and Warren (2009); García-Lizana and Sarría-Santamera (2007); Klersy, De Silvestri, Gabutti, Regoli, and Auricchio (2009); Paré, Jaana, and Sicotte (2007); Paré, Moqadem, Pineau, and St-Hilaire (2010); Samoocha, Bruinvels, Elbers, Anema, and van der Beek (2010). For economic analyses, see Klersy et al. (2011); Polisena, Coyle, Coyle, and McGill (2009); and Seto (2008).

[54] Alberta's Netcare system, which provides electronic access to diagnostic imaging and laboratory results, is one success (Mayes & Mador, 2010).

[55] The exception being the need for common communication standards (see, for example, the Health Level Seven International website, retrieved 15 August 2011 from http://www.hl7.org/

[56] Hughes, Joshi, and Wareham (2008) in fact proffered this as a definition of Medicine 2.0 but noted that it also applied to Health 2.0. Van De Belt, Engelen, Berben, and Schoonhoven (2010) found 46 unique definitions of Health 2.0/Medicine 2.0.

[57] The published data mostly report trends for all physicians and by specialty (family practice not separately identified), but it appears from the most recent data from the national physician database that family physicians have similar take-up of

alternative remuneration models as specialists although there are significant inter-provincial differences; see Canadian Institute for Health Information (2008a, Table 2).

[58] Data in this section are drawn from the Canadian Medical Association's 2007 National Physician Survey, retrieved 15 August 2011 from http://www.nationalphysiciansurvey.ca/nps/2007_Survey/Results/ENG/National/pdf/Final%20Posted%20National%20Level%20Table%20Set/NPS.2007.National.Results.Binder.Final.pdf. There are significant differences between rural and urban settings in the structure of family practice and in the scope of work of family physicians (Wong & Stewart, 2010).

[59] Task assigning role relationship and task initiating role relationship are Jaques's (2006) terms. Jaques has attempted to describe clearly many managerial relation-ships. See also Rowbottom (1973).

[60] A common term used for this type of concept is "medical home." There are a host of different definitions of this term, as well as different lists of defining elements (Vest et al., 2010).

[61] The term "social animation," which I first came across in Quebec, provides an apt description of what is required (Doré, 1985).

[62] Some of the adverse effects of the different remuneration arrangements may be mitigated by self-selection of physicians into different remuneration structures (Devlin & Sarma, 2008), although physicians remunerated on other than fee-for-service contracts still see fewer patients (Sarma, Devlin, & Hogg, 2010).

[63] For example, Bruni, Nobilio, and Ugolini (2009) show reduced hospitalizations for hyperglycaemic emergencies in an Italian setting; and Scott, Schurer, Jensen, and Sivey (2009) found that an incentive program increased by 20 percent the probability of an HbA1c test being ordered as part of diabetes care.

[64] This was my experience in Alberta. Alberta Health Services released a discussion paper on primary care reform that was well received in consultations with physician and other stakeholders, but discussion of its implications for the fee structure was deferred in the negotiation process of the 2011 trilateral agreement (Jacobs, Moffatt, Rapoport, & Bell, 2010).

[65] Sometimes called "meso-level" structures (Epping-Jordan, Pruitt, Bengoa, & Wagner, 2004); Alberta's "primary care networks" are an example.

[66] The proposals are contentious (see Pollock & Price, 2011; Walshe & Ham, 2011).

[67] This approach was canvassed in a discussion paper on primary care models released for consultations with stakeholders by Alberta Health Services in February 2010; see Jacobs et al. (2010).

[68] Data in this section are drawn from Canadian Institute for Health Information (2010a).

[69] See also an earlier paper by one of the coauthors (Hollis, 2009) that incorporated similar suggestions for provincial reform in Alberta.

[70] The Australian National Health and Medical Research Council has started a similar process; see Kingwell et al. (2006).

[71] I prefer the term "research transformation" to research translation, especially for bringing research into implemented policy: the latter term de-emphasizes the magnitude of what needs to be done to make research policy implementable (see Gibson, 2003).

[72] Clinical research here includes research into population health (the fourth pillar) and into clinical services (third pillar).

[73] In my recent experience, discharges from one major hospital were delayed on Thursdays because curriculum timetabling meant students and junior doctors were not available to do the tasks normally assigned to them.

[74] Although in an interesting note, the OECD (2010a, p. 153) reported that "presently, marketing activities account for a larger share of industry costs than does pharmaceutical R&D."

[75] An allusion to a famous Australian children's story about a self-regenerating pudding, a.k.a. dessert (Lindsay, 1918).

[76] Institute of Medicine web page, retrieved 15 August 2011 from http://www.iom.edu/Reports/2011/~/media/Files/Activity%20Files/Quality/VSRT/Core%20Documents/LearningHealthSystem.pdf

[77] In addition to the publication and interpretation bias exhibited in studies funded by the pharmaceutical industry (Golder & Loke, 2008; Lexchin et al., 2003; Neumann, Sandberg, Bell, Stone, & Chapman, 2000).

[78] This latter weakness can be overcome by using "intent to treat" as the basis for analysis.

[79] The reality is that different thresholds appear to exist for different conditions (Martin et al., 2008).

[80] Quality-adjusted life years (QALYs) are a standard interval-level metric for measuring health outcomes. Essentially QALYs discount life years gained from a treatment by whether they are years of full health or associated with some impairment and pain (McKie, Richardson, Singer, & Kuhse, 1998).

[81] Peer reviewed articles can also be subtly "hyped" (Bubela & Caulfield, 2004).

[82] I faced one public example of this in my time at Alberta Health Services; with media mobilized to condemn our failure to take over funding immediately, the manufacturer's "generosity" ceased.

[83] I stimulated introduction of such a process as chair of a board of a group of hospitals in Melbourne, where new technologies were assessed in terms of their financial impact on the organization.

[84] Statistics Canada (2011), *Residential Care Facilities 2008/2009*. This is the source of information in this section. The term "residential care facilities" as used by Statistics Canada refers to "facilities with four beds or more that are funded, licensed or approved by provincial/territorial departments of health and/or social services." It does not include lodges and other facilities that do not provide care.

[85] Data on these patients are taken from Canadian Institute for Health Information (2009a), *Alternate Level of Care in Canada*.

[86] Data in this paragraph are from a multivariate analysis by Trottier, Martel, Houle, Berthelot, and Légaré (2000).

[87] The choice of terms is primarily influenced by Statistics Canada, which uses residential care facility as its term for residential services for the aged and for those with mental illness.

[88] The same is true of mental health care.

[89] Inter-RAI is an international network of researchers based at the University of Michigan who have an interest in developing standardized assessment instruments for use in non-acute care settings; see www.interrai.org, retrieved 13 August 2011.

[90] Although this and many other proposals in this chapter are phrased as applying to the seniors population, many would apply with equal force to people with disabilities.

[91] Retrieved 15 August 2011 from http://www.medicare.gov/NHCompare/Include/DataSection/Questions/ProximitySearch.asp

[92] This provides another argument for the expansion of assisted living facilities, which generally allow residents more autonomy.

[93] Their delightfully named article proposes moving beyond the problem of "comparing apples, oranges, and broccoli."

[94] To be fair, Shapiro and Tate (1995) also examined subcategories but found no differences.

[95] Canadian Institute for Health Information, "Resource Utilization Groups III (RUG-III)," retrieved 15 August 2011 from http://www.cihi.ca/CIHI-ext- portal/internet/en/document/standards+and+data+submission/standards/case+mix/casemix_rug. See Hirdes, Sinclair, King, Tuttle, and McKinley (2003) for an account of the implementation of Resource Utilization Groups in Ontario.

[96] This is the Alberta version: http://www.hqca.ca/assets/pdf/User%20Guide%20R290506.pdf, retrieved 12 August 2011 from the Health Quality Council of Alberta website; see Raleigh and Foot (2010) for a comparison of lists of a range or organizations.

[97] For instance, what is not preventable today might be preventable with new knowledge, and what is not preventable in one setting might be in another with different access to diagnostic technologies.

[98] A common metaphor for this "web of causation" is a block of Swiss cheese (Perneger, 2005): essentially, a mistake can only occur (get through the Swiss cheese) if all the holes (causative factors) are in alignment. The Swiss cheese metaphor leads to the idea that erecting more barriers will reduce safety incidents, although as McNutt and Hasler (2011) point out, adding complexity also adds to risk.

[99] Many health care organizations offer patient safety training to staff, elements of which emphasize a just and trusting culture. At one point in my career, I was lucky enough to serve with a Minister for Health who undertook such training and so understood these issues better (Stephen Robertson, Queensland Health Minister 2005–09).

[100] The Australian-developed Classification of Hospital Acquired Diagnoses (CHADx) is the first such classification. See http://www.health.gov.au/internet/safety/publishing.nsf/Content/8368C7AFFADDFA44CA2575AB008380B7/$File/35566-CHADx.pdf, retrieved 15 August 2011.

[101] There is good work at the provincial level: the Institute for Clinical Evaluative Sciences has undertaken work on practice variations in Ontario (see, for example, Goel et al., 1996), as has the Manitoba Centre for Health Policy (Fransoo et al., 2009).

[102] This is the 1990 reported "extremal quotient" (rate in highest area vs. rate in lowest area). The extremal quotient declined over time; in 1984 it was 8.2.

[103] For example, patient decision aids are available commercially at Health Dialog, http://www.healthdialog.com, retrieved 15 August 2011.

[104] The graphical portrayal is described as an example of a "Stacey diagram" (Stacey, 2007, 2010).

[105] Standard sets of investigations to order for particular types of patients.

[106] Items to be added to the Medicare fee schedule in Australia are assessed by an independent Medical Services Advisory Committee (MSAC), which advises the federal minister who makes the final decision about listing. The committee is required to take cost-effectiveness into account in its considerations; see the MSAC "About Us" web page, retrieved 27 August 2011 from http://www.msac.gov.au/internet/msac/publishing.nsf/Content/about-us-lp-1

[107] Roemer's original phrasing was softer, referring to the "central importance of the supply of beds in determining the hospital utilization rate" (Roemer, 1961, p. 42).

[108] Retrieved 15 August 2011 from the Western Canada Waiting List Project website, http://www.wcwl.org.

[109] Computerized utilization management software is also available to facilitate this; see, for example, the medworxx.com web page, retrieved 6 September 2011 from http://www.medworxx.com/Site_Published/medworxx_com/prod_UMS.aspx

[110] See also the caveats in the Canadian Institute for Health Information's (2010) "Wait Times Tables – A Comparison by Province, 2010," retrieved 15 August 2011 from http://secure.cihi.ca/cihiweb/products/wait_times_tables_2010_e.pdf

[111] The others are revenue-increasing strategies.

[112] Data extracted from CIHI Health Indicator reports, retrieved 20 August 2011 from http://secure.cihi.ca/hireports/search.jspa?language=en&healthIndicatorSelection=ACSC

[113] The importance of thinking about provision of acute care beyond hospital walls is why the title of this chapter refers to "hospitals and acute care."

[114] For family medicine the list is: Don't do imaging for low back pain within the first six weeks unless identified red flags are present; Don't routinely prescribe antibiotics for acute mild to moderate sinusitis unless designated symptoms last for 7 or more days or symptoms worsen after initial clinical improvement; Don't order annual ECGs or any other cardiac screening for asymptomatic, low-risk patients; Don't perform Pap tests on patients younger than 21 years or in women status post-hysterectomy for benign disease; Don't use dual energy x-ray absorptiometry screening for osteoporosis in women under age 65 years or men under 70 years with no risk factors.

[115] In terms of this latter point, this occurred in Alberta where post-budget supplements were allocated to the larger regions outside the funding formula almost every year.

[116] The term "activity-based funding" is preferred as it is a more accurate description.

[117] A recent RAND review identified 90 separate payment reform proposals, grouped into 11 categories (Schneider, Hussey, & Schnyer, 2011).

[118] Royal College of Physicians and Surgeons of Canada, "About CanMEDS" web page, retrieved 15 August 2011 from http://rcpsc.medical.org/canmeds/

[119] While I was chief executive officer of Alberta Health Services, the College and Association of Registered Nurses in Alberta mounted a campaign against care model redesign at the University of Alberta Hospital. The union, United Nurses of Alberta, has a more legitimate role in protecting the interests of their members and also initially opposed the project. The project, nevertheless, was implemented and anecdotal evidence suggests that considerable productivity gains have been achieved, supported by staff. Previous quality-improvement initiatives at the University of Alberta Hospital have also been contested (Reshef & Lam, 1999).

[120] Of course, workforce planning is not alone with a track record of poor forecasting (Gardner, 2011).

[121] Statistics Canada, "Population Estimates and Projections" (2010), retrieved 16 August 2011 from http://www40.statcan.ca/l01/cst01/demo23a-eng.htm

[122] This quinquennial approach should cover, at least, nursing and medicine.

[123] Statistics Canada, "Population Estimates and Projections" (2010), retrieved 16 August 2011 from http://www40.statcan.ca/l01/cst01/demo23a-eng.htm

[124] Government of Alberta, "Health Care Aide Programs in Alberta" (updated 2010), retrieved 16 August 2011 from http://www.health.alberta.ca/professionals/health-care-aide-programs.html

[125] The national Coordinating Council on Entry to Practice Credentials has established a process to assess professions' bids for upgrading credentials required for entry into practice (see Health Canada, "Entry-to-Practice Credentials Assessment Process" [2010], retrieved 27 August 2011 from http://www.hc-sc.gc.ca/hcs-sss/hhr-rhs/committee-comite-hdhr-ssrh/practice-practique-eng.php), but this does not appear to have been an effective use of health sector power (see S. Lewis, "Degrees of Separation: Do Higher Credentials Make Health Care Better?" [Web log post, 5 November 2009], retrieved 27 August 2011 from http://longwoodessays.blogspot.com/2009/11/degrees-of-separation-do-higher.html

[126] http://www.ait-aci.ca/index_en.htm, retrieved 16 August 2011.

[127] The *ex post* reality of the English implementation was far different from the prior aspirations, with the creation of a purchaser function appearing to drive little change (Le Grand et al., 1998; Lewis, Smith, & Harrison, 2009).

[128] http://wildrosealliance.ca/policy-text/health-care/

[129] Similar results were found following changes to pharmaceutical copayments in Australia: use of both "essential" and "discretionary" drugs reduced, although prescription of essential drugs returned to pre-change levels over a two-year period (McManus et al., 1996).

[130] My experience in Alberta revealed very poorly written contracts (see Dranove et al., 2009, for one example) that resembled a "provider entitlement program," to use Cooper and Vladeck's (2000) phrase.

[131] For example, compare the data available on the two national health information bodies' websites, the Canadian Institute for Health Information at www.Canadian Institute for Health Information.ca and the Australian Institute of Health and Welfare at www.aihw.gov.au, retrieved 16 August 2011.

[132] Manitoba Centre for Health Policy website, retrieved 16 August 2011 from http://umanitoba.ca/faculties/medicine/units/community_health_sciences/departmental_units/mchp/

[133] Institute for Clinical Evaluative Sciences website, retrieved 16 August 2011 from http://www.ices.on.ca/

[134] Institute of Medicine, "The Learning Health System Series," retrieved 16 August 2011 from http://www.iom.edu/Reports/2011/~/media/Files/Activity%20Files/Quality/VSRT/Core%20Documents/LearningHealthSystem.pdf

[135] See Smith and Pell (2003).

[136] "IAP2 Spectrum of Public Participation" (2007), retrieved 16 August 2011 from http://www.iap2.org/associations/4748/files/IAP2%20Spectrum_vertical.pdf

[137] From Ambrose Bierce's *Devil's Dictionary*: "Politics: A strife of interests masquerading as a contest of principles. The conduct of public affairs for private advantage," brought to my attention in the title of a book about health care in Australia by Sid Sax (1984).

# REFERENCES

Aaron, H. J., & Ginsburg, P. B. (2009). Is health spending excessive? If so, what can we do about it? *Health Affairs, 28*(5), 1260-1275.

Abbott, A. (1988). *The system of professions: An essay on the division of expert labor.* Chicago: University of Chicago Press.

Abdullah, A., Wolfe, R., Stoelwinder, J. U., de Courten, M., Stevenson, C., Walls, H. L., et al. (2011). The number of years lived with obesity and the risk of all-cause and cause-specific mortality. *International Journal of Epidemiology, 40*(4), 985-996.

Abelson, J., Miller, F. A., & Giacomini, M. (2009). What does it mean to trust a health system? A qualitative study of Canadian health care values. *Health Policy, 91*(1), 63-70.

Adams, C. P., & Brantner, V. V. (2010). Spending on new drug development. *Health Economics, 19*(2), 130-141.

Adams, S. A. (2011). Sourcing the crowd for health services improvement: The reflexive patient and "share-your-experience" websites. *Social Science & Medicine, 72*(7), 1069-1076.

Addicott, R., McGivern, G., & Ferlie, E. (2006). Networks, organizational learning and knowledge management: NHS Cancer Networks. *Public Money & Management, 26*(2), 87-94.

Addicott, R., McGivern, G., & Ferlie, E. (2007). The distortion of a managerial technique? The case of clinical networks in UK health care. *British Journal of Management, 18*(1), 93-105.

Adler, N. E., & Stewart, J. (2009). Reducing obesity: Motivating action while not blaming the victim. *Milbank Quarterly, 87*(1), 49-70.

Aghion, P., Howitt, P., & Murtin, F. (2010). *The relationship between health and growth: When Lucas meets Nelson-Phelps.* National Bureau of Economic Research Working Paper Series (No. 15813).

Aglukkaq, L. (2011). Minister of Health speech – Canadian Medical Association annual general assembly. 22 August, St. John's. Retrieved 25 August 2011 from http://www.hc-sc.gc.ca/ahc-asc/minist/speeches-discours/_2011/2011_08_22-eng.php

Ahern, J., Jones, M. R., Bakshis, E., & Galea, S. (2008). Revisiting Rose: Comparing the benefits and costs of population-wide and targeted interventions. *Milbank Quarterly, 86*(4), 581-600.

Aiken, L. H., Cheung, R. B., & Olds, D. M. (2009). Education policy initiatives to address the nurse shortage in the United States. *Health Affairs, 28*(4), w646-w656.

Alberta Health Services. (2009). Engaging the patient in healthcare: An overview of personal health record systems and implications for Alberta. Retrieved 15 August 2011 from http://www.albertahealthservices.ca/org/ahs-org-ehr.pdf

Alberta Ombudsman. (2009). *Prescription for fairness: Out of country health services (Special report)*. Edmonton, AB: Author.

Albrecht, D. (1998). Community health centres in Canada. *Leadership in Health Services, 11*(1), 5-10.

Aldana, S. G. (2001). Financial impact of health promotion programs: A comprehensive review of the literature. *American Journal of Health Promotion, 15*(5), 296-320.

Al-Delaimy, W. K., Pierce, J. P., Messer, K., White, M. M., Trinidad, D. R., & Gilpin, E. A. (2007). The California Tobacco Control Program's effect on adult smokers: (2) Daily cigarette consumption levels. *Tobacco Control, 16*(2), 91-95.

Allan, J. D., & Aldebron, J. (2008). A systematic assessment of strategies to address the nursing faculty shortage. *Nursing Outlook, 56*(6), 286-297.

Allard, M., Jelovac, I., & Léger, P. T. (2011). Treatment and referral decisions under different physician payment mechanisms. *Journal of Health Economics, 30*(5), 880-893.

Allareddy, V., Ward, M. M., Allareddy, V., & Konety, B. R. (2010). Effect of meeting leapfrog volume thresholds on complication rates following complex surgical procedures. *Annals of Surgery, 251*(2), 377-383.

Allin, S. (2006). *Equity in the use of health services in Canada* (No. LSE Health Working Paper 3/2006). London: London School of Economics and Political Science.

Allin, S. (2008). Does equity in healthcare use vary across Canadian provinces? *Healthcare Policy, 3*(4), 83-99.

Altman, S., Tompkins, C. P., Eilat, E., & Glavin, M. P. V. (2003). Escalating health care spending: Is it desirable or inevitable? *Health Affairs* (Web exclusive), w3-1–w3-14.

Alvaro, C., Jackson, L. A., Kirk, S., McHugh, T. L., Hughes, J., Chircop, A., et al. (2011). Moving Canadian governmental policies beyond a focus on individual lifestyle: Some insights from complexity and critical theories. *Health Promotion International, 26*(1), 91-99.

Anand, S. S., & Yusuf, S. (2011). Stemming the global tsunami of cardiovascular disease. *The Lancet, 377*(9765), 529-532.

Anderson, G. F., Reinhardt, U. E., Hussey, P. S., & Petrosyan, V. (2003). It's the prices, stupid. Why the United States is so different from other countries. *Health Affairs, 22*(3), 89-105.

Anderson, L. M., Shinn, C., Fullilove, M. T., Scrimshaw, S. C., Fielding, J. E., Normand, J., et al. (2003). The effectiveness of early childhood development programs: A systematic review. *American Journal of Preventive Medicine, 24*(3), 32-46.

Andrews, G. (2000). Meeting the unmet need with disease management. In G. Andrews & S. Anderson (Eds.), *Unmet need in psychiatry*. Cambridge: Cambridge University Press.

Angell, M. (2004). Excess in the pharmaceutical industry. *Canadian Medical Association Journal, 171*(12), 1451-1453.

Annemans, L., Boeckxstaens, P., Borgermans, L., De Smedt, D., Duchesnes, C., Heyrman, J., et al. (2009). *Advantages, disadvantages and feasibility of the introduction of 'Pay for Quality' programmes in Belgium*. Brussels: Federaal Kenniscentrum voor de gezondheiszorg, Centre fédéral d'expertise des soins de santé, Belgian Health Care Knowledge Centre.

Ansari, Z. (2007). The concept and usefulness of ambulatory care sensitive conditions as indicators of qualty and access to primary health care. *Australian Journal of Primary Health, 13*(3), 91-110.

Ansari, Z., Laditka, J. N., & Laditka, S. B. (2006). Access to health care and hospitalization for ambulatory care sensitive conditions. *Medical Care Research & Review, 63*(6), 719-741.

Antonazzo, E., Scott, A., Skatun, D., & Elliott, R. F. (2003). The labour market for nursing: A review of the labour supply literature. *Health Economics, 12*(6), 465-478.

Appleby, J. (2011). What's happening to waiting times? *BMJ, 342*, 526-529.

Arah, O., & Westert, G. (2005). Correlates of health and healthcare performance: Applying the Canadian health indicators framework at the provincial-territorial level. *BMC Health Services Research, 5*(76).

Arellano, L. E., Willett, J. M., & Borry, P. (2011). International survey on attitudes toward ethics in health technology assessment: An exploratory study. *International Journal of Technology Assessment in Health Care, 27*(1), 50-54.

Armitage, G., Suter, E., Oelke, N., & Adair, C. (2009). Health systems integration: State of the evidence. *International Journal of Integrated Care, 17*(9).

Armstrong, B. (1990). Morbidity and mortality in Australia: How much is preventable. In J. McNeil, R. King, G. Jennings, & J. Powles (Eds.), *A textbook of preventive medicine*. Melbourne: Edward Arnold.

Armstrong, P. W. (2009). What do we know? Limitations of the two methods most commonly used to estimate the length of the prospective wait. *Health Services Management Research, 22*(1), 8-16.

Armstrong, P. W. (2010a). One question, two answers: Do the two most commonly used methods of sampling describe the length of the prospective wait for admission to hospital? *Health Services Management Research, 23*(1), 18-24.

Armstrong, P. W. (2010b). Spotting the pantomime villain: Do the usual approaches correctly indicate when waiting times got shorter? *Health Services Management Research, 23*(3), 103-115.

Armstrong, P., & Banerjee, A. (2009). Challenging questions: Designing long-term residential care with women in mind. In P. Armstrong et al. (Eds.), *A place to call home: Long-term care in Canada*. Halifax: Fernwood.

Arrow, K. J. (1963). Uncertainty and the welfare economics of medical care. *American Economic Review, 53*, 941-973.

Audit Commission. (2011). *Reducing spending on low clinical value treatments*. London: Author.

Averill, R. F., Goldfield, N. I., Hughes, J. S., Eisenhandler, J., & Vertrees, J. C. (2009). Developing a prospective payment system based on episodes of care. *Journal of Ambulatory Care Management, 32*(3), 241-251.

Averill, R. F., Hughes, J. S., & Goldfield, N. I. (2011). Paying for outcomes, not performance: Lessons from the Medicare inpatient prospective payment system. *Joint Commission Journal on Quality and Patient Safety, 37*(4), 184-192.

Averill, R. F., Vertrees, J., McCullough, E., Hughes, J., & Goldfield, N. (2006). Redesigning Medicare inpatient PPS to adjust payment for post-admission Complications. *Health Care Financing Review, 27*(3), 83-93.

Aylin, P., Bottle, A., & Majeed, A. (2007). Pay-for-performance: Will the latest payment trend improve care? *Journal of the American Medical Association, 297*(February 21), 740-744.

Bach, P. B., Mirkin, J. N., & Luke, J. J. (2011). Episode-based payment for cancer care: A proposed pilot for Medicare. *Health Affairs, 30*(3), 500-509.

Bachrach, L. L. (1980). Is the least restrictive environment always the best? Sociological and semantic implications. *Hospital & Community Psychiatry, 31*(2), 97-103.

Bahl, V., Thompson, M. A., Kau, T.-Y., Hu, H. M., & Campbell, D. A. J. (2008). Do the AHRQ patient safety indicators flag conditions that are present at the time of hospital admission? *Medical Care, 46*(5), 516-522.

Baicker, K., & Goldman, D. (2011). Patient cost-sharing and healthcare spending growth. *Journal of Economic Perspectives, 25*(2), 47-68.

Baker, G. R., Denis, J.-L., Pomey, M.-P., & Macintosh-Murray, A. (2010). *Effective governance for quality and patient safety in Canadian healthcare organizations: A report to the Canadian Health Services Research Foundation and the Canadian Patient Safety Institute.* Ottawa: Canadian Health Services Research Foundation and Canadian Patient Safety Institute.

Baker, G. R., Norton, P. G., Flintoft, V., Blais, R., Brown, A., Cox, J., et al. (2004). The Canadian adverse events study: The incidence of adverse events among hospital patients in Canada. *Canadian Medical Association Journal, 170*(11), 1678-1686.

Balch, G. I. (1980). The stick, the carrot, and other strategies: A theoretical analysis of governmental intervention. *Law & Policy, 2*(1), 35-60.

Baliunas, D., Patra, J., Rehm, J., Popova, S., Kaiserman, M., & Taylor, B. (2007). Smoking-attributable mortality and expected years of life lost in Canada 2002: Conclusions for prevention and policy. *Chronic Diseases in Canada, 27*(4), 154-162.

Ballinger, G., Zhang, J., Hicks, V. A., & Gyorfi-Dyke, C. (2003). *Monitoring the feasibility of reporting home care estimates in national health expenditures.* Ottawa: Canadian Institute for Health Information.

Banta, H. D., & de Wit, G. A. (2008). Public health services and cost-effectiveness analysis. *Annual Review of Public Health, 29*(1), 383-397.

Banting, K. (2005). Community federalism and fiscal arrangements in Canada. In H. Lazar (Ed.), *Canadian fiscal arrangements: What works, what might work better.* Montreal and Kingston: McGill-Queen's University Press.

Barber, P., & Lopez-Valcarcel, B. (2010). Forecasting the need for medical specialists in Spain: Application of a system dynamics model. *Human Resources for Health, 8*(24).

Barbera, L., Taylor, C., & Dudgeon, D. (2010). Why do patients with cancer visit the emergency department near the end of life? *Canadian Medical Association Journal, 182*(6), 563-568.

Barer, M. L., Bhatla, V., Evans, R. G., & Stoddard, G. L. (1993). *Who are the zombie masters, and what do they want?* Health Policy Research Unit, HPRU 93:13D. Vancouver: University of British Columbia.

Barer, M. L., Evans, R. G., & Hertzman, C. (1995). Avalanche or glacier? health care and the demographic rhetoric. *Canadian Journal on Aging, 14*(2), 193-224.

Barer, M. L., Evans, R. G., & Labelle, R. J. (1988). Fee controls as cost control: Tales from the frozen north. *Milbank Quarterly, 66*(1), 1-64.

Barer, M. L., Lomas, J., & Sanmartin, C. (1996). Re-minding our Ps and Qs: Medical cost controls in Canada. *Health Affairs, 15*(2), 216-234.

Barlow, J., Singh, D., Bayer, S., & Curry, R. (2007). A systematic review of the benefits of home telecare for frail elderly people and those with long-term conditions. *Journal of Telemedicine and Telecare, 13*(4), 172-179.

Barnas, K. (2011). ThedaCare's business performance system: Sustaining continuous daily improvement through hospital management in a lean environment. *Joint Commission Journal on Quality and Patient Safety, 37*(9), 387-399.

Barnoya, J., & Glantz, S. (2004). Association of the California Tobacco Control Program with declines in lung cancer incidence. *Cancer Causes and Control, 15*(7), 689-695.

Barr, N. (2001). *The welfare state as piggy bank information, risk, uncertainty, and the role of the state.* Oxford: Oxford University Press.

Barrett, R., Kuzawa, C. W., McDade, T., & Armelagos, G. J. (1998). Emerging and re-emerging infectious diseases: The third epidemiologic transition. *Annual Review of Anthropology, 27*(1), 247-271.

Barry, C. L., Brescoll, V. L., Brownell, K. D., & Schlesinger, M. (2009). Obesity metaphors: How beliefs about the causes of obesity affect support for public policy. *Milbank Quarterly, 87*(1), 7-47.

Battersby, M., Von Korff, M., Schaeffer, J., Davis, C., Ludman, E., Greene, S. M., et al. (2010). Twelve evidence-based principles for implementing self-management support in primary care. *Joint Commission Journal on Quality and Patient Safety, 36*(12), 561-570.

Baumol, W. J. (1967). Macroeconomics of unbalanced growth: The anatomy of urban crisis. *American Economic Review, 57*(3), 415-426.

Bayer, A., & Tadd, W. (2000). Unjustified exclusion of elderly people from studies submitted to research ethics committee for approval: Descriptive study. *British Medical Journal, 321*(October), 992-993.

Beach, M., Gary, T., Price, E., Robinson, K., Gozu, A., Palacio, A., et al. (2006). Improving health care quality for racial/ethnic minorities: A systematic review of the best evidence regarding provider and organisation interventions. *BMC Public Health, 6*(104), 1-11.

Beaulieu, M.-D., Rioux, M., Rocher, G., Samson, L., & Boucher, L. (2008). Family practice: Professional identity in transition. A case study of family medicine in Canada. *Social Science & Medicine, 67*(7), 1153-1163.

Beckfield, J., & Krieger, N. (2009). Epi + demos + cracy: Linking political systems and priorities to the magnitude of health inequities – Evidence, gaps, and a research agenda. *Epidemiologic Reviews, 31*(1), 152-177.

Béland, F. (2007). Arithmetic failure and the myth of the unsustainability of universal health insurance. *Canadian Medical Association Journal, 177*(1), 54-56.

Béland, F., Bergman, H., Lebel, P., Clarfield, A. M., Tousignant, P., Contandriopoulos, A.-P., et al. (2006). A system of integrated care for older persons with disabilities in Canada: Results from a randomized controlled trial. *The Journals of Gerontology Series A: Biological Sciences and Medical Sciences, 61*(4), 367-373.

Bélanger, E., & Rodríguez, C. (2008). More than the sum of its parts? A qualitative research synthesis on multi-disciplinary primary care teams. *Journal of Interprofessional Care, 22*(6), 587-597.

Bell, C. M., Brener, S. S., Gunraj, N., Huo, C., Bierman, A. S., Scales, D. C., Bajcar, J., Zwarenstein, M., & Urbach, D. R. (2011). Association of ICU or hospital admission with unintentional discontinuation of medications for chronic diseases. *JAMA, 306*(8), 840-847.

Benach, J., Malmusi, D., Yasui, Y., Martínez, J., & Muntaner, C. (2011). Beyond Rose's strategies: A typology of scenarios of policy impact on population health and health inequalities. *International Journal of Health Services, 41*(1), 1-9.

Benning, A., Dixon-Woods, M., Nwulu, U., Ghaleb, M., Dawson, J., Barber, N., et al. (2011). Multiple component patient safety intervention in English hospitals: Controlled evaluation of second phase. *BMJ, 342.*

Benning, A., Ghaleb, M., Suokas, A., Dixon-Woods, M., Dawson, J., Barber, N., et al. (2011). Large scale organisational intervention to improve patient safety in four UK hospitals: Mixed method evaluation. *BMJ, 342.*

Bensink, M., Hailey, D., & Wootton, R. (2006). A systematic review of successes and failures in home telehealth: Preliminary results. *Journal of Telemedince and Telecare, 12*(Suppl. 3), 8-16.

Bensink, M., Hailey, D., & Wootton, R. (2007). A systematic review of successes and failures in home telehealth. Part 2: Final quality rating results. *Journal of Telemedicine and Telecare, 13*(Suppl. 3), 10-14.

Bentley, T. G. K., Effros, R. M., Palar, K., & Keeler, E. B. (2008). Waste in the U.S. health care system: A conceptual framework. *Milbank Quarterly, 86*(4), 629-659.

Berlin, L. E., & Sechrist, K. R. (2002). The shortage of doctorally prepared nursing faculty: A dire situation. *Nursing Outlook, 50*(2), 50-56.

Berta, W., Laporte, A., Zarnett, D., Valdmanis, V., & Anderson, G. (2006). A pan-Canadian perspective on institutional long-term care. *Health Policy, 79*(2), 175-194.

Berwick, D. M. (2009). Measuring physicians' quality and performance. *JAMA, 302*(22), 2485-2486.

Best, A., Saul, J., Carroll, S., Bitz, J., Higgins, C., Greenhalgh, T., et al. (2010). *Knowledge and action for system transformation (KAST): A systematic realist review and evidence synthesis of the role of government policy in coordinating large system transformation.* Vancouver, BC: Centre for Clinical Epidemiology and Evaluation, Vancouver Coastal Health Research Institute.

Bhattacharya, J., & Sood, N. (2011). Who pays for obesity? *Journal of Economic Perspectives, 25*(1), 139-158.

Bickerton, J. (2010). Deconstructing the new federalism. *Canadian Political Science Review, 4*(2-3), 56-72.

Bigelow, J. H., Fonkych, K., Fung, C., & Wang, J. (2005). *Analysis of healthcare interventions that change patient trajectories.* Santa Monica: RAND Corporation.

Biorn, E., Hagen, T. P., Iversen, T., & Magnussen, J. (2010). How different are hospitals' responses to a financial reform? The impact on efficiency of activity-based financing. *Health Care Management Science, 13*(1), 1-16.

Birch, S., & Gafni, A. (2005). Achievements and challenges of Medicare in Canada: Are we there yet? Are we on course? *International Journal of Health Services, 35*(3), 443-463.

Birch, S., & Gafni, A. (2006). The biggest bang for the buck or bigger bucks for the bang: The fallacy of the cost-effectiveness threshold. *Journal of Health Services Research and Policy, 11*(1), 46-51.

Birch, S., Kephart, G., Tomblin-Murphy, G., O'Brien-Pallas, L., Alder, R., & MacKenzie, A. (2008). Health human resources planning and the production of health: A needs-based analytical framework. *Canadian Public Policy, 33*(1), 1-16.

Birkmeyer, J. D., Hamby, L. S., Birkmeyer, C. M., Decker, M. V., Karon, N. M., & Dow, R. W. (2001). Is unplanned return to the operating room a useful quality indicator in general surgery? *Archives of Surgery, 136*(4), 405-411.

Black, N. (2001). Evidence-based policy: Proceed with care. *BMJ, 323*(4 August), 275-279.

Blackmore, C. C., Mecklenburg, R. S., & Kaplan, G. S. (2011). At Virginia Mason, collaboration among providers, employers, and health plans to transform care cut costs and improved quality. *Health Affairs, 30*(9), 1680-1687.

Bleich, S. N., Cutler, D., Murray, C., & Adams, A. (2008). Why is the developed world obese? *Annual Review of Public Health, 29*(1), 273-295.

Blishen, B. R. (1969). *Doctors and doctrines: The ideology of medical care in Canada.* Toronto, ON: University of Toronto Press.

Bliss, M. (2010). *Critical condition: A historian's prognosis on Canada's aging health-care system.* Toronto, ON: C.D. Howe Institute.

Block, L. M., Claffey, C., Korow, M. K., & McCaffrey, R. (2005). The value of mentorship within nursing organizations. *Nursing Forum, 40*(4), 134-140.

Blomqvist, Å. (2008). Social health insurance: Government funding of health care. In M. Lu & E. Jonsson (Eds.), *Financing health care new ideas for a changing society.* Weinheim: Wiley-VCH.

Bloor, K., & Maynard, A. (2003). *Planning human resources in health care: Towards an economic approach. An international comparative review.* Ottawa: Canadian Health Services Research Foundation.

Blustein, J., Borden, W. B., & Valentine, M. (2010). Hospital performance, the local economy, and the local workforce: Findings from a US national longitudinal study. *PLoS Medicine, 7*(6), e1000297.

Bodenheimer, T., Wagner, E. H., & Grumbach, K. (2002a). Improving primary care for patients with chronic illness. *JAMA, 288*(14), 1775-1779.

Bodenheimer, T., Wagner, E. H., & Grumbach, K. (2002b). Improving primary care for patients with chronic illness: The chronic care model Part 2. *JAMA, 288*(15), 1909-1914.

Bohm, P. (1987). *Social efficiency: A concise introduction to welfare economics.* London: Macmillan Education.

Bohmer, R., & Sepucha, K. R. (2005). Shared decision making. Case number: 9-604-001. Harvard Business School.

Boismenu, G., & Graefe, P. (2004). The new federal tool belt: Attempts to rebuild social policy leadership. *Canadian Public Policy, 30*(1), 71-89.

Boockvar, K., Brodie, H. D., & Lachs, M. (2000). Nursing assistants detect behaviour changes in nursing home residents that precede acute illness: Development and validation of an illness warning instrument. *Journal of the American Geriatrics Society, 48*(9), 1086-1091.

Boon, H., Verhoef, M., O'Hara, D., & Findlay, B. (2004). From parallel practice to integrative health care: A conceptual framework. *BMC Health Services Research, 4*, 15-19.

Boonen, L. H. H. M., & Schut, F. T. (2011). Preferred providers and the credible commitment problem in health insurance: First experiences with the implementation of managed competition in the Dutch health care system. *Health Economics, Policy and Law, 6*(2), 219-235.

Bordignon, M., & Turati, G. (2009). Bailing out expectations and public health expenditure. *Journal of Health Economics, 28*(2), 305-321.

Bosch, M., Faber, M. J., Cruijsberg, J., Voerman, G. E., Leatherman, S., Grol, R. P. T. M., et al. (2009). Effectiveness of patient care teams and the role of clinical expertise and coordination. *Medical Care Research and Review, 66*(Suppl. 6), 5S-35S.

Bower, A. G. (2005). *The diffusion and value of healthcare information technology.* Santa Monica: RAND Corporation.

Boychuk, G. W. (2008a). *National health insurance in the United States and Canada: Race, territory, and the roots of difference.* Washington, DC: Georgetown University Press.

Boychuk, G. W. (2008b). *The regulation of private health insurance in Alberta under the Canada Health Act: A comparative cross-provincial perspective.* Calgary, AB: School of Public Policy, University of Calgary.

Boychuk Duchscher, J. E., & Cowin, L. S. (2004). The experience of marginalization in new nursing graduates. *Nursing Outlook, 52*(6), 289-296.

Braën, A. (2002). *Health and the distribution of powers in Canada.* Saskatoon, SK: Commission on the Future of Health Care in Canada.

Braën, A. (2004). Health and the distribution of powers in Canada. In T. A. McIntosh, P.-G. Forest, & G. P. Marchildon (Eds.), *The governance of health care in Canada. Romanow papers, Vol. 3.* Toronto, ON: University of Toronto Press.

Braithwaite, J., Makkai, T., & Braithwaite, V. A. (2007). *Regulating aged care: Ritualism and the new pyramid.* Cheltenham, UK, and Northampton, MA: Edward Elgar.

Braithwaite, R. S., Meltzer, D. O., King, J. T. J., Leslie, D., & Roberts, M. S. (2008). What does the value of modern medicine say about the $50,000 per quality-adjusted life-year decision rule? *Medical Care, 46*(4), 349-356.

Braithwaite, J., Travaglia, J., & Corbett, A. (2011). Can questions of the privatization and corporatization, and the autonomy and accountability of public hospitals, ever be resolved? *Health Care Analysis, 19*(2), 133-153.

Braithwaite, J., Westbrook, J., & Iedema, R. (2005). Restructuring as gratification. *Journal of the Royal Society of Medicine, 98*(12), 542-544.

Branch, L. G. (2001). Community long-term care services. *The Gerontologist, 41*(3), 305-306.

Brandeis, L. D. (1914). *Other people's money: And how the bankers use it.* New York: Frederick A. Stokes Co.

Braveman, P., Egerter, S., & Williams, D. R. (2011). The social determinants of health: Coming of age. *Annual Review of Public Health, 32*(1), 381-398.

Bravo, G., De Wals, P., Dubois, M. F., & Charpentier, M. (1999). Correlates of care quality in long-term care facilities: A multilevel analysis. *The Journals of Gerontology. Series B, Psychological Sciences and Social Sciences, 54*(3), 180-188.

Bravo, G., Raiche, M., Dubois, M., & Hebert, R. (2008). Assessing the impact of integrated delivery systems: Practical advice from three experiments conducted in Quebec. *Journal of Integrated Care, 16*, 9-18.

Braybrooke, D., & Lindblom, C. E. (1970). *A strategy of decision: Policy evaluation as a social process.* New York: Free Press.

Brennan, T. A., Gawande, A., Thomas, E., & Studdert, D. (2005). Accidental deaths, saved lives, and improved quality. *New England Journal of Medicine, 353*(13), 1405-1409.

Brennan, N., Mattick, K., & Ellis, T. (2010). The map of medicine: A review of evidence for its impact on healthcare. *Health Information & Libraries Journal, 28*(2), 93-100.

Breslow, L. (2004). The third revolution in health. *Annual Review of Public Health, 25*(1).

Breslow, L. (2006). Health measurement in the third era of health. *American Journal of Public Health, 96*(1), 17-19.

Breton, E., Richard, L., Gagnon, F., Jacques, M., & Bergeron, P. (2006). Fighting a tobacco-tax rollback: A political analysis of the 1994 cigarette contraband crisis in Canada. *Journal of Public Health Policy, 27*(1), 77-99.

Breyer, F., Costa-Font, J., & Felder, S. (2011). Ageing, health, and health care. *Oxford Review of Economic Policy, 26*(4), 674-690.

Briner, R. B., Denyer, D., & Rousseau, D. M. (2009). Evidence-based management: Concept cleanup time? *Academy of Management Perspectives, 23*(4), 19-32.

Brook, R. H., & Lohr, K. N. (1986). Will we need to ration effective health care? *Issues in Science and Technology, 3*(1), 68-77.

Brook, R. H., & Lohr, K. N. (1991). *Will we need to ration effective health care?* Santa Monica, CA: RAND.

Broome, J. (1999). *Ethics out of economics.* Cambridge: University of Cambridge.

Brousselle, A., & Lessard, C. (2011). Economic evaluation to inform health care decision-making: Promise, pitfalls and a proposal for an alternative path. *Social Science & Medicine, 72*(6), 832-839.

Brownell, K. D., Farley, T., Willett, W. C., Popkin, B. M., Chaloupka, F. J., Thompson, J. W., et al. (2009). The public health and economic benefits of taxing sugar-sweetened beverages. *New England Journal of Medicine, 361*(16), 1599-1605.

Brownell, K. D., & Warner, K. E. (2009). The perils of ignoring history: Big tobacco played dirty and millions died. How similar is big food? *Milbank Quarterly, 87*(1), 259-294.

Brownson, R., Haire-Joshu, D., & Luke, D. (2006). Shaping the context of health: A review of environmental and policy approaches in the prevention of chronic diseases. *Annual Review of Public Health, 27*, 341-370.

Brumley, R. D., Enguidanos, S., & Cherin, D. A. (2003). Effectiveness of a home-based palliative care program for end-of-life. *Journal of Palliative Medicine, 6*(5), 715-724.

Bruni, R., Laupacis, A., Levinson, W., & Martin, D. (2010). Public views on a wait time management initiative: A matter of communication. *BMC Health Services Research, 10*(228).

Bruni, M. L., Nobilio, L., & Ugolini, C. (2009). Economic incentives in general practice: The impact of pay-for-participation and pay-for-compliance programs on diabetes care. *Health Policy, 90*(2-3), 140-148.

Bryant, R. (2007). Contradictions in the concept of professional culpability. *Health Care Analysis, 15*(2), 137-152.

Bryant, T., Raphael, D., Schrecker, T., & Labonte, R. (2011). Canada: A land of missed opportunity for addressing the social determinants of health. *Health Policy, 101*(1), 44-58.

Bubela, T. M., & Caulfield, T. A. (2004). Do the print media "hype" genetic research? A comparison of newspaper stories and peer-reviewed research papers. *Canadian Medical Association Journal, 170*(9), 1399-1407.

Buchan, J., & Dal Poz, M. R. (2002). Skill mix in the health care workforce: Reviewing the evidence. *Bulletin of the World Health Organization, 80*(7), 575-580.

Buchan, J., & O'May, F. (2000). Determining skill mix: Practical guidelines for managers and health professionals. *Human Resources Development Journal, 4*(2), 111-118.

Buerhaus, P. I., & Needleman, J. (2000). Policy implications of research on nurse staffing and quality of patient care. *Policy, Politics, & Nursing Practice, 1*(1), 5-15.

Bunn, F., Byrne, G., & Kendall, S. (2004). Telephone consultation and triage: Effects on health care use and patient satisfaction. *Cochrane Database of Systematic Reviews (Online)*(4).

Burge, F., Lawson, B., & Putnam, W. (2011). Assessing the acceptability of quality indicators and linkages to payment in primary care in Nova Scotia. *Healthcare Policy, 6*(4), 72-87.

Busato, A., & von Below, G. (2010). The implementation of DRG-based hospital reimbursement in Switzerland: A population-based perspective. *Health Research Policy and Systems, 8*(31).

Busby, C., & Robson, W. R. B. (2011). *A social insurance model for Pharmacare: Ontario's options for a more sustainable, cost-effective drug program.* Toronto, ON: C.D. Howe Institute.

Buxton, M., & Chambers, J. (2011). What values do the public want their health care systems to use in evaluating technologies? *European Journal of Health Economics, 12*(4), 285-288.

Buxton, M., Hanney, S., & Jones, T. (2004). Estimating the economic value to societies of the impact of health research: A critical review. *Bulletin of the World Health Organization, 82*, 733-739.

Buyx, A. M., Friedrich, D. R., & Schöne-Seifert, B. (2011). Ethics and effectiveness: Rationing healthcare by thresholds of minimum effectiveness. *BMJ, 342*.

Cacace, M., & Schmid, A. (2008). The healthcare systems of the USA and Canada: Forever on divergent paths? *Social Policy & Administration, 42*(4), 396-417.

Callen, J., Georgiou, A., Li, J., & Westbrook, J. I. (2011). The safety implications of missed test results for hospitalised patients: A systematic review. *BMJ Quality & Safety, 20*(2), 194-199.

Callender, C., & Jackson, J. (2005). Does the fear of debt deter students from higher education? *Journal of Social Policy, 34*(4), 509-540.

Callender, C., & Jackson, J. (2008). Does the fear of debt constrain choice of university and subject of study? *Studies in Higher Education, 33*(4), 405-429.

Callinan, J. E., Clarke, A., Doherty, K., & Kelleher, C. (2010). Legislative smoking bans for reducing secondhand smoke exposure, smoking prevalence and tobacco consumption. *Cochrane Database of Systematic Reviews, 14*(4), CD005992.

Campbell, J. L., Richards, S. H., Dickens, A., Greco, M., Narayanan, A., & Brearley, S. (2008). Assessing the professional performance of UK doctors: An evaluation of the utility of the General Medical Council patient and colleague questionnaires. *Quality and Safety in Health Care, 17*(3), 187-193.

Canadian Academy of Health Sciences. Panel on the Return on Investments in Health Research. (2009). *Making an impact: A preferred framework and indicators to measure returns on investment in health research.* Ottawa: Author.

Canadian Centre for Elder Law. (2008). *Discussion paper on assisted living: Past, present and future legal trends in Canada.* Vancouver, BC: Author.

Canadian Healthcare Association. (2010). *Tomorrow's health system, today: A sustainable, high quality publicly funded health system in Canada.* Ottawa: Author.

Canadian Heart Health Strategy and Action Plan. (2009). *Building a heart healthy Canada.* Ottawa: Author.

Canadian Institute for Health Information. (2007a). *Canada's health care providers, 2007.* Ottawa: Author.

Canadian Institute for Health Information. (2007b). *Trends in acute inpatient hospitalizations and day surgery visits in Canada, 1995–1996 to 2005–2006.* Ottawa: Author.

Canadian Institute for Health Information. (2008a). *Physicians in Canada: The status of alternative payment programs, 2005–2006.* Ottawa: Author.

Canadian Institute for Health Information. (2008b). *Reducing gaps in health: A focus on socio-economic status in urban Canada.* Ottawa: Author.

Canadian Institute for Health Information. (2009a). *Alternate level of care in Canada.* Ottawa: Author.

Canadian Institute for Health Information. (2009b). *Health care in Canada 2009: A decade in review.* Ottawa: Author.

Canadian Institute for Health Information. (2010a). *Drug expenditure in Canada 1985 to 2009.* Ottawa: Author.

Canadian Institute for Health Information. (2010b). *National health expenditure trends, 1975 to 2010.* Ottawa: Author.

Canadian Institute for Health Information. (2010c). *Regulated nurses: Canadian trends, 2005 to 2009.* Ottawa: Author.

Canadian Institute for Health Information. (2010d). *Supply, distribution and migration of Canadian physicians in Canada, 2009.* Ottawa: Author.

Canadian Institute for Health Information. (2011). Seniors and the health care system: What is the impact of multiple chronic conditions? Retrieved 15 August 2011 from http://secure.Canadian Institute for Health Information.ca/Canadian Institute for Health Informationweb/products/air-chronic_disease_aib_en.pdf

Canadian Medical Association. (2010). *Health care transformation in Canada: Change that works, care that lasts.* Ottawa: Author.

Canadian Population Health Initiative. (2003). *Obesity in Canada – Identifying policy priorities: Proceedings of a round table.* Ottawa: Canadian Institute for Health Information.

Canadian Public Health Association. (2005). *Public health goals for Canada: A federal, provincial and territorial commitment to Canadians.* Retrieved 15 August 2011 from http://www.phac-aspc.gc.ca/hgc-osc/pdf/BkgrndDisc.pdf

Cantrell, J., & Shelley, D. (2009). Implementing a fax referral program for quitline smoking cessation services in urban health centers: A qualitative study. *BMC Family Practice, 10*(81).

Cardoen, B., Demeulemeester, E., & Beliën, J. (2010). Operating room planning and scheduling: A literature review. *European Journal of Operational Research, 201*(3), 921-932.

Carlson, E. M. (2010). Trends and tips in long-term care: Who benefits – or loses – from expanded choices? *The Elder Law Journal, 18*(1), 191-212.

Carlton, A.-L. (2006). National models for regulation of the health professions. *Law in Context, 23*(2), 21-51.

Carnes, B. A., & Olshansky, S. J. (2001). Heterogeneity and its biodemographic implications for longevity and mortality. *Experimental Gerontology, 36*(3), 419-430.

Carnes, B. A., Olshansky, S. J., & Grahn, D. (1996). Continuing the search for a law of mortality. *Population and Development Review, 22*(2), 231-264.

Carrell, S. E., Hoekstra, M., & West, J. E. (2011). Is poor fitness contagious? Evidence from randomly assigned friends. *Journal of Public Economics, 95*(7-8), 657-663.

Carrière, G. (2006). Seniors' use of home care. *Health Reports, 17*(4), 43-47.

Carrière, Y. (2000). The impact of population aging and hospital days. In J. M. Ellen & G. M. Gutman (Eds.), *The overselling of population aging: Apocalyptic demography, intergenerational challenges, and social policy.* Toronto, ON: Oxford University Press.

Carrin, G., & Hanvoravongchai, P. (2003). Provider payments and patient charges as policy tools for cost-containment: How successful are they in high-income countries? *Human Resources for Health, 1*(6).

Carroll, D. L., Greenwood, R., Lynch, K. E., Sullivan, J. K., Ready, C. H., & Fitzmaurice, J. B. (1997). Barriers and facilitators to the utilization of nursing research. *Clinical Nurse Specialist, 11*(5), 207-212.

Carroll, R., McLean, J., & Walsh, M. K. (2003). Reporting hospital adverse events using The Alfred Hospital's morbidity data. *Australian Health Review, 26*(2), 100-105.

Carter, S., Garside, P., & Black, A. (2003). Multidisciplinary team working, clinical networks, and chambers: Opportunities to work differently in the NHS. *Quality and Safety in Health Care, 12*(Suppl. 1), i25-i28.

Casamatta, G., Cremer, H., & Pestieau, P. (2000). Political sustainability and the design of social insurance. *Journal of Public Economics, 75*(3), 341-364.

Casebeer, A. (2004). Regionalizing Canadian healthcare: The good – the bad – the ugly. *HealthcarePapers, 5*(1), 88-93.

Cash, S. B., & Lacanilao, R. D. (2007). Taxing food to improve health: Economic evidence and arguments. *Agricultural and Resource Economics Review, 36*(2), 174-182.

Castelli, A., Laudicella, M., Street, A., & Ward, P. (2011). Getting out what we put in: Productivity of the English National Health Service. *Health Economics, Policy and Law, 6,* 313-335.

Castelli, A., & Nizalova, O. (2011). *Avoidable mortality: What it means and how it is measured.* York, UK: Centre for Health Economics, University of York.

Castle, N. G. (2003). Searching for and selecting a nursing facility. *Medical Care Research and Review, 60*(2), 223-247.

Castle, N. G. (2009). The Nursing Home Compare report card: Consumers' use and understanding. *Journal of Aging & Social Policy, 21*(2), 187.

Castle, N. G., Engberg, J., & Liu, D. (2007). Have Nursing Home Compare quality measure scores changed over time in response to competition? *Quality and Safety in Health Care, 16*(3), 185-191.

Castle, N. G., & Ferguson, J. C. (2010). What is nursing home quality and how is it measured? *The Gerontologist, 50*(4), 426-442.

Catalano, R., Goldman-Mellor, S., Saxton, K., Margerison-Zilko, C., Subbaraman, M., LeWinn, K., et al. (2011). The health effects of economic decline. *Annual Review of Public Health, 32*(1), 431-450.

Caulfield, T. A. (1996). Wishful thinking: Defining "medically necessary" in Canada. *Health Law Journal, 4,* 63-85.

Chafe, R., Culyer, A., Dobrow, M., Coyte, P. C., Sawka, C., O'Reilly, S., et al. (2011). Access to cancer drugs in Canada: Looking beyond coverage decisions. *Healthcare Policy, 6*(3), 27-35.

Chafe, R., Merali, F., Laupacis, A., Levinson, W., & Martin, D. (2010). Does the public think it is reasonable to wait for more evidence before funding innovative health technologies? The case of PET scanning in Ontario. *International Journal of Technology Assessment in Health Care, 26*(2), 192-197.

Chaiton, M. O., Cohen, J. E., & Frank, J. (2008). Population health and the hardcore smoker: Geoffrey Rose revisited. *Journal of Public Health Policy, 29*(3), 307-318.

Chaix-Couturier, C., Durand-Zaleski, I., Jolly, D., & Durieux, P. (2000). Effects of financial incentives on medical practice: Results from a systematic review of the literature and methodological issues. *International Journal for Quality in Health Care, 12*(2), 133-142.

Chalkidou, K., Tunis, S., Lopert, R., Rochaix, L., Sawicki, P. T., Nasser, M., et al. (2009). Comparative effectiveness research and evidence-based health policy: Experience from four countries. *Milbank Quarterly, 87*(2), 339-367.

Chalkley, M., & McVicar, D. (2008). Choice of contracts in the British National Health Service: An empirical study. *Journal of Health Economics, 27*(5), 1155-1167.

Chan, M., Campo, E., Estève, D., & Fourniols, J.-Y. (2009). Smart homes – Current features and future perspectives. *Maturitas, 64*(2), 90-97.

Chandra, A., & Skinner, J. S. (2011). *Technology growth and expenditure growth in health care.* National Bureau of Economic Research Working Paper Series, No. 16953.

Chang, R.-K. R., Joyce, J. J., Castillo, J., Ceja, J., Quan, P., & Klitzner, T. S. (2004). Parental preference regarding hospitals for children undergoing surgery: A trade-off between travel distance and potential outcome improvement. *Canadian Journal of Cardiology, 20*(9), 877-882.

Chaoulli v. Quebec (Attorney General), [2005] 1 S.C.R. 791, 2005 SCC 35 2005.

Chapman, B., & Ryan, C. (2005). The access implications of income-contingent charges for higher education: Lessons from Australia. *Economics of Education Review, 24*(5), 491-512.

Chappell, N. L., Dlitt, B. H., Hollander, M. J., Miller, J. A., & McWilliam, C. (2004). Comparative costs of home care and residential care. *The Gerontologist, 44*(3), 389-400.

Chappell, N. L., & Hollander, M. J. (2011). An evidence-based policy prescription for an aging population. *HealthcarePapers, 11*(1), 8-18.

Chappell, N. L., McDonald, L., & Stones, M. (2008). *Aging in Contemporary Canada* (2nd ed.). Toronto, ON: Pearson Education Canada.

Charles, C., Lomas, J., & Giacomini, M. (1997). Medical necessity in Canadian health policy: Four meanings and ... a funeral? *Milbank Quarterly, 75*(3), 365-394.

Chen, L. M., Jha, A. K., Guterman, S., Ridgway, A. B., Orav, E. J., & Epstein, A. M. (2010). Hospital cost of care, quality of care, and readmission rates: Penny wise and pound foolish? *Archives of Internal Medicine, 170*(4), 340-346.

Chernichovsky, D. (1995). Health system reforms in industrialized democracies: An emerging paradigm. *Milbank Quarterly, 73*(3), 339-372.

Chiolero, A., & Paccaud, F. (2009). An obesity epidemic booga booga? *The European Journal of Public Health, 19*(6), 568-569.

Chodosh, J., Morton, S. C., Mojica, W., Maglione, M., Suttorp, M. J., Hilton, L., et al. (2005). Meta-analysis: Chronic disease self-management programs for older adults. *Annals of Internal Medicine, 143*(6), 427-438.

Choudhry, S. (2000). Bill 11, the *Canada Health Act* and the Social Union: The need for institutions. *Osgoode Hall Law Journal, 38*(1), 39-76.

Christakis, N. A., & Fowler, J. H. (2007). The spread of obesity in a large social network over 32 years. *New England Journal of Medicine, 357*(4), 370-379.

Christensen, C. M. (1997). *The innovator's dilemma: When new technologies cause great firms to fail.* Cambridge, MA: Harvard University Press.

Christensen, C. M., Grossman, J. H., & Hwang, J. (2009). *The innovator's prescription: A disruptive solution for health care.* New York: McGraw Hill.

Christianson, J. B., Leatherman, S., & Sutherland, K. (2008). Lessons from evaluations of purchaser pay-for-performance programs. *Medical Care Research and Review, 65*(Suppl. 6), 5S-35S.

Church, J., & Smith, N. (2006). Health reform and privatization in Alberta. *Canadian Public Administration, 49*(4), 486-505.

Clark, D. O., Frankel, R. M., Morgan, D. L., Ricketts, G., Bair, M. J., Nyland, K. A., & Callahan, C. M. (2008). The meaning and significance of self-management among socioeconomically vulnerable older adults. *The Journals of Gerontology Series B: Psychological Sciences and Social Sciences, 63,* S312-S319.

Clark, R. A., Inglis, S. C., McAlister, F. A., Cleland, J. G. F., & Stewart, S. (2007). Telemonitoring or structured telephone support programmes for patients with chronic heart failure: Systematic review and meta-analysis. *BMJ, 334*(7600), 942.

Clarke, J. (2006). Consumers, clients or citizens? Politics, policy and practice in the reform of social care. *European Societies, 8*(3), 423-442.

Clarke, S. (2006). The relationship between safety climate and safety performance: A meta-analytic review. *Journal of Occupational Health Psychology, 11*(4), 315-327.

Clarke, M., Shah, A., & Sharma, U. (2011). Systematic review of studies on telemonitoring of patients with congestive heart failure: A meta-analysis. *Journal of Telemedicine and Telecare, 17*(1), 7-14.

Clarke, S. P., & Donaldson, N. E. (2008). Nurse staffing and patient care quality and safety. In R. G. Hughes (Ed.), *Patient safety and quality: An evidence-based handbook for nurses* (Vol. AHRQ Publication No. 08-0043.). Rockville, MD: Agency for Healthcare Research and Quality.

Clavier, C. (2010). Bottom up policy convergence: A sociology of the reception of policy transfer in public health policies in Europe. *Journal of Comparative Policy Analysis: Research and Practice, 12*(5), 451-466.

Cleemput, I., Neyt, M., Thiry, N., De Laet, C., & Leys, M. (2011). Using threshold values for cost per quality-adjusted life-year gained in healthcare decisions. *International Journal of Technology Assessment in Health Care, 27*(1), 71-76.

Clement, F. M., Harris, A., Li, J. J., Yong, K., Lee, K. M., & Manns, B. J. (2009). Using effectiveness and cost-effectiveness to make drug coverage decisions. *JAMA, 302*(13), 1437-1443.

Clements, D., Dault, M., & Priest, A. (2007). Effective teamwork in healthcare: Research and reality. *HealthcarePapers, 7*(Suppl.), 26-34.

Clough, R. (1999). Scandalous care: Interpreting public enquiry reports of scandals in residential care. *Journal of Elder Abuse & Neglect, 10*(1/2), 13.

CMAJ Editorial. (2000). Time for a new Canada Health Act. *Canadian Medical Association Journal, 163*(6), 689.

Coast, J. (1997). Rationing within the NHS should be explicit: The case against. In B. New (Ed.), *Rationing: Talk and action in health care* (pp. 149-156). London: BMJ Publishing.

Coast, J. (2001). Citizens, their agents and health care rationing: An exploratory study using qualitative methods. *Health Economics, 10*(2), 159-174.

Cochrane, C. (2010). Left/right ideology and Canadian politics. *Canadian Journal of Political Science, 43*(3), 583-605.

Cohen, A., Restuccia, J., Shwartz, M., Drake, J., Kang, R., Kralovec, P., et al. (2008). A survey of hospital quality improvement activities. *Medical Care Research and Review, 65*(5), 571-595.

Cohen, J. T., Neumann, P. J., & Weinstein, M. C. (2008). Does preventive care save money? Health economics and the presidential candidates. *New England Journal of Medicine, 358*(7), 661-663.

Cohen, L. (1993). Quebec, Ontario battle over cross-border health care charges. *Canadian Medical Association Journal, 148*(7), 1206-1209.

Cohen, M. D., & Hilligoss, P. B. (2010). The published literature on handoffs in hospitals: Deficiencies identified in an extensive review. *Quality and Safety in Health Care, 19*(6), 493-497.

Cohen-Cole, E., & Fletcher, J. M. (2008). Is obesity contagious? Social networks vs. environmental factors in the obesity epidemic. *Journal of Health Economics, 27*(5), 1382-1387.

Coiera, E. (2011). Why system inertia makes health reform so difficult. *BMJ, 342.*

Cole, B. L., & Fielding, J. E. (2007). Health impact assessment: A tool to help policy makers understand health beyond health care. *Annual Review of Public Health, 28*(1), 393-412.

Coleman, K., Austin, B. T., Brach, C., & Wagner, E. H. (2009). Evidence on the chronic care model in the new millennium. *Health Affairs, 28*(1), 75-85.

Colla, J. B., Bracken, A. C., Kinney, L. M., & Weeks, W. B. (2005). Measuring patient safety climate: A review of surveys. *Quality & Safety in Health Care, 14*(5), 364-366.

College of Family Physicians of Canada. (2009). *Patient-centred primary care in Canada – Bring it on home.* Discussion Paper. Ottawa: Author.

Collier, R. (2008). Activity-based hospital funding: Boon or boondoggle? *Canadian Medical Association Journal, 178*(11), 1407-1408.

Collins, P., & Hayes, M. (2010). The role of urban municipal governments in reducing health inequities: A meta-narrative mapping analysis. *International Journal for Equity in Health, 9*(13).

Colombo, F., Llena-nozal, A., Mercier, J., & Tjadens, F. (2011). *Help wanted? Providing and paying for long-term care.* Paris: OECD.

Colombo, F., & Tapay, N. (2004). *Health insurance in OECD countries: Benefits and costs for individuals and health systems* (Vol. 15). Paris: OECD.

Commission on Education of Health Professionals for the 21st Century. (2010). *Health professionals for a new century: Transforming education to strengthen health systems in an interdependent world.* Cambridge, MA: Harvard University Press.

Commission on the Future of Health Care in Canada. (2002). *Building on values: The future of health care in Canada.* Final report. Roy Romanow, chair. Ottawa.

Comondore, V. R., Devereaux, P. J., Zhou, Q., Stone, S. B., Busse, J. W., Ravindran, N. C., et al. (2009). Quality of care in for-profit and not-for-profit nursing homes: Systematic review and meta-analysis. *BMJ, 339.*

Conference Board of Canada. (2004). *Understanding health care cost drivers and escalators.* Ottawa: Author.

Conrad, D., & Christianson, J. (2004). Penetrating the "black box": Financial incentives for enhancing the quality of physician services. *Medical Care Research and Review, 61*(3), 37s-68s.

Conrad, D. A., & Perry, L. (2009). Quality-based financial incentives in health care: Can we improve quality by paying for it? *Annual Review of Public Health, 30*(1), 357-371.

Conrad, L., & Guven Uslu, P. (2011). Investigation of the impact of "payment by results" on performance measurement and management in NHS Trusts. *Management Accounting Research, 22*(1), 46-55.

Constant, A., Petersen, S., Mallory, C. D., & Major, J. (2011). *Research synthesis on cost drivers In the health sector and proposed policy options.* Ottawa: Canadian Health Services Research Foundation.

Contandriopoulos, D., & Bilodeau, H. (2009). The political use of poll results about public support for a privatized healthcare system in Canada. *Health Policy, 90*(1), 104-112.

Contandriopoulos, D., & Brouselle, A. (2010). Reliable in their failure: An anaylsis of healthcare reform policies in public systems. *Health Policy, 95*, 144-152.

Cooke, P. (2003). Biotechnology clusters, "big pharma" and the knowledge-driven economy. *International Journal of Technology Management, 25*(1), 65-80.

Cooper, B. S., & Vladeck, B. C. (2000). Bringing competitive pricing to medicare. *Health Affairs, 19*(5), 49-54.

Costa-Font, J., Gemmill, M., & Rubert, G. (2011). Biases in the healthcare luxury good hypothesis? A meta-regression analysis. *Journal of the Royal Statistical Society: Series A (Statistics in Society), 174*(1), 95-107.

Coulam, R. F., Feldman, R. D., & Dowd, B. E. (2011). Competitive pricing and the challenge of cost control in Medicare. *Journal of Health Politics, Policy and Law, 36*(4), 649-689.

Courchene, T. J. (2003). Medicare as a moral enterprise: The Romanow and Kirby perspectives. *Policy Matters, 4*(1), 1-20.

Courchene, T. J. (2010). Intergovernmental transfers and Canadian values: Retrospect and prospect. *Policy Options, 31*(5), 32-40.

Coutts, J. (2010). *Experts and evidence: Opportunities in nursing* (No. 9780978409876 0978409876). Ottawa: Canadian Federation of Nurses Unions.

Coutts, J., & Thornhill, J. (2009). Service-based funding and pay for performance: Will incentive payments give Canadian healthcare the quality boost it needs? *Healthcare Quarterly, 12*(3), 18-21.

Coye, M. J., Haselkorn, A., & DeMello, S. (2009). Remote patient management: Technology-enabled innovation and evolving business models for chronic disease care. *Health Affairs, 28*(1), 126-135.

Coyte, P. C., & McKeever, P. (2001). Home care in Canada: Passing the buck. *Canadian Journal of Nursing Research, 33*(2), 11-25.

Coyte, P., Wang, P. P., Hawker, G., & Wright, J. G. (1997). The relationship between variations in knee replacement utilization rates and the reported prevalence of arthritis in Ontario, Canada. *Journal of Rheumatology, 24*(12), 2403-2412.

Creighton, J. L. (2005). *The public participation handbook: Making better decisions through citizen involvement.* San Francisco, CA: Jossey-Bass.

Crichton, A., Hsu, D. H.-S., & Tsang, S. (1994). *Canada's health care system: Its funding and organization.* Ottawa: CHA Press.

Cropper, S., Hopper, A., & Spencer, S. A. (2002). Managed clinical networks: Multilateral collaboration as a basis for the future organisation of paediatric services? *Archives of Disease in Childhood, 87*(1), 1-4.

Crossley, T. F., Hurley, J., & Jeon, S.-H. (2009). Physician labour supply in Canada: A cohort analysis. *Health Economics, 18*(4), 437-456.

Cuff, K., Hurley, J., Mestelman, S., Muller, A., & Nuscheler, R. (in press). Public and private health-care financing with alternate public rationing rules. *Health Economics.*

Currie, G., Donaldson, C., & Lu, M. (2003). What does Canada profit from the for-profit debate on health care? *Canadian Public Policy, 24*(2), 227-251.

Currie, J. (2009). Healthy, wealthy, and wise: Socioeconomic status, poor health in childhood, and human capital development. *Journal of Economic Literature, 47*, 87-122.

Curtis, L. J., & MacMinn, W. J. (2008). Health care utilization in Canada: Twenty-five years of evidence. *Canadian Public Policy, 34*(1), 65-87.

Custers, T., Hurley, J., Klazinga, N., & Brown, A. (2008). Selecting effective incentive structures in health care: A decision framework to support health care purchasers in finding the right incentives to drive performance. *BMC Health Services Research, 8*, 66.

Cutler, D. M. (2010). *Where are the health care entrepreneurs? The failure of organizational innovation in health care.* Cambridge, MA: National Bureau of Economic Research.

Cutler, D. M., Deaton, A., & Lleras-Muney, A. 2006. The determinants of mortality. *Journal of Economic Perspectives, 20*, 97-120.

Cutler, D. M., & Ly, D. P. (2011). The (paper)work of medicine: Understanding international medical costs. *Journal of Economic Perspectives, 25*(2), 3-25.

Cutler, D. M., & McClellan, M. (2001). Is technological change in medicine worth it? *Health Affairs, 20*(5), 11-29.

Da Roit, B., & Le Bihan, B. (2010). Similar and yet so different: Cash-for-care in six European countries' long-term care policies. *Milbank Quarterly, 88*(3), 286-309.

Daatland, S., & Lowenstein, A. (2005). Intergenerational solidarity and the family–welfare state balance. *European Journal of Ageing, 2*(3), 174-182.

Dabhadkar, K. C., Kulshreshtha, A., Ali, M. K., & Venkat Narayan, K. M. (2011). Prospects for a cardiovascular disease prevention polypill. *Annual Review of Public Health, 32*(1), 23-38.

Dagger, T. S., Sweeney, J. C., & Johnson, L. W. (2007). A hierarchical model of health service quality. *Journal of Service Research, 10*(2), 123-142.

Dai, S., Robitaille, C., Bancej, C., Loukine, L., Waters, C., & Baclic, O. (2010). Report from the Canadian Chronic Disease Surveillance System: Hypertension in Canada, 2010. *Chronic Diseases Canada, 31*(1), 46-47.

Dalby, D., Hirdes, J., & Fries, B. (2005). Risk adjustment methods for Home Care Quality Indicators (HCQIs) based on the minimum data set for home care. *BMC Health Services Research, 5*(7).

Daly, S., Campbell, D. A., & Cameron, P. A. (2003). Short-stay units and observation medicine: A systematic review. *Medical Journal of Australia, 178*(11), 559-563.

Danaei, G., Rimm, E. B., Oza, S., Kulkarni, S. C., Murray, C. J. L., & Ezzati, M. (2010). The promise of prevention: The effects of four preventable risk factors on national life expectancy and life expectancy disparities by race and county in the United States. *PLoS Medicine, 7*(3), e1000248.

Dang, S., Dimmick, S., & Kelkar, G. (2009). Evaluating the evidence base for the use of home telehealth remote monitoring in elderly with heart failure. *Telemedicine and e-Health, 15*(8), 783-796.

Davidoff, F. M. D., Goodspeed, R. M. D., & Clive, J. P. (1989). Changing test ordering behavior: A randomized controlled trial comparing probabilistic reasoning with cost-containment education. *Medical Care, 27*(1), 45-58.

Davidson, A. (2004). Dynamics without change: Continuity of Canadian health policy. *Canadian Public Administration, 47*(3), 251-279.

Davis, K. (2007). Paying for care episodes and care coordination. *New England Journal of Medicine, 356*(11), 1166-1168.

de Brantes, F., Rastogi, A., & Painter, M. (2010). Reducing potentially avoidable complications in patients with chronic diseases: The Prometheus payment approach. *Health Services Research, 45*(6 Pt. 2), 1854-1871.

de Jong, J., Westert, G., Lagoe, R., & Groenewegen, P. (2006). Variation in hospital length of stay: Do physicians adapt their length of stay decisions to what is usual in the hospital where they work? *Health Services Research, 41*(2), 374-394.

De Maio, F. (2010). Immigration as pathogenic: A systematic review of the health of immigrants to Canada. *International Journal for Equity in Health, 9*(27).

de Vries, E. N., Ramrattan, M. A., Smorenburg, S. M., Gouma, D. J., & Boermeester, M. A. (2008). The incidence and nature of in-hospital adverse events: A systematic review. *Quality and Safety in Health Care, 17*(3), 216-223.

Deber, R. (2006). Rethinking and rebalancing: The changing role of hospitals in the Canadian health care system. In D. Goyette, D. W. Magill, & J. Denis (Eds.), *Survival strategies: The life, death and renaissance of a Canadian teaching hospital.* Toronto, ON: Canadian Scholars' Press.

Deber, R., Hollander, M. J., & Jacobs, P. (2008). Models of funding and reimbursement in health care: A conceptual framework. *Canadian Public Administration, 51*(3), 381-405.

DeCicca, P., & McLeod, L. (2008). Cigarette taxes and older adult smoking: Evidence from recent large tax increases. *Journal of Health Economics, 27*(4), 918-929.

Decker, C., Arnold, S., Olabiyi, O., Ahmad, H., Gialde, E., Luark, J., et al. (2008). Implementing an innovative consent form: The PREDICT experience. *Implementation Science, 3*, 58.

Decter, M. (2007). Chronic disease: Our growing challenge. In J. Dorland & M. A. McColl (Eds.), *Emerging approaches to chronic disease management in primary health care.* Montreal and Kingston: McGill-Queen's University Press.

Degos, L., & Rodwin, V. G. (2011). Two faces of patient safety and care quality: A Franco-American comparison. *Health Economics, Policy and Law, 6*(3), 287-294.

Delamaire, M.-L., & Lafortune, G. (2010). Nurses in advanced roles: A description and evaluation of experiences in 12 developed countries. *OECD Health Working Papers* (Vol. 54). Paris: OECD Directorate for Employment, Labour and Social Affairs.

Delbanco, T., & Bell, S. (2007). Guilty, afraid and alone – struggling with medical error. *New England Journal of Medicine, 357*(17), 1682-1683.

DelliFraine, J. L., & Dansky, K. H. (2008). Home-based telehealth: A review and meta-analysis. *Journal of Telemedicine and Telecare, 14*(2), 62-66.

DelliFraine, J. L., Langabeer, J. R., & Nembhard, I. M. (2010). Assessing the evidence of Six Sigma and Lean in the health care industry. *Quality Management in Health Care, 19*(3), 211-225.

Deming, W. E. (1993). *The new economics for industry, government, education.* Cambridge, MA: Massachusetts Institute of Technology, Center for Advanced Engineering Study.

Dennis, S., May, J., Perkins, D., Zwar, N., Sibbald, B., & Hasan, I. (2009). What evidence is there to support skill mix changes between GPs, pharmacists and practice nurses in the care of elderly people living in the community? *Australia and New Zealand Health Policy, 6*(23).

Denton, F. T., & Spencer, B. G. (2010). Chronic health conditions: Changing prevalence in an aging population and some implications for the delivery of health care services. *Canadian Journal on Aging, 29*(1), 11-21.

Dentzer, S. (2006). Media mistakes in coverage of the Institute of Medicine's error report. *Effective Clinical Practice, 3*(6), 305-308.

Deom, M., Agoritsas, T., Bovier, P., & Perneger, T. (2010). What doctors think about the impact of managed care tools on quality of care, costs, autonomy, and relations with patients. *BMC Health Services Research, 10*(331).

Deshong, D., & Henderson, A. (2010). The trainee assistant in nursing: A pilot exercise in building and retaining a workforce. *Australian Health Review, 34*(1), 41-43.

Detering, K. M., Hancock, A. D., Reade, M. C., & Silvester, W. (2010). The impact of advance care planning on end of life care in elderly patients: Randomised controlled trial. *BMJ, 340*.

Detsky, A. S., & Naylor, C. D. (2003). Canada's health care system: Reform delayed. *New England Journal of Medicine, 349*(8), 804-810.

Devereaux, P. J., Choi, P. T. L., Lacchetti, C., Weaver, B., Schunemann, H. J., Haines, T., et al. (2002). A systematic review and meta-analysis of studies comparing mortality rates of private for-profit and private not-for-profit hospitals. *Canadian Medical Association Journal, 166*(11), 1399-1406.

Devlin, R. A., & Sarma, S. (2008). Do physician remuneration schemes matter? The case of Canadian family physicians. *Journal of Health Economics, 27*(5), 1168-1181.

Dhalla, I. (2007). Canada's health care system and the sustainability paradox. *Canadian Medical Association Journal, 177*(1), 51-53.

Dhalla, I. A., Guyatt, G. H., Stabile, M., & Bayoumi, A. M. (2011). Broadening the base of publicly funded health care. *Canadian Medical Association Journal, 183*, E296-305.

Dhalla, I. A., Kwong, J. C., Streiner, D. L., Baddour, R. E., Waddell, A. E., & Johnson, I. L. (2002). Characteristics of first-year students in Canadian medical schools. *Canadian Medical Association Journal, 166*(8), 1029-1035.

Di Matteo, L. (2003). The income elasticity of health care spending. *European Journal of Health Economics, 4*(1), 20-29.

Di Matteo, L. (2009). Policy choice or economic fundamentals: What drives the public-private health expenditure balance in Canada? *Health Economics, Policy and Law, 4*(1), 29-53.

Di Matteo, L. (2010). The sustainability of public health expenditures: Evidence from the Canadian federation. *European Journal of Health Economics, 11*(6), 569-584.

Diamond, C. C., & Shirky, C. (2008). Health information technology: A few years of magical thinking? *Health Affairs, 27*(5), w383-w390.

DiCenso, A., Bourgeault, I., Abelson, J., Martin-Misener, R., Kaasalainen, S., Carter, N., et al. (2011). Utilization of nurse practitioners to increase patient access to primary healthcare in Canada – Thinking outside the box. *Nursing Leadership, 23*[Special Issue], 239-259.

DiCenso, A., Martin-Misener, R., Bryant-Lukosius, D., Bourgeault, I., Kilpatrick, K., Donald, F., et al. (2011). Advanced practice nursing in Canada: Overview of a decision support synthesis. *Nursing Leadership, 23*[Special Issue], 15-34.

Dickson, M., & Gagnon, J. P. (2004). Key factors in the rising cost of new drug discovery and development. *Nature Reviews Drug Discovery, 3*(5), 417-429.

Dimick, J. B., & Welch, H. G. (2008). The zero mortality paradox in surgery. *Journal of American College of Surgeons, 206*(1), 13-16.

Dixon-Woods, M., Bosk, C. L., Aveling, E. L., Goeschel, C. A., & Pronovost, P. J. (2011). Explaining Michigan: Developing an ex post theory of a quality improvement program. *Milbank Quarterly, 89*(2), 167-205.

Djulbegovic, B., & Paul, A. (2011). From efficacy to effectiveness in the face of uncertainty. *JAMA, 305*(19), 2005-2006.

Do, N. V., Barnhill, R., Heermann-Do, K. A., Salzman, K. L., & Gimbel, R. W. (2011). The military health system's personal health record pilot with Microsoft HealthVault and Google Health. *Journal of the American Medical Informatics Association, 18*(2), 118-124.

Dodge, D. A., & Dion, R. (2011). *Chronic healthcare spending disease: A macro diagnosis and prognosis.* Toronto, ON: C.D. Howe Institute.

Donald, F., Martin-Misener, R., Bryant-Lukosius, D., Kilpatrick, K., Kaasalainen, S., Carter, N., et al. (2011). The primary healthcare nurse practitioner role in Canada. *Nursing Leadership, 23*[Special Issue], 88-113.

Doran, T., Fullwood, C., Kontopantelis, E., & Reeves, D. (2008). Effect of financial incentives on inequalities in the delivery of primary clinical care in England: Analysis of clinical activity indicators for the quality and outcomes framework. *The Lancet, 372*(9640), 728-736.

Doré, G. (1985). L'organisation communautaire : définition et paradigme. *Service social, 34*, 210-230.

Dormont, B., Grignon, M., & Huber, H. (2006). Health expenditure growth: Reassessing the threat of ageing. *Health Economics, 15*(9), 947-963.

Dougherty, D., & Conway, P. (2008). The "3T's" road map to transform US health care: The "how" of high-quality care. *JAMA, 299*(19), 2319-2321.

Douglas, T. (1979). Tommy Douglas – 1979 S.O.S. Medicare Conference, Ottawa. [Video file]. Posted by Health Coalition, 19 November 2009. Retrieved 11 August 2011 http://www.youtube.com/watch?v=V1A0vrz36Sc

Dranove, D. (2003). *What's your life worth? Health care rationing ... who lives? who dies? who decides?* Upper Saddle River, NJ: FT Prentice Hall.

Dranove, D. (2008). *Code red: An economist explains how to revive the healthcare system without destroying it.* Princeton: Princeton University Press.

Dranove, D., Capps, C., & Dafny, L. (2009). *A competitive process for procuring health services a review of principles with an application to cataract services.* Calgary, AB: School of Public Policy, University of Calgary.

Draper, A. K., Hewitt, G., & Rifkin, S. (2010). Chasing the dragon: Developing indicators for the assessment of community participation in health programmes. *Social Science & Medicine, 71*(6), 1102-1109.

Dror, D. M., & Preker, A. S. (Eds.). (2002). *Social reinsurance: A new approach to sustainable community health financing.* Washington DC: World Bank.

Drummond, D., & Burleton, D. (2010). *Charting a path to sustainable health care in Ontario: 10 proposals to restrain cost growth without compromising quality of care.* Toronto, ON: TD Bank Financial Group.

Dubois, C.-A., & McKee, M. (2006). Cross-national comparisons of human resources for health – What can we learn? *Health Economics, Policy and Law, 1*(1), 59-78.

Dubois, C.-A., & Singh, D. (2009). From staff-mix to skill-mix and beyond: Towards a systemic approach to health workforce management. *Human Resources for Health, 7*(87).

Dückers, M., Faber, M., Cruijsberg, J., Grol, R., Schoonhoven, L., & Wensing, M. (2009). Safety and risk management interventions in hospitals. *Medical Care Research and Review, 66*(Suppl. 6), 90S-119S.

Duckett, S. (1995). Hospital payment arrangements to encourage efficiency: The case of Victoria, Australia. *Health Policy, 34*, 113-134.

Duckett, S. (2005a). Living in the parallel universe in Australia: Public Medicare and private hospitals. *Canadian Medical Association Journal, 173*(7), 745-747.

Duckett, S. (2005b). Private care and public waiting. *Australian Health Review, 29*(1), 87-93.

Duckett, S. (2007). A new approach to clinical governance in Queensland. *Australian Health Review, 31*(Suppl. 1), S16-S19.

Duckett, S. (2008). Design of price incentives for adjunct policy goals in formula funding for hospitals and health services. *BMC Health Services Research, 8*(72).

Duckett, S. (2009). Interdependence of the health and education sectors in meeting health human resource needs. *HealthcarePapers, 9*(2), 30-34.

Duckett, S. (2011). Getting the foundations right: Alberta's approach to health-care reform. *Healthcare Policy, 6*(3), 22-26.

Duckett, S., Hatcher, J., Murphy, K., & Richards, H. (2011). *Policy choices in developing casemix payment weights for hospital care in Canada*. Ottawa: Canadian Institute for Health Information.

Duckett, S., & Kempton, A. (2012). Canadians' views about health system performance. *Healthcare Policy, 7*(3), 88-104.

Duckett, S., Kramer, G., & Sarnecki, L. (2012). Alberta's health spending challenge: A policy-oriented analysis of inter and intra-provincial differences in health expenditure. In D. Ryan (Ed.), *Boom and bust again: Policy challenges for a commodity based economy*. Edmonton: University of Alberta Press.

Duckett, S., Sarnecki, L., & Kramer, G. (2011, October). Implementation of activity based funding for long-term care in Alberta. Paper presented to 27th Patient Classification Systems International (PCSI) Conference, Montreal.

Duckett, S., & Ward, M. (2008). Developing "robust performance benchmarks" for the next Australian Health Care Agreement: The need for a new framework. *Australian and New Zealand Health Policy, 5*(1).

Duckett, S., & Willcox, S. (2011). *The Australian health care system*. Melbourne: Oxford University Press.

Duffin, J. (2011). The impact of single-payer health care on physician income in Canada, 1850–2005. *American Journal of Public Health, 101*(7), 1198-1208.

Dunt, D., Wilson, R., Day, S., Kelaher, M., & Gurrin, L. (2007). Impact of telephone triage on emergency after hours GP Medicare usage: A time-series analysis. *Australia and New Zealand Health Policy, 4*(21).

Durand, C. P., Andalib, M., Dunton, G. F., Wolch, J., & Pentz, M. A. (2011). A systematic review of built environment factors related to physical activity and obesity risk: Implications for smart growth urban planning. *Obesity Reviews, 12*(5), e173-e182.

Durier-Copp, M., & Wranik, D. (2005). Barriers and solutions to implementation strategies to improve health human resource models in Canada. In C. M. Beach, R. P. Chaykowski, S. Shortt, F. St-Hilaire, & A. Sweetman (Eds.), *Health services restructuring in Canada: New evidence and new directions*. Kingston, ON: John Deutsch Institute for the Study of Economic Policy, Queen's University.

Duthie, K., & Bond, K. (2011). Improving ethics analysis in health technology assessment. *International Journal of Technology Assessment in Health Care, 27*(1), 64-70.

Dyment, J. E., & Bell, A. C. (2008). Grounds for movement: Green school grounds as sites for promoting physical activity. *Health Education Research, 23*(6), 952-962.

Earle, C. C., Park, E. R., Lai, B., Weeks, J. C., Ayanian, J. Z., & Block, S. (2003). Identifying potential indicators of the quality of end-of-life cancer care from administrative data. *Journal of Clinical Oncology, 21*(6), 1133-1138.

Easton, D. (1979). *A systems analysis of political life.* Chicago: University of Chicago Press.

Eckel, C. C., Johnson, C., Montmarquette, C., & Rojas, C. (2007). Debt aversion and the demand for loans for postsecondary education. *Public Finance Review, 35*(2), 233-262.

Edelman, M. (1988). *Constructing the political spectacle.* Chicago: University of Chicago Press.

Edwards, N. (2002). Clinical networks. *BMJ, 324*(7329), 63.

Edwards, N. (2010). *The triumph of hope over experience: Lessons from the history of reorganisation.* London: NHS Confederation.

Egan, M., Wells, J., Byrne, K., Jaglal, S., Stolee, P., Chesworth, B. M., et al. (2009). The process of decision-making in home-care case management: Implications for the introduction of universal assessment and information technology. *Health and Social Care in the Community, 17*(4), 371-378.

Egger de Campo, M. (2007). Exit and voice: An investigation of care service users in Austria, Belgium, Italy, and Northern Ireland. *European Journal of Ageing, 4*(2), 59-69.

Eichler, H.-G., Kong, S. X., Gerth, W. C., Mavros, P., & Jönsson, B. (2004). Use of cost-effectiveness analysis in health-care resource allocation decision-making: How are cost-effectiveness thresholds expected to emerge? *Value in Health, 7*(5), 518-528.

Eisenberg, M. J., Atallah, R., Grandi, S. M., Windle, S. B., & Berry, E. M. (2011). Legislative approaches to tackling the obesity epidemic. *Canadian Medical Association Journal, 183*(13), 1496-1500.

Ekeland, A. G., Bowes, A., & Flottorp, S. (2010). Effectiveness of telemedicine: A systematic review of reviews. *International Journal of Medical Informatics, 79*(11), 736-771.

El Ansari, W. (2011). When meanings blur, do differences matter? Initiatives for improving the quality and integration of care: Conceptual matrix or measurement maze? *Journal of Integrated Care, 19,* 5-22.

El Emam, K., Paton, D., Dankar, F., & Koru, G. (2011). De-identifying a public use microdata file from the Canadian National Discharge Abstract Database. *BMC Medical Informatics and Decision Making, 11*(53).

Ellis, R. P., & Miller, M. M. (2008). Provider payment methods and incentives. In K. Heggenhougen & S. R. Quah (Eds.), *International encyclopedia of public health.* Amsterdam and Boston: Elsevier/Academic Press.

Elshaug, A. G., & Garber, A. M. (2011). How CER could pay for itself – Insights from vertebral fracture treatments. *New England Journal of Medicine, 364*(15), 1390-1393.

Elshaug, A. G., Watt, A. M., Moss, J. R., & Hiller, J. E. (2009). *Policy perspectives on the obsolescence of health technologies in Canada.* Canadian Agency for Drugs and Technologies in Health.

Encinosa, W., Bernard, D., & Dor, A. (2010). *Does prescription drug adherence reduce hospitalizations and costs?* National Bureau of Economic Research Working Paper Series, No. 15691.

Engström, S., Foldevi, M., & Borgquist, L. (2001). Is general practice effective? A systematic literature review. *Scandinavian Journal of Primary Health Care, 19*(2), 131-144.

Epping-Jordan, J. E., Pruitt, S. D., Bengoa, R., & Wagner, E. H. (2004). Improving the quality of health care for chronic conditions. *Quality and Safety in Health Care, 13,* 299-305. .

Epps, T., & Flood, C. M. (2002). Have we traded away the opportunity for innovative health care reform? The implications of the NAFTA for Medicare. *McGill Law Journal, 47*(4), 747-790.

Esserman, L., Shieh, Y., & Thompson, I. (2009). Rethinking screening for breast cancer and prostate cancer. *JAMA, 302*(15), 1685-1692.

Estes, C. L., Lohrer, S. P., Goldberg, S., Grossman, B. R., Nelson, M., Koren, M. J., et al. (2010). Factors associated with perceived effectiveness of local long-term care ombudsman programs in New York and California. *Journal of Aging and Health, 22*(6), 772-803.

Etheredge, L. M. (2007). A rapid-learning health system. *Health Affairs, 26*(2), w107-w118.

Etowa, J. B., Foster, S., Vukic, A. R., Wittstock, L., & Youden, S. (2005). Recruitment and retention of minority students: Diversity in nursing education. *International Journal of Nursing Education Scholarship, 2*(1).

Evans, R. G. (1990a). Tension, compression, and shear: Directions, stresses, and outcomes of health care cost control. *Journal of Health Politics, Policy and Law, 15*(1), 101-128.

Evans, R. G. (1990b). The dog in the night-time: Medical practice variations and health policy. In T. F. Andersen & G. Mooney (Eds.), *The challenges of medical practice variations* (pp. 117-152). London: MacMillan Press.

Evans, R. G. (1997). Going for the gold: The redistributive agenda behind market-based health care reform. *Journal of Health Politics, Policy and Law, 22*(2), 427-465.

Evans, R. G. (2002). *Interpreting and addressing inequalities in health: From Black to Acheson to Blair...?* London: Office of Health Economics.

Evans, R. G. (2009). The iron chancellor and the fabian. *Healthcare Policy, 5*(1), 16-24.

Evans, R. G. (2010). The TSX gives a short course in health economics: It's the prices, stupid! *Healthcare Policy, 6*(2), 13-23.

Evans, R.G., & Stoddart, G.L. (1990). Producing health, consuming health care. *Social Science & Medicine, 31,* 1347-1363.

Evans, R. G., & Stoddart, G. L. (2003). Consuming research, producing policy? *American Journal of Public Health, 93*(3), 371-379.

Evans, R. G., Barer, M. L., & Stoddart, G. L. (1995). User fees for health care: Why a bad idea keeps coming back (or, what's health got to do with it?). *Canadian Journal on Aging, 14*(2), 360-390.

Evans, R. G., Barer, M., Stoddart, G. L., & Bhatia, V. (1994). *Who are the zombie masters, and what do they want?* Toronto, ON: Premier's Council on Health, Well-Being and Social Justice.

Evans, R. G., Schneider, D., & Barer, M. L. (2010). *Health human resources productivity: What it is, how it's measured, why (how you measure) it matters, and who's thinking about it.* Ottawa: Canadian Health Services Research Foundation.

Eveleens, J. L., & Verhoef, C. (2010). The rise and fall of the Chaos report figures. *IEEE Software, 27*(1), 30-36.

Evensen, A., Sanson-Fisher, R., D'Este, C., & Fitzgerald, M. (2010). Trends in publications regarding evidence-practice gaps: A literature review. *Implementation Science, 5*(11).

Falit, B. P. (2008). Twisting the truth: Tinkering with patient decision aids to reduce health care expenditures. *Yale Journal of Biology and Medicine, 81*(1), 43-47.

Fang, R., & Millar, J. S. (2009). Canada's global position in life expectancy: A longitudinal comparison with the healthiest countries in the world. *Canadian Journal of Public Health, 100*(1), 9-13.

Farrelly, M. C., Pechacek, T. F., & Chaloupka, F. J. (2003). The impact of tobacco control program expenditures on aggregate cigarette sales: 1981–2000. *Journal of Health Economics, 22*(5), 843-859.

Felder, S., Werblow, A., & Zweifel, P. (2010). Do red herrings swim in circles? Controlling for the endogeneity of time to death. *Journal of Health Economics, 29*(2), 205-212.

Felitti, V. J., Anda, R. F., Nordenberg, D., Williamson, D. F., Spitz, A. M., Edwards, V., et al. (1998). Relationship of childhood abuse and household dysfunction to many of the leading causes of death in adults: The adverse childhood experiences (ACE) study. *American Journal of Preventive Medicine, 14*(4), 245-258.

Fernandes, N., & Spencer, B. G. (2010). The private cost of long-term care in Canada: Where you live matters. *Canadian Journal on Aging, 29*(3), 307-316.

Fichtenberg, C. M., & Glantz, S. A. (2000). Association of the California Tobacco Control Program with declines in cigarette consumption and mortality from heart disease. *New England Journal of Medicine, 343*(24), 1772-1777.

Finks, J. F., Osborne, N. H., & Birkmeyer, J. D. (2011). Trends in hospital volume and operative mortality for high-risk surgery. *New England Journal of Medicine, 364*(22), 2128-2137.

Finlayson, S. R. G., Birkmeyer, J. D., Tosteson, A. N. A., & Nease, R. F. (1999). Patient preferences for location of care: Implications for regionalization. *Medical Care, 37*(2), 204-209.

Finnie, R. (2002). Student loans, student financial aid and post-secondary education in Canada. *Journal of Higher Education Policy and Management, 24*(2), 155-170.

Finocchio, L. J., Dower, C. M., McMahon, T., Gragnola, C. M., & Pew Health Professions Commission – Taskforce on Health Care Workforce Regulation. (1995). *Reforming health care workforce regulation: Policy considerations for the 21st century.* San Francisco, CA: Pew Health Professions Commission.

Finucane, M. M., Stevens, G. A., Cowan, M. J., Danaei, G., Lin, J. K., Paciorek, C. J., et al. (2011). National, regional, and global trends in body-mass index since 1980: Systematic analysis of health examination surveys and epidemiological studies with 960 country-years and 9.1 million participants. *The Lancet, 377*(9765), 557-567.

Fisher, E. S., Bynum, J. P., & Skinner, J. S. (2009). Slowing the growth of health care costs: Lessons from regional variation. *New England Journal of Medicine, 360*(9), 849-852.

Fitzpatrick, R. (2009). Patient reported outcome measures and performance measurement. In P. Smith, E. Mossialos, I. Papanicolas, & S. Leatherman (Eds.), *Performance measurement for health system improvement: Experiences, challenges, and prospects.* Cambridge and New York: Cambridge University Press.

Fletcher, A., Bonell, C., & Sorhaindo, A. (2011). You are what your friends eat: Systematic review of social network analyses of young people's eating behaviours and bodyweight. *Journal of Epidemiology and Community Health, 65*(6), 548-555.

Flexner, A. (1910). *Medical education in the United States and Canada: A report to the Carnegie Foundation for the Advancement of Teaching.* New York: Carnegie Foundation for the Advancement of Teaching.

Flood, C. M., & Archibald, T. (2001). The illegality of private health care in Canada. *Canadian Medical Association Journal, 164*(6), 825-830.

Flood, C. M., & Choudhry, S. (2002). *Strengthening the foundations modernizing the* Canada Health Act. Saskatoon, SK: Commission on the Future of Health Care in Canada.

Flood, C. M., & Choudhry, S. (2004). Strengthening the foundations: Modernizing the *Canada Health Act.* In T. A. McIntosh, P.-G. Forest, & G. P. Marchildon (Eds.), *The governance of health care in Canada. Romanow papers, Vol. 3.* Toronto, ON: University of Toronto Press.

Flood, C. M., & Erdman, J. N. (2004). The boundaries of Medicare: Tensions in the dual role of Ontario's Physician Services Review Committee. *Health Law Journal, 12*, 1-16.

Flood, C. M., & Sinclair, D. (2004). Devolution – a Solution for Ontario: Could the lone wolf lead the pack? *HealthcarePapers, 5*(1), 63-68.

Flood, C. M., Stabile, M., & Tuohy, C. (2008a). *Defining the Medicare "basket."* Ottawa: Canadian Health Services Research Foundation.

Flood, C. M., Stabile, M., & Tuohy, C. J. (Eds.). (2008b). *Exploring social insurance: Can a dose of Europe cure Canadian health care finance?* Montreal and Kingston: McGill-Queen's University Press.

Flood, C. M., Stabile, M., & Tuohy, C. (2008c). Seeking the Grail: Financing for quality, accessibility, and sustainability in the health care system. In C. M. Flood, M. Stabile, & C. Tuohy (Eds.), *Exploring social insurance: Can a dose of Europe cure Canadian health care finance?* Montreal and Kingston: McGill-Queen's University Press.

Flood, C. M., & Thomas, B. (2011). Searching for the sweet spot: How do we trade-off research benefits with health information privacy concerns? In C. M. Flood (Ed.), *Data data everywhere: Access and accountability?* Montreal and Kingston: McGill-Queen's University Press.

Flood, C. M., Tuohy, C., & Stabile, M. (2006). What is in and out of Medicare? Who decides? In C. M. Flood (Ed.), *Just Medicare: What's in, what's out, how we decide.* Toronto, ON: University of Toronto Press.

Flynn, K. E., & Smith, M. A. (2002). From physician to consumer: The effectiveness of strategies to manage health care utilization. *Medical Care Research and Review, 59*(4), 455-481.

Fojo, T., & Grady, C. (2009). How much is life worth: Cetuximab, non-small cell lung cancer, and the $440 billion question. *Journal of the National Cancer Institute, 101*(15), 1044-1048.

Follett, M. P. (1926). The giving of orders. In P. Graham (Ed.), *Mary Parker Follett, prophet of management: A celebration of writings from the 1920s.* Cambridge, MA: Harvard Business School Press.

Fontaine, P., Jacques, J., Gillain, D., Sermeus, W., Kolh, P., & Gillet, P. (2011). Assessing the causes inducing lengthening of hospital stays by means of the Appropriateness Evaluation Protocol. *Health Policy, 99*(1), 66-71.

Foote, S. B. (1992). *Managing the medical arms race: Public policy and medical device innovation.* Berkeley: University of California Press.

Ford, E. S., & Capewell, S. (2011). Proportion of the decline in cardiovascular mortality disease due to prevention versus treatment: Public health versus clinical care. *Annual Review of Public Health, 32*(1), 5-22.

Forget, C. E. (2002). Comprehensiveness in public health care: An impediment to effective restructuring. *Policy Matters, 3*(11), 1-23.

Foster, G., Taylor, S. J., Eldridge, S., Ramsay, J., & Griffiths, C. J. (2007). Self-management education programmes by lay leaders for people with chronic conditions. *Cochrane Database of Systematic Reviews* (4).

Fotaki, M. (2010). Why do public policies fail so often? Exploring health policy-making as an imaginary and symbolic construction. *Organization, 17*(6), 703-720.

Fowler, J. H., & Christakis, N. A. (2008). Estimating peer effects on health in social networks: A response to Cohen-Cole and Fletcher; and Trogdon, Nonnemaker, and Pais. *Journal of Health Economics, 27*(5), 1400-1405.

Fox, D. M. (2006). The determinants of policy for population health. *Health Economics, Policy and Law, 1*(4), 395-407.

Fox, D. M., & Markel, H. (2010). Is history relevant to implementing health reform? *JAMA, 303*(17), 1749-1750.

Fralick, P. C., & President and Chief Executive Officer Canadian Healthcare Association. (2011, February). Common prescriptions. Presentation to Southwestern Ontario Chapter of the Canadian College of Health Leaders.

Franco, Á., Álvarez-Dardet, C., & Ruiz, M. (2004). Effect of democracy on health: Ecological study. *BMJ, 329*, 1421-1424.

Frank, L. D., Andresen, M. A., & Schmid, T. L. (2004). Obesity relationships with community design, physical activity, and time spent in cars. *American Journal of Preventive Medicine, 27*(2), 87-96.

Frank, C., Marshall, D., Faris, P., & Smith, C. (2011). Improving access to hip and knee replacement and its quality by adopting a new model of care in Alberta. *Canadian Medical Association Journal, 183*(6), E347-350.

Fransoo, R., Martens, P., Burland, E., The Need to Know Team, Prior, H., & Burchill, C. (2009). *Manitoba RHA indicators atlas 2009.* Winnipeg: Manitoba Centre for Health Policy. Retrieved 24 August 2011 from http://mchp-appserv.cpe.umanitoba.ca/reference/RHA_Atlas_Report.pdf

Freedman, V. A., Hodgson, N., Lynn, J., Spillman, B. C., Waidmann, T., Wilkinson, A. M., et al. (2006). Promoting declines in the prevalence of late-life disability: Comparisons of three potentially high-impact interventions. *Milbank Quarterly, 84*(3), 493-520.

Freeman, B. (2011). Tobacco plain packaging legislation: A content analysis of commentary posted on Australian online news. *Tobacco Control, 20*(5), 361-366.

Freeman, R., & Frisina, L. (2010). Health care systems and the problem of classification. *Journal of Comparative Policy Analysis: Research and Practice, 12*(1), 163-178.

Freidson, E. (1970). *Profession of medicine: A study of the sociology of applied knowledge.* New York: Dodd, Mead.

Friedberg, M. W., Hussey, P. S., & Schneider, E. C. (2010). Primary care: A critical review of the evidence on quality and costs of health care. *Health Affairs, 29*(5), 766-772.

Fries, J. F. (1983). The compression of morbidity. *Milbank Memorial Fund Quarterly, 61*(3), 397-419.

Fries, J. F. (2005). The compression of morbidity. *Milbank Quarterly, 83*(4), 801-823.

Frogner, B. K. (2010). The missing technology: An international comparison of human capital investment in healthcare. *Applied Health Economics and Health Policy, 8*(6), 361-371.

Frogner, B. K., Anderson, G. F., Cohen, R. A., & Abrams, C. (2011). Incorporating new research into Medicare risk adjustment. *Medical Care, 49*, 295-300.

Frohlich, K., & Potvin, L. (2008). The inequality paradox: The population approach and vulnerable populations. *Government, Politics, and Law, 98*(2), 216-221.

Frølich, A., Talavera, J. A., Broadhead, P., & Dudley, R. A. (2007). A behavioral model of clinician responses to incentives to improve quality. *Health Policy, 80*(1), 179-193.

Frost, J. H., & Massagli, M. P. (2008). Social uses of personal health information within PatientsLikeMe, an online patient community: What can happen when patients have access to one another's data. *Journal of Medical Internet Research, 10*(3), e15.

Frueh, F. W. (2009). Back to the future: Why randomized controlled trials cannot be the answer to pharmacogenomics and personalized medicine. *Pharmacogenomics, 10*(7), 1077-1081.

Fuchs, V. R. (1998). *Who shall live? Health, economics and social choice.* Singapore: World Scientific Publishing.

Fuchs, V. R., & Milstein, A. (2011). The $640 billion question: Why does cost-effective care diffuse so slowly? *New England Journal of Medicine, 364*(21), 1985-1987.

Fung, C. H., Lim, Y.-W., Mattke, S., Damberg, C., & Shekelle, P. G. (2008). Systematic review: The evidence that publishing patient care performance data improves quality of care. *Annals of Internal Medicine, 148*(2), 111-123.

Gagnon, M.-A. (2010). *The economic case for universal pharmacare: Costs and benefits of publicly funded drug coverage for all Canadians.* Ottawa and Montreal: Canadian Centre for Policy Alternatives and Institut de recherche et d'informations socio-économiques.

Gagnon, M.-P., Desmartis, M., Lepage-Savary, D., Gagnon, J., St-Pierre, M., Rhainds, M., et al. (2011). Introducing patients' and the public's perspectives to health technology assessment: A systematic review of international experiences. *International Journal of Technology Assessment in Health Care, 27*(1), 31-42.

Gaikwad, R., & Warren, J. (2009). The role of home-based information and communications technology interventions in chronic disease management: A systematic literature review. *Health Informatics Journal, 15*(2), 122-146.

Galarneau, D. (2003). Health care professionals. *Perspectives on Labour and Income, 4*(12), 14-27.

Galbraith, J. W., & Kaiserman, M. (1997). Taxation, smuggling and demand for cigarettes in Canada: Evidence from time-series data. *Journal of Health Economics, 16*(3), 287-301.

Gao, J., Moran, E., Almenoff, P. L., Render, M. L., Campbell, J., & Jha, A. K. (2011). Variations in efficiency and the relationship to quality of care in the veterans health system. *Health Affairs, 30*(4), 655-663.

Garattini, L., & van de Vooren, K. (2011). Budget impact analysis in economic evaluation: A proposal for a clearer definition. *European Journal of Health Economics, 12*, 499-502.

García-Lizana, F., & Sarria-Santamera, A. (2007). New technologies for chronic disease management and control: A systematic review. *Journal of Telemedicine and Telecare, 13*(2), 62-68.

Gardner, D. (2011). *Future babble: Why expert predictions are next to worthless, and you can do better.* New York: Dutton.

Garg, A. X., Adhikari, N. K. J., McDonald, H., Rosas-Arellano, M. P., Devereaux, P. J., Beyene, J., et al. (2005). Effects of computerized clinical decision support systems on practitioner performance and patient outcomes. *JAMA, 293*(10), 1223-1238.

Garner, S., & Littlejohns, P. (2011). Disinvestment from low value clinical interventions: NICEly done? *BMJ, 343.*

Garvin, D. A. (1980). *The economics of university behavior.* New York: Academic Press.

Gauvin, F.-P., Abelson, J., Giacomini, M., Eyles, J., & Lavis, J. N. (2010). "It all depends": Conceptualizing public involvement in the context of health technology assessment agencies. *Social Science & Medicine, 70*(10), 1518-1526.

Gauvin, F.-P., Abelson, J., Giacomini, M., Eyles, J., & Lavis, J. N. (2011). Moving cautiously: Public involvement and the health technology assessment community. *International Journal of Technology Assessment in Health Care, 27*(1), 43-49.

Gawande, A. (2009a). *The checklist manifesto: How to get things right.* New York: Metropolitan Books.

Gawande, A. (2009b). The cost conundrum – What a Texas town can teach us about health care. *The New Yorker,* 1 June, pp. 36-40.

Gee, E. M. (2000). Population and politics: Voodoo demography, population aging, and Canadian social policy. In E. M. Gee & G. M. Gutman (Eds.), *The overselling of population aging: Apolcalyptic demography, intergenerational challenges, and social policy* (pp. 5-25). Toronto, ON: Oxford University Press.

Gertman, P. M., & Restuccia, J. D. (1981). The Appropriateness Evaluation Protocol: A technique for assessing unnecessary days of hospital care. *Medical Care, 19*(8), 855-871.

Gérvas, J., Starfield, B., & Heath, I. (2008). Is clinical prevention better than cure? *The Lancet, 372,* 1997-1999.

Getzen, T. E. (2000, July). Aggregation and the measurement of health care costs. Paper presented to 57th HESG meeting, University of Nottingham.

Ghemawat, P., & Ricart I Costa, J. E. (1993). The organizational tension between static and dynamic efficiency. *Strategic Management Journal, 14,* 59-73.

Giacomini, M. K. (1999). The which-hunt: Assembling health technologies for assessment and rationing. *Journal of Health Politics, Policy & Law, 24*(4), 715.

Giacomini, M., Kenny, N., & DeJean, D. (2008). Ethics frameworks in Canadian health policies: Foundation, scaffolding, or window dressing? *Health Policy, 89*(1), 58-71.

Gibson, D. (1996). The *Canada Health Act* and the constitution. *Health Law Journal, 4,* 1-33.

Gibson, B. J. J. (2003). *From transfer to transformation: Rethinking the relationship between research and policy.* Australian National University.

Gibson, D., & Goodin, R. E. (1999). The veil of vagueness: A model of institutional design. In M. Egeberg & P. Laegreid (Eds.), *Organizational and institutional factors in political life: Essays in honour of Yohan P. Olsen.* Oslo: Scandinavian University Press.

Gilbert, J. H. V. (2008). Abraham Flexner and the roots of interprofessional educa-tion. *Journal of Continuing Education in the Health Professions, 28*(S1), 11-14.

Gill, L., & White, L. (2009). A critical review of patient satisfaction. *Leadership in Health Services, 22*(1), 8-19.

Ginsburg, L., Gilin, D., Tregunno, D., Norton, P. G., Flemons, W., & Fleming, M. (2009). Advancing measurement of patient safety culture. *Health Services Re-search, 44*(1), 205-224.

Giskes, K., Van Lenthe, F., Avendano-Pabon, M., & Brug, J. (2011). A systematic review of environmental factors and obesogenic dietary intakes among adults: Are we getting closer to understanding obesogenic environments? *Obesity Re-views, 12*(5), e95-e106.

Glance, L. G., Dick, A. W., Osler, T. M., Meredith, W., & Mukamel, D. B. (2010). The association between cost and quality in trauma: Is greater spending associated with higher-quality care? *Annals of Surgery, 252*(2), 217-222.

Glasby, J., & Littlechild, R. (2009). *Direct payments and personal budgets: Putting personalisation into practice.* Bristol: Policy Press.

Glasgow, J. M., Scott-Caziewell, J. R., & Kaboli, P. J. (2010). Guiding inpatient qual-ity improvement: A systematic review of Lean and Six Sigma. *Joint Commission Journal on Quality and Patient Safety, 36*(12), 533-540.

Glassman, P. A., Model, K. E., Kahan, J. P., Jacobson, P. D., & Peabody, J. W. (1997). The role of medical necessity and cost-effectiveness in making medical decisions. *Annals of Internal Medicine, 126*(2), 152-156.

Glasziou, P., & Haynes, B. (2005). The paths from research to improved health outcomes. *Evidence Based Medicine, 10*(1), 4-7.

Glazier, R. H., Klein-Geltink, J., Kopp, A., & Sibley, L. M. (2009). Capitation and enhanced fee-for-service models for primary care reform: A population-based evaluation. *Canadian Medical Association Journal, 180*(11), E72-E81.

Glazier, R. H., Moineddin, R., Agha, M., Zagorski, B., Hall, R., Manuel, D., et al. (2008). *The impact of not having a primary care physician among people with chronic conditions.* Toronto, ON: Institute for Clinical Evaluative Sciences.

Glazier, R. H., & Redelmeier, D. A. (2010). Building the patient-centered medical home in Ontario. *JAMA, 303*(21), 2186-2187.

Glied, S. (2008a). Health care financing: Efficiency and equity. In C. M. Flood, M. Stabile, & C. Tuohy (Eds.), *Exploring social insurance: Can a dose of Europe cure Canadian health care finance?* Montreal and Kingston: McGill-Queen's University Press.

Glied, S. (2008b). Universal public health insurance and private coverage: Exter-nalities in health care consumption. *Canadian Public Policy, 34*(3), 345-357.

Glouberman, S., & Millar, J. (2003). Evolution of the determinant of health policy, and health information systems in Canada. *American Journal of Public Health, 93*(3), 388-392.

Glouberman, S., & Zimmerman, B. (2002). *Complicated and complex systems: What would successful reform of Medicare look like?* Saskatoon, SK: Commission on the Future of Health Care in Canada.

Glouberman, S., & Zimmerman, B. (2004). Complicated and complex systems: What would successful reform of Medicare look like? In P.-G. Forest, G. P. Marchildon, & T. McIntosh (Eds.), *Changing health care in Canada: The Romanow papers, Vol. 2.* Toronto, ON: University of Toronto Press.

Glover, S., Rivers, P. A., Asoh, D. A., Piper, C. N., & Murph, K. (2010). Data mining for health executive decision support: An imperative with a daunting future! *Health Services Management Research, 23*(1), 42-46.

Goddard, M., Hauck, K., Preker, A., & Smith, P. (2006). Priority setting in health – A political economy perspective. *Health Economics, Policy and Law, 1*, 79-90.

Goel, V., Williams, J., Anderson, G., Blackstien-Hirsch, P., Fooks, C., & Naylor, D. (1996). *Patterns of health care in Ontario* (2nd ed.). Institute for Clinical Evaluative Sciences. Retrieved 24 August 2011 from http://www.ices.on.ca/webpage. cfm?site_id=1&org_id=67&morg_id=0&gsec_id=0&item_id=1411&type=atlas

Goeree, R., He, J., O'Reilly, D., Tarride, J.-E., Xie, F., Lim, M., et al. (2011). Transferability of health technology assessments and economic evaluations: A systematic review of approaches for assessment and application. *ClinicoEconomics and Outcomes Research, 3*, 89-104.

Gold, M. R. (Ed.). (1996). *Cost-effectiveness in health and medicine: Report to the U.S. Public Health Service, by the Panel on Cost-Effectiveness in Health and Medicine*. New York: Oxford University Press.

Gold, M., Helms, D., & Guterman, S. (2011). *Identifying, monitoring, and assessing promising innovations: Using evaluation to support rapid-cycle change*. New York: Commonwealth Fund.

Golder, S., & Loke, Y. K. (2008). Is there evidence for biased reporting of published adverse effects data in pharmaceutical industry-funded studies? *British Journal of Clinical Pharmacology, 66*(6), 767-773.

Goldmann, D. (2010). Five puzzle pieces, ten cautionary notes. *International Journal of Care Pathways, 14*(1), 33-35.

Goldsmith, L., Hutchison, B., & Hurley, J. (2006). *Economic evaluation across the four faces of prevention: A Canadian perspective*. Hamilton, ON: Centre for Health Economics and Policy Analysis (CHEPA), McMaster University.

Goldzweig, C. L., Towfigh, A., Maglione, M., & Shekelle, P. G. (2009). Costs and benefits of health information technology: New trends from the literature. *Health Affairs, 28*(2), w282-w293.

Gooch, K. L., Smith, D., Wasylak, T., Faris, P. D., Marshall, D. A., Khong, H., et al. (2009). The Alberta hip and knee replacement project: A model for health technology assessment based on comparative effectiveness of clinical pathways. *International Journal of Technology Assessment in Health Care, 25*(2), 113-123.

Good Stewardship Working Group. (2011). The "top 5" lists in primary care: Meeting the responsibility of professionalism. *Archives of Internal Medicine, 71(15), 1385-1390.*

Goodman, D., & Fisher, E. S. (2008). Physician workforce crisis? Wrong diagnosis, wrong prescription. *New England Journal of Medicine, 358*(16), 1658-1657.

Goodwin, S. (2007). Telephone nursing: An emerging practice area. *Nursing Leadership, 20*(4), 38-46.

Gortmaker, S. L., Swinburn, B. A., Levy, D., Carter, R., Mabry, P. L., Finegood, D. T., et al. (2011). Changing the future of obesity: Science, policy, and action. *The Lancet, 378*(9793), 838-847.

Gosden, T., Forland, F., Kristiansen, I. S., Sutton, M., Leese, B., Giuffrida, A., et al. (2001). Impact of payment method on behaviour of primary care physicians: A systematic review. *Journal of Health Services Research and Policy, 6*(1), 44-55.

Gospodinov, N., & Irvine, I. (2009). Tobacco taxes and regressivity. *Journal of Health Economics, 28*(2), 375-384.

Grabowski, D. C. (2006). The cost-effectiveness of noninstitutional long-term care services: Review and synthesis of the most recent evidence. *Medical Care Research and Review, 63*(1), 3-28.

Grabowski, D. C., Orfaly Cadigan, R., Miller, E. A., Stevenson, D. G., Clark, M., & Mor, V. (2010). Supporting home- and community-based care: Views of long-term care specialists. *Medical Care Research and Review, 67*(Suppl. 4), 82S-101S.

Grabowski, D. C., Stewart, K., Broderick, S., & Coots, L. (2008). Predictors of nursing home hospitalization: A review of the literature. *Medical Care Research and Review, 65*(1), 3-39.

Graefe, P., & Bourns, A. (2009). The gradual defederalization of Canadian health policy. *Publius: The Journal of Federalism, 39*(1), 187-209.

Graff Zivin, J., & Neidell, M. (2010). Medical technology adoption, uncertainty, and irreversibilities: Is a bird in the hand really worth more than in the bush? *Health Economics, 19*(2), 142-153.

Graham, H. (2004). Social determinants and their unequal distribution: Clarifying policy understandings. *Milbank Quarterly, 82*(1), 101-124.

Grandchamp, C., & Gardiol, L. (2011). Does a mandatory telemedicine call prior to visiting a physician reduce costs or simply attract good risks? *Health Economics*.

Gray, J. A. M. (1999). Postmodern medicine. *The Lancet, 354*(9189), 1550-1553.

Gray, L., Berg, K., Fries, B., Henrard, J.-C., Hirdes, J., Steel, K., et al. (2009). Sharing clinical information across care settings: The birth of an integrated assessment system. *BMC Health Services Research, 9*(71).

Gray, L., & Wootton, R. (2008). Innovations in aged care comprehensive geriatric assessment "online." *Australasian Journal of Ageing, 27*(4), 205-208.

Greaves, C., Sheppard, K., Abraham, C., Hardeman, W., Roden, M., Evans, P., et al. (2011). Systematic review of reviews of intervention components associated with increased effectiveness in dietary and physical activity interventions. *BMC Public Health, 11*(119).

Greenfield, D., Nugus, P., Travaglia, J., & Braithwaite, J. (2011). Factors that shape the development of interprofessional improvement initiatives in health organisations. *BMJ Quality & Safety, 20*(4), 332-337.

Greenhalgh, T., Potts, H. W. W., Wong, G., Bark, P., & Swinglehurst, D. (2009). Tensions and paradoxes in electronic patient record research: A systematic literature review using the meta-narrative method. *Milbank Quarterly, 87*(4), 729-788.

Greenhalgh, T., Robert, G., MacFarlane, F., Bate, P., & Kyriakidou, O. (2004). Diffusion of innovations in service organizations: Systematic review and recommendations. *Milbank Quarterly, 82*(4), 581-629.

Greß, S., Delnoij, D. M. J., & Groenewegen, P. P. (2006). Managing primary care behaviour through payment systems and financial incentives. In R. B. Saltman, A. Rico, & W. Boerma (Eds.), *Primary care in the driver's seat? Organizational reform in European primary care*. Maidenhead: Open University Press.

Griener, G. (2002). Defining medical necessity: Challenges and implications (Canada). *Health Law Review, 10*(3), 6-8.

Grignon, M., Paris, V., & Polton, D. (2002). *Influence of physician payment methods on the efficiency of the health care system*. Saskatoon, SK: Commission on the Future of Health Care in Canada.

Grignon, M., Paris, V., & Polton, D. (2004). Influence of physician payment methods on the efficiency of the health care system. In P.-G. Forest, G. P. Marchildon, & T.

McIntosh (Eds.), *Changing health care in Canada: The Romanow papers, Vol. 2.* Toronto, ON: University of Toronto Press.

Grimshaw, J., Shirran, L., Thomas, R., Mowatt, G., Fraser, C., Bero, L., et al. (2001). Changing provider behaviour: An overview of systematic reviews of interventions. *Medical Care, 39*(8 Suppl. 2), II-2-II-45.

Grogan, C. M. (2011). Political moments and persistent policy questions: Pricing, volume, and organs. *Journal of Health Politics, Policy and Law, 36*(4), 643-647.

Grol, R. P. T. M., Bosch, M. C., Hulscher, M. E. J. L., Eccles, M. P., & Wensing, M. (2007). Planning and studying improvement in patient care: The use of theoretical perspectives. *Milbank Quarterly, 85*(1), 93-138.

Grootendorst, P., & Hollis, A. (2011). *Managing pharmaceutical expenditure: Overview and options for Canada.* Ottawa: Canadian Health Services Research Foundation.

Grosse, S. D., Teutsch, S. M., & Haddix, A. C. (2007). Lessons from cost-effectiveness research for United States public health policy. *Annual Review of Public Health, 28*(1), 365-391.

Grossmann, C., Goolsby, A. W., Olsen, L., & McGinnis, J. M. (Eds.). (2010). *Clinical data as the basic staple of health learning: Creating and protecting a public good* [Workshop summary]. Washington, DC: National Academies Press.

Gruber, J., Sen, A., & Stabile, M. (2003). Estimating price elasticities when there is smuggling: The sensitivity of smoking to price in Canada. *Journal of Health Economics, 22*(5), 821-842.

Gruen, R. L., Pearson, S. D., & Brennan, T. A. (2004). Physician-citizens: Public roles and professional obligations. *JAMA, 291*(1), 94-98.

Guldenmund, F. W. (2000). The nature of safety culture: A review of theory and research. *Safety Science, 34*(1-3), 215-257.

Guven-Uslu, P. (2006). Uses of performance metrics in clinical and managerial networks. *Public Money & Management, 26*(2), 95-100.

Hacker, J. S. (2004). Dismantling the health care state? Political institutions, public policies and the comparative politics of health reform. *British Journal of Political Science, 34*(4), 693-724.

Haggerty, J. L., Pineault, R., Beaulieu, M.-D., Brunelle, Y., Gauthier, J., Goulet, F., et al. (2008). Practice features associated with patient-reported accessibility, continuity, and coordination of primary health care. *Annals of Family Medicine, 6*(2), 116-123.

Halfon, P., Eggli, Y., Pretre-Rochrbach, I., Meylan, D., Marazzi, A., & Burnand, B. (2006). Validation of the potentially avoidable hospital readmission rate as a routine indicator of the quality of hospital care. *Medical Care, 44*(11), 972-981.

Hallam, A. (2008). *The effectiveness of interventions to address health inequalities in the early years: A review of relevant literature.* Edinburgh: Scottish Government.

Halligan, M., & Zecevic, A. (2011). Safety culture in healthcare: A review of concepts, dimensions, measures and progress. *BMJ Quality & Safety, 20*(4), 338-343.

Ham, C. (2010). The ten characteristics of the high-performing chronic care system. *Health Economics, Policy and Law, 5*(1), 71-90.

Hamburg, M. A., & Collins, F. S. (2010). The path to personalized medicine. *New England Journal of Medicine, 363*(4), 301-304.

Hancock, T. (1986). Lalonde and beyond: Looking back at "A New Perspective on the Health of Canadians." *Health Promotion International, 1*, 93-100.

Hankivsky, O., Friesen, J., Varcoe, C., MacPhail, F., Greaves, L., & Spencer, C. (2004). Expanding economic costing in health care: Values, gender and diversity. *Canadian Public Policy, 30*(3), 257-282.

Hanley, G. E., & Morgan, S. (2009). Chronic catastrophes: Exploring the concentration and sustained nature of ambulatory prescription drug expenditures in the population of British Columbia, Canada. *Social Science & Medicine, 68*(5), 919-924.

Harper, S., Lynch, J., & Smith, G. D. (2011). Social determinants and the decline of cardiovascular diseases: Understanding the links. *Annual Review of Public Health, 32*(1), 39-69.

Hartwig, J. (2008). What drives health care expenditure? Baumol's model of "unbalanced growth" revisited. *Journal of Health Economics, 27*(3), 603-623.

Harvey, S., Rowan, K., Harrison, D., & Black, N. (2010). Using clinical databases to evaluate healthcare interventions. *International Journal of Technology Assessment in Health Care, 26*(1), 86-94.

Hassan, T. B. (2003). Clinical decision units in the emergency department: Old concepts, new paradigms, and refined gate keeping. *Emergency Medicine Journal, 20*(2), 123-125.

Hauck, K., & Street, A. (2006). Performance assessment in the context of multiple objectives: A multivariate multilevel analysis. *Journal of Health Economics, 25*(2006), 1029-1048.

Hauck, K., & Street, A. (2007). Do targets matter? A comparison of English and Welsh national health priorities. *Health Economics, 16*(3), 275-290.

Hawe, P., & Shiell, A. (1995). Preserving innovation under increasing accountability pressures: The health promotion investment portfolio approach. *Health Promotion Journal of Australia, 5*(1), 4-9.

Hawes, C., & Phillips, C. D. (2007). Defining quality in assisted living: Comparing apples, oranges, and broccoli. *The Gerontologist, 47*(Suppl. 1), 40-50.

Hawker, G. A., Wright, J. G., Coyte, P. C., Williams, J. I., Harvey, B., Glazier, R., et al. (2001). Determining the need for hip and knee arthroplasty: The role of clinical severity and patients' preferences. *Medical Care, 39*(3), 206-216.

Haynes, B., & Haines, A. (1998). Barriers and bridges to evidence based clinical practice. *BMJ, 317*(7153), 273-276.

Häyrinen, K., Saranto, K., & Nykänen, P. (2008). Definition, structure, content, use and impacts of electronic health records: A review of the research literature. *International Journal of Medical Informatics, 77*(5), 291-304.

Health Canada. (2004). *A 10-year plan to strengthen health care.* Retrieved 15 November 2011 from http://www.hc-sc.gc.ca/hcs-sss/delivery-prestation/fptcollab/2004-fmm-rpm/index-eng.php

Health Canada. (2008a). Administration and compliance. In *Canada Health Act annual report, 2007–2008* (Chapter 2). Retrieved from http://www.hc-sc.gc.ca/hcs-sss/pubs/cha-lcs/2008-cha-lcs-ar-ra/index-eng.php#Chapt2

Health Canada. (2008b). *Healthy Canadians: A federal report on comparable health indicators.* Retrieved 25 August 2011 from http://www.hc-sc.gc.ca/hcs-sss/alt_formats/hpb-dgps/pdf/pubs/system-regime/2008-fed-comp-indicat/index-eng.pdf

Health Canada. (2010). *Canada Health Act annual report, 2009–2010.* Retrieved from http://www.hc-sc.gc.ca/hcs-sss/pubs/cha-lcs/2010-cha-lcs-ar-ra/index-eng.php

Health Council of Canada. (2009a). Getting it right: Case studies of effective management of chronic disease using primary health care teams. Toronto, ON: Author. Retrieved 15 August 2011 from http://www.healthcouncilcanada.ca/docs/rpts/2009/CaseStudies_FINAL.pdf

Health Council of Canada. (2009b). *Value for money: Making Canadian health care stronger.* Retrieved from http://www.healthcouncilcanada.ca/docs/rpts/2009/HCC_VFMReport_WEB.pdf

Health Economics Research Group, Office of Health Economics, & Rand Europe. (2008). *Medical research: What's it worth? Estimating the economic benefits from medical research in the UK.* Uxbridge, Middlesex: Brunel University, Health Economics Research Group.

Hébert, R. (2011). Public long-term care insurance: A way to ensure sustainable continuity of care for frail older people. *HealthcarePapers, 11*(1), 69-75.

Heiber, S., & Deber, R. (1987). Banning extra-billing in Canada: Just what the doctor didn't order. *Canadian Public Policy, 13*(1), 62-74.

Heller, R. F., Gemmell, I., Wilson, E. C. F., Fordham, R., & Smith, R. D. (2006). Using economic analyses for local priority setting: The population cost-impact approach. *Applied Health Economics and Health Policy, 5*(1), 45-54.

Hepburn, C. (2006). Regulation by prices, quantities, or both: A review of instrument choice. *Oxford Review of Economic Policy, 22*(2), 226-247.

Hernandez, M. (2005). Assisted living in all of its guises. *Generations, 29*(4), 16-23.

Herr, A. (2008). Cost and technical efficiency of German hospitals: Does ownership matter? *Health Economics, 17*(9), 1057-1071.

Herr, A., Schmitz, H., & Augurzky, B. (2011). Profit efficiency and ownership of German hospitals. *Health Economics, 20*(6), 660-674.

Herring, L. (2009). Lean experience in primary care. *Quality in Primary Care, 17*(4), 271-275.

Hewett, D. G., Watson, B. M., Gallois, C., Ward, M., & Leggett, B. A. (2009). Communication in medical records. *Journal of Language and Social Psychology, 28*(2), 119-138.

Hirdes, J. P. (2001). Long-term care funding in Canada: A policy mosaic. *Journal of Aging and Social Policy, 13*(2/3), 69.

Hirdes, J. P. (2006). Addressing the health needs of frail elderly people: Ontario's experience with an integrated health information system. *Age and Ageing, 35*(4), 329-331.

Hirdes, J. P., Frijters, D. H., & Teare, G. F. (2003). The MDS-CHESS Scale: A new measure to predict mortality in institutionalized older people. *Journal of the American Geriatrics Society, 51*(1), 96-100.

Hirdes, J., Ljunggren, G., Morris, J., Frijters, D., Finne Soveri, H., Gray, L., et al. (2008). Reliability of the InterRAI suite of assessment instruments: A 12-country study of an integrated health information system. *BMC Health Services Research, 8*(277).

Hirdes, J., Poss, J., & Curtin-Telegdi, N. (2008). The method for assigning priority levels (MAPLe): A new decision-support system for allocating home care resources. *BMC Medicine, 6*(9).

Hirdes, J., Sinclair, D. G., King, J., Tuttle, P., & McKinley, J. (2003). From anecdotes to evidence: Complex continuing care at the dawn of the information age in Ontario. In B. E. Fries (Ed.), *Implementing the resident assessment instrument: Case studies of policymaking for long-term care in eight countries.* New York: Milbank Memorial Fund.

Hoff, T., Jameson, L., Hannan, E., & Flink, E. (2004). A review of the literature examining linkages between organizational factors, medical errors, and patient safety. *Medical Care Research and Review, 61*(1), 3-37.

Hoff, T. J., & Soerensen, C. (2011). No payment for preventable complications: Reviewing the early literature for content, guidance, and impressions. *Quality Management in Health Care, 20*(1), 62-75.

Hoffman, A., & Pearson, S. D. (2009). "Marginal medicine": Targeting comparative effectiveness research to reduce waste. *Health Affairs, 28*(4), w710-w718.

Hofmann, B. M. (2008). Why ethics should be part of health technology assessment. *International Journal of Technology Assessment in Health Care, 24*(4), 423-429.

Hogan, S., & Hogan, S. (2004). How an ageing population will affect health care. In G. P. Marchildon, T. A. McIntosh, & P.-G. Forest (Eds.), *The fiscal sustainability of health care in Canada. Romanow Papers, Vol. 1.* Toronto, ON: University of Toronto Press.

Hollander, M. J. (1995). The continuum of care: An integrated system of service delivery. In E. Sawyer & M. Stephenson (Eds.), *Continuing the care: The issues and challenges for long-term care.* Ottawa: CHA Press.

Hollander, M. J., & Chappell, N. L. (2007). A comparative analysis of costs to government for home care and long-term residential care services, standardized for client care needs. *Canadian Journal on Aging, 26*(Suppl. S1), 149-161.

Hollander, M. J., & Walker, E. R. (1998). *Report of continuing care organization and terminology* (No. 0662274911 9780662274919). Ottawa: Federal/Provincial/Territorial Committee of Officials.

Hollingsworth, B. (2008). The measurement of efficiency and productivity of health care delivery. *Health Economics, 17,* 1107-1128.

Hollis, A. (2009). *Generic drug pricing and procurement a policy for Alberta.* Calgary, AB: University of Calgary, School of Policy Studies.

Hollis, A. (2010). *Generic drug pricing in Canada: Components of the value chain.* Calgary, AB: University of Calgary.

Hollis, A., & Law, S. (2004). A national formulary for Canada. *Canadian Public Policy/Analyse de politiques, 30*(4), 445-452.

Homer, J., & Hirsch, G. (2006). System dynamics modeling for public health: Background and opportunities. *American Journal of Public Health, 96,* 452-458.

Hood, C. (2002). The risk game and the blame game. *Government and Opposition, 37*(1), 15-37.

Hopkins, M. M., Martin, P. A., Nightingale, P., Kraft, A., & Mahdi, S. (2007). The myth of the biotech revolution: An assessment of technological, clinical and organisational change. *Research Policy, 36*(4), 566-589.

Houston, C. S. (2002). *Steps on the road to Medicare: Why Saskatchewan led the way.* Montreal: McGill-Queen's University Press.

Howard, M., Goertzen, J., Hutchison, B., Kaczorowski, J., & Morris, K. (2007). Patient satisfaction with care for urgent health problems: A survey of family practice patients. *Annals of Family Medicine, 5*(5), 419-424.

Howlett, M. (2009). Policy analytical capacity and evidence-based policy-making: Lessons from Canada. *Canadian Public Administration, 52*(2), 153-175.

Huerta, T. R., Thompson, M. A., & Ford, E. W. (2011). The role of safe practices in hospitals' total factor productivity. *Journal of Healthcare Leadership, 3,* 1-7.

Hughes, B., Joshi, I., & Wareham, J. (2008). Health 2.0 and Medicine 2.0: Tensions and controversies in the field. *Journal of Medical Internet Research, 10*(3), e23.

Hughes, S. L., Ulasevich, A., Weaver, F. M., Henderson, W., Manheim, L., Kubal, J. D., et al. (1997). Impact of home care on hospital days: A meta analysis. *Health Services Research, 32*(4), 415-432.

Hunter, S., & Ritchie, P. (Eds.). (2007). *Co-production and personalisation in social care: Changing relationships in the provision of social care.* London: Jessica Kingsley Publishers.

Hurley, J., & Card, R. (1996). Global physician budgets as common-property resources: Some implications for physicians and medical associations. *Canadian Medical Association Journal, 154*(8), 1161-1168.

Hurley, J. E., Vaithianathan, R., Crossley, T. F., & Cobb-Clark, D. (2001). *Parallel private health insurance in Australia: A cautionary tale and lessons for Canada.* Hamilton, ON: Centre for Health Economics and Policy Analysis, McMaster University.

Hurst, J. (2010). Effective ways to realise policy reforms in health systems. In OECD (Ed.), *OECD health working paper* (Vol. 50). Paris: OECD.

Husereau, D., Boucher, M., & Noorani, H. (2010). Priority setting for health technology assessment at CADTH. *International Journal of Technology Assessment in Health Care, 26*(3), 341-347.

Hussey, P. S., De Vries, H., Romley, J., Wang, M. C., Chen, S. S., Shekelle, P. G., et al. (2009). A systematic review of health care efficiency measures. *Health Services Research, 44*(3), 784-805.

Hussey, P. S., Sorbero, M. E., Mehrotra, A., Liu, H., & Damberg, C. L. (2009). Episode-based performance measurement and payment: Making it a reality. *Health Affairs, 28*(5), 1406-1417.

Hutchison, B., Abelson, J., & Lavis, J. (2001). Primary care in Canada: So much innovation, so little change. *Health Affairs, 20*(1), 116-131.

Hutchison, B., Levesque, J.-F., Strumpf, E., & Coyle, N. (2011). Primary health care in Canada: Systems in motion. *Milbank Quarterly, 89*(2), 256-288.

Ibargoyen-Roteta, N., Gutierrez-Ibarluzea, I., Asua, J., Benguria-Arrate, G., & Galnares-Cordero, L. (2009). Scanning the horizon of obsolete technologies: Possible sources for their identification. *International Journal of Technology Assessment in Health Care, 25*(3), 249-254.

Iliffe, S., & Shepperd, S. (2002). What do we know about hospital at home? Lessons from international experience. *Applied Health Economics and Health Policy, 1*(3), 141-147.

Imai, M. (1997). *Gemba kaizen: A common sense low-cost approach to management.* Retrieved from http://www.netlibrary.com/urlapi.asp?action=summaryan dv=1andbookid=6975

Isaacs, A. J., Critchley, J. A., Tai, S. S., Buckingham, K., Westley, D., Harridge, S. D., et al. (2007). Exercise Evaluation Randomised Trial (EXERT): A randomised trial comparing GP referral for leisure centre-based exercise, community-based walking and advice only. *Health Technology Assessment, 11*(10), 1-165.

Iversen, T. (1997). The effect of a private sector on the waiting time in a national health service. *Journal of Health Economics, 16*, 381-396.

Jack, B. W., Chetty, V. K., Johnson, A. E., Forsythe, S. R., O'Donnell, J. K., Manasseh, C., et al. (2009). A reengineered hospital discharge program to decrease rehospitalization: A randomized trial. *Annals of Internal Medicine, 150*(3), 178-187.

Jackman, M. (1994). Regulation of private health care under the Canada Health Act and the Canadian Charter. *Constitutional Forum, 6*, 54-60.

Jackson, T. (1985). On the limitations of health promotion. *Community Health Studies, 9*(1), 1-9.

Jackson, T. J., Michel, J. L., Roberts, R. F., Jorm, C. M., & Wakefield, J. G. (2009). A classification of hospital-acquired diagnoses for use with routine hospital data. *Medical Journal of Australia, 191*(10), 544-548.

Jacobs, P., Moffatt, J., Rapoport, J., & Bell, N. (2010). *Primary care economics.* Edmonton, AB: Institute of Health Economics. Retrieved 15 August 2011 from http://www.ihe.ca/documents/Primary%20Care%20Economics%20Final%20Report.pdf

James, P. D., Wilkins, R., Detsky, A. S., Tugwell, P., & Manuel, D. G. (2007). Avoidable mortality by neighbourhood income in Canada: 25 years after the establishment of universal health insurance. *Journal of Epidemiology and Community Health, 61*(4), 287-296.

Jansen, I. (2011). Residential long-term care: Public solutions to access and quality problems. *HealthcarePapers, 10*(1), 8-22.

Jaques, E. (2006). *Requisite organization: A total system for effective managerial organization and managerial leadership for the 21st century.* Arlington, VA: Cason Hall.

Järvinen, T. L. N., Sievänen, H., Kannus, P., Jokihaara, J., & Khan, K. M. (2011). The true cost of pharmacological disease prevention. *BMJ, 342.*

Jayadev, A., & Stiglitz, J. (2009). Two ideas to increase innovation and reduce pharmaceutical costs and prices. *Health Affairs, 28*(1), w165-w168.

Jegers, M., Kesteloot, K., De Graeve, D., & Gilles, W. (2002). A typology for provider payment systems in health care. *Health Policy, 60(3),* 255-273.

Jérôme-Forget, M., White, J., & Wiener, J. M. (Eds.). (1995). *Health care reform through internal markets: Experience and proposals.* Montreal and Washington: Institute for Research on Public Policy / Brookings Institution.

Jha, A. K., Chan, D. C., Ridgway, A. B., Franz, C., & Bates, D. W. (2009). Improving safety and eliminating redundant tests: Cutting costs in U.S. hospitals. *Health Affairs, 28*(5), 1475-1484.

Johansson, T., & Wild, C. (2010). Telemedicine in acute stroke management: Systematic review. *International Journal of Technology Assessment in Health Care, 26*(2), 149-155.

Johansson, T., & Wild, C. (2011). Telerehabilitation in stroke care: A systematic review. *Journal of Telemedicine and Telecare, 17,* 1-6.

Johnston, L., Lardner, C., & Jepson, R. (2008). *Overview of evidence relating to shifting the balance of care: A contribution to the knowledge base.* Edinburgh: Scottish Government Social Research.

Johri, M., Béland, F., & Bergman, H. (2003). International experiments in integrated care for the elderly: A synthesis of the evidence. *International Journal of Geriatric Psychiatry, 18*(3), 222-235.

Jordan, J. (2009). Federalism and health care cost containment in comparative perspective. *Publius: The Journal of Federalism, 39*(1), 164-186.

Joshi, N. P., Stahnisch, F. W., & Noseworthy, T. W. (2009). *Reassessment of health technologies obsolescence and waste.* Ottawa: Canadian Agency for Drugs and Technologies in Health.

Joumard, I., André, C., & Nicq, C. (2010). Health care systems: Efficiency and institutions. *OECD Economics Department Working Papers, 769.*

Joumard, I., Andre, C., Nicq, C., & Chatal, O. (2008). Health status determinants: Lifestyle, environment, health care resources and efficiency. *OECD Economics Department Working Papers, 627.*

Joumard, I., Hoeller, P., André, C., & Nicq, C. (2010). *Health care systems: Efficiency and policy settings.* Paris: OECD.

Kalisch, B. J., Friese, C., Choi, S. H., & Rochman, M. (2011). Hospital nurse staffing: Choice of measure matters. *Medical Care, 49*(8), 775-779.

Kane, R., Shamliyan, T., Mueller, C., Duval, S., & Wilt, T. (2007). The Association of Registered Nurse staffing levels and patient outcomes: Systematic review and meta-analysis. *Medical Care, 45*(12), 1195-1204.

Kantarevic, J., Kralj, B., & Weinkauf, D. (2011). Enhanced fee-for-service model and physician productivity: Evidence from family health groups in Ontario. *Journal of Health Economics, 30*(1), 99-111.

Kapczynski, A., Chaifetz, S., Katz, Z., & Benkler, Y. (2005). Addressing global health inequities: An open licensing approach for university innovations. *Berkeley Technology Law Journal, 20*(2), 1031-1114.

Kaplan, H. C., Brady, P. W., Dritz, M. C., Hooper, D. K., Linam, W. M., Froehle, C. M., et al. (2010). The influence of context on quality improvement success in health care: A systematic review of the literature. *Milbank Quarterly, 88*(4), 500-559.

Kaptchuk, T. J. (2001). The double-blind, randomized, placebo-controlled trial: Gold standard or golden calf? *Journal of Clinical Epidemiology, 54*(6), 541-549.

Karnieli-Miller, O., Vu, T. R., Holtman, M. C., Clyman, S. G., & Inui, T. S. (2010). Medical students' professionalism narratives: A window on the informal and hidden curriculum. *Academic Medicine, 85*(1), 124-133.

Katz, S. J., Charles, C., Lomas, J., & Welch, H. G. (1997). Physician relations in Canada: Shooting inward as the circle closes. *Journal of Health Politics Policy and Law, 22*(6), 1413-1431.

Katz, A., Glazier, R. H., & Vijayaraghavan, J. (2009). *The health and economic consequences of achieving a high-quality primary healthcare system in Canada. Applying what works in Canada: Closing the gap.* Ottawa: Canadian Health Services Research Foundation.

Katzmarzyk, P. T., & Janssen, I. (2004). The economic costs associated with physical inactivity and obesity in Canada: An update. *Canadian Journal of Applied Physiology, 29*(1), 90-115.

Kaufman, H. (1975). The natural history of human organizations. *Administration and Society, 7*(2), 131-149.

Kaufman, H. (1976). *Are government organizations immortal?* Washington: Brookings Institution.

Kaufman, H. (1991). *Time, chance, and organizations: Natural selection in a perilous environment.* Chatham, NJ: Chatham House Publishers.

Kearns, N., & Pursell, L. (2011). Time for a paradigm change? Tracing the institutionalisation of health impact assessment in the Republic of Ireland across health and environmental sectors. *Health Policy, 99*(2), 91-96.

Keefe, J., & Rajnovich, B. (2007). To pay or not to pay: Examining underlying principles in the debate on financial support for family caregivers. *Canadian Journal on Aging, 26*(Suppl. S1), 77-89.

Kelley, J. M., & Kaptchuk, T. J. (2010). Group analysis versus individual response: The inferential limits of randomized controlled trials. *Contemporary Clinical Trials, 31*(5), 423-428.

Kelly, M., Morgan, A., Ellis, S., Younger, T., Huntley, J., & Swann, C. (2010). Evidence-based public health: A review of the experience of the National Institute of Health and Clinical Excellence (NICE) of developing public health guidance in England. *Social Science & Medicine, 71*(6), 1056-1062.

Kempe, A., Bunik, M., Ellis, J., Magid, D., Hegarty, T., Dickinson, L. M., et al. (2006). How safe is triage by an after-hours telephone call center? *Pediatrics, 118*(2), 457-463.

Kennedy, I. (2001). *The report of the public inquiry into children's heart surgery at the Bristol Royal Infirmary 1984-1995: Learning from Bristol.* Norwich, UK: The Stationery Office.

Kent, T. (2004). Paul Martin's sugar-daddy federalism, donating to a favoured cause – health care. *Policy Options, 25*(10), 29-34.

Kershaw, P., Warburton, B., Anderson, L., Hertzman, C., Irwin, L. G., & Forer, B. (2010). The economic costs of early vulnerability in Canada. *Canadian Journal of Public Health, 101*(6), S8-11.

Keyhani, S., Kim, A., Mann, M., & Korenstein, D. (2011). A new independent authority is needed to issue national health care guidelines. *Health Affairs, 30*(2), 256-265.

Kickbusch, I. (2010). Health in all policies: Where to from here? *Health Promotion International, 25*(3), 261-264.

Killburn, M. R., & Karoly, L. A. (2008). *The economics of early childhood policy: What the dismal science has to say about investing in children.* Santa Monica: RAND Corporation.

Kimberly, J. R., & de Pouvourville, G. (1993). Managerial innovation, migration, and DRGs. In J. R. Kimberly & G. de Pouvourville and Associates (Eds.), *The migration of managerial innovation: Diagnosis related groups and health care administration in Western Europe.* San Francisco: Jossey-Bass.

Kimberly, J. R., de Pouvourville, G., & D'Aunno, T. (Eds.). (2008). *The globalization of managerial innovation in health care.* Cambridge: Cambridge University Press.

King, L., Gill, T., Allender, S., & Swinburn, B. (2011). Best practice principles for community-based obesity prevention: Development, content and application. *Obesity Reviews, 12*(5), 329-338.

Kingwell, B. A., Anderson, G. P., Duckett, S. J., Hoole, E. A., Jackson-Pulver, L. R., Khachigian, L. M., et al. (2006). Evaluation of NHMRC funded research completed in 1992, 1997 and 2003: Gains in knowledge, health and wealth. *Medical Journal of Australia, 184*(6), 282-286.

Kirch, D. G. (2010). The Flexnerian legacy in the 21st century. *Academic Medicine, 85*(2), 190-192.

Klersy, C., De Silvestri, A., Gabutti, G., Raisaro, A., Curti, M., Regoli, F. O., et al. (2011). Economic impact of remote patient monitoring: An integrated economic model derived from a meta-analysis of randomized controlled trials in heart failure. *European Journal of Heart Failure, 13*(4), 450-459.

Klersy, C., De Silvestri, A., Gabutti, G., Regoli, F., & Auricchio, A. (2009). A meta-analysis of remote monitoring of heart failure patients. *Journal of the American College of Cardiology, 54*(18), 1683-1694.

Klomp, J., & de Haan, J. (2009). Is the political system really related to health? *Social Science & Medicine, 69*(1), 36-46.

Ko, H., Turner, T., & Finnigan, M. (2011). Systematic review of safety checklists for use by medical care teams in acute hospital settings – limited evidence of effectiveness. *BMC Health Services Research, 11*(211).

Kohn, L. T., Corrigan, J. M., & Donaldson, M. S. (Eds.). (2000). *To err is human: Building a safer health system.* Washington, DC: National Academy Press.

Kondo, N., Sembajwe, G., Kawachi, I., van Dam, R. M., Subramanian, S. V., & Yamagata, Z. (2009). Income inequality, mortality, and self rated health: Meta-analysis of multilevel studies. *BMJ, 339*, b4471.

Konetzka, R., Spector, W., & Limcangco, M. (2008). Reducing hospitalizations from long-term care settings. *Medical Care Research and Review, 65*(1), 40-66.

Korp, P. (2008). The symbolic power of "healthy lifestyles." *Health Sociology Review, 17*(1), 18-26.

Kraut, A., Walld, R., Tate, R., & Mustard, C. (2001). Impact of diabetes on employment and income in Manitóba, Canada. *Diabetes Care, 24*(1), 64-68.

Kreindler, S. A. (2010). Policy strategies to reduce waits for elective care: A synthesis of international evidence. *British Medical Bulletin, 95*(1), 7-32.

Krieger, N. (2001). Theories for social epidemiology in the 21st century: An ecosocial perspective. *International Journal of Epidemiology, 30*(4), 668-677.

Kringos, D., Boerma, W., Hutchinson, A., van der Zee, J., & Groenewegen, P. (2010). The breadth of primary care: A systematic literature review of its core dimensions. *BMC Health Services Research, 10*(65).

Kronebusch, K. (2009). Quality information and fragmented markets: Patient responses to hospital volume thresholds. *Journal of Health Politics Policy and Law, 34*(5), 777-827.

Laffont, J.-J., & Tirole, J. (1993). *A theory of incentives in procurement and regulation.* Cambridge, MA: The MIT Press.

Laframboise, H. L. (1973). Health policy: Breaking the problem down into more manageable segments. *Canadian Medical Association Journal, 108*(3), 388-391.

Lagu, T., Rothberg, M. B., Nathanson, B. H., Pekow, P. S., Steingrub, J. S., & Lindenauer, P. K. (2011). The relationship between hospital spending and mortality in patients with sepsis. *Archives of Internal Medicine, 171*(4), 292-299.

Laing, A., Hogg, G., & Winkelman, D. (2004). Healthcare and the information revolution: Re-configuring the healthcare service encounter. *Health Service Management Research, 17*, 188-199.

Lalonde, M. (1974). *A new perspective on the health of Canadians: A working document.* Ottawa: Health and Welfare.

Lamb, S. E., Bartlett, H. P., Ashley, A., & Bird, W. (2002). Can lay-led walking programmes increase physical activity in middle aged adults? A randomised controlled trial. *Journal of Epidemiology and Community Health, 56*(4), 246-252.

Lambooij, M. S., Engelfriet, P., & Westert, G. P. (2010). Diffusion of innovations in health care: Does the structural context determine its direction? *International Journal of Technology Assessment in Health Care, 26*(4), 415-420.

Landon, S., McMillan, M. L., Muralidharan, V., & Parsons, M. (2006). Does healthcare spending crowd out other provincial government expenditures? *Canadian Public Policy, 32*(2), 121-141.

Landon, S., & Ryan, D. L. (1997). The political costs of taxes and government spending. *Canadian Journal of Economics, 30*(1), 85-111.

Lane, D., & Husemann, E. (2007). System dynamics mapping of acute patient flows. *Journal of the Operational Research Society, 59*(2), 213-224.

Lang, T., Hodge, M., Olson, V., Romano, P., & Kravitz, R. (2004). Nurse-patient ratios: A systematic review on the effects of nurse staffing on patient, nurse employee, and hospital outcomes. *Journal of Nursing Administration, 34*(7-8), 326-337.

Langley, G. J., Moen, R., Nolan, K. M., Nolan, T. W., Norman, C. L., & Provost, L. P. (2009). *The improvement guide: A practical approach to enhancing organizational performance* (2nd ed.). San Francisco: Jossey-Bass.

Lanham, H. J., McDaniel, R. R., Jr., Crabtree, B. F., Miller, W. L., Stange, K. C., Tallia, A. F., et al. (2009). How improving practice relationships among clinicians and nonclinicians can improve quality in primary care. *Joint Commission Journal on Quality and Patient Safety, 35*(9), 457-466.

Lankshear, A. J., Sheldon, T. A., & Maynard, A. (2005). Nurse staffing and healthcare outcomes: A systematic review of the international research evidence. *Advances in Nursing Science, 28*(2), 163-174.

Laporte, A., Nauenberg, E., & Shen, L. (2008). Aging, social capital, and health care utilization in Canada. *Health Economics, Policy and Law, 3*(4), 393-411.

Laurant, M., Harmsen, M., Wollersheim, H., Grol, R., Faber, M., & Sibbald, B. (2009). The impact of nonphysician clinicians: Do they improve the quality and cost-effectiveness of health care services? *Medical Care Research & Review, 66*(Suppl. 6), 36S-89S.

Lavieri, M., & Puterman, M. (2009). Optimizing nursing human resource planning in British Columbia. *Health Care Management Science, 12*(2), 119-128.

Lavis, J. N., Wilson, M. G., Grimshaw, J. M., Haynes, R. B., Ouimet, M., Raina, P., et al. (2010). Supporting the use of health technology assessments in policy making about health systems. *International Journal of Technology Assessment in Health Care, 26*(4), 405-414.

Lavoie, J. G., Forget, E. L., Dahl, M., Martens, P. J., & O'Neil, J. D. (2011). Is it worthwhile to invest in home care? *Healthcare Policy, 6*(4), 35-48.

Law, M. R., & Morgan, S. G. (2011). Purchasing prescription drugs in Canada: Hang together or hang separately? *Healthcare Policy, 6*(4), 22-26.

Lawn, S., Battersby, M., Lindner, H., Mathews, R., Morris, S., Wells, L., et al. (2009). What skills do primary health care professionals need to provide effective self-management support? Seeking consumer perspectives. *Australian Journal of Primary Health, 15*(1), 37-44.

Lazar, H., St-Hilaire, F., & Tremblay, J.-F. (2004). Vertical fiscal imbalance: Myth or reality? In H. Lazar & F. St-Hilaire (Eds.), *Money, politics and health care: Reconstructing the federal-provincial partnership.* Montreal and Kingston: Institute for Research on Public Policy and Institute of Intergovernmental Relations.

Le Goff, P. (2004). *Home care sector in Canada: Economic problems.* Ottawa: Parliamentary Research Branch.

Le Grand, J. (2003). *Motivation, agency and public policy: Of knights and knaves, pawns and queens.* Oxford: Oxford University Press.

Le Grand, J., Mays, N., & Mulligan, J.-A. (Eds.). (1998). *Learning from the NHS internal market. A review of the evidence.* London: Kings Fund.

Leatherman, S., & Warrick, L. (2008). Effectiveness of decision aids a review of the evidence. *Medical Care Research and Review, 65*(6), 79S-116S.

Lee, R. C., Marshall, D., Waddell, C., Hailey, D., & Juzwishin, D. (2003). Health technology assessment, research, and implementation within a health region in Alberta, Canada. *International Journal of Technology Assessment in Health Care, 19*(3), 513-520.

Lee, T. H. (2004). "Me-too" products – Friend or foe? *New England Journal of Medicine, 350*(3), 211-212.

Leeson, H. A. (2002). *Constitutional jurisdiction over health and health care services in Canada.* Saskatoon, SK: Commission on the Future of Health Care in Canada.

Leeson, H. A. (2004). Constitutional jurisdiction over health and health care services in Canada. In T. A. McIntosh, P.-G. Forest, & G. P. Marchildon (Eds.), *The governance of health care in Canada. Romanow papers, Vol. 3.* Toronto, ON: University of Toronto Press.

Légaré, F., Ratté, S., Stacey, D., Kryworuchko, J., Gravel, K., Graham, I., et al. (2010). Interventions for improving the adoption of shared decision making by healthcare. *Cochrane Database of Systematic Reviews, 5.*

Léger, P.-T. (2011). *Physician payment mechanisms: Overview and options for Canada.* Ottawa: Canadian Health Services Research Foundation.

Leggat, S. (2007). Effective healthcare teams require effective team members: Defining teamwork competencies. *BMC Health Services Research, 7*(1), 17.

Lehoux, P., Williams-Jones, B., Miller, F., Urbach, D., & Tailliez, S. (2008). What leads to better health care innovation? Arguments for an integrated policy-oriented research agenda. *Journal of Health Services Research and Policy, 13*(4), 251-254.

Leicester, A., & Windmeijer, F. (2004). *The "fat tax": Economic incentives to reduce obesity.* London: Institute for Fiscal Studies.

Leichter, H. (2003). "Evil habits" and "personal choices": Assigning responsibility for health in the 20th century. *Milbank Quarterly, 81*(4), 603-625.

Leijon, M., Bendtsen, P., Nilsen, P., Ekberg, K., & Stahle, A. (2008). Physical activity referrals in Swedish primary health care: Prescriber and patient characteristics, reasons for prescriptions, and prescribed activities. *BMC Health Services Research, 8*(201).

Leistikow, I. P., Kalkman, C. J., & de Bruijn, H. (2011). Why patient safety is such a tough nut to crack. *BMJ, 342.*

Lemieux-Charles, L., & McGuire, W. (2006). What do we know about health care team effectivness? A review of the literature. *Medical Care Research and Review, 63*(3), 263-300.

Léonard, C., Stordeur, S., & Roberfroid, D. (2009). Association between physician density and health care consumption: A systematic review of the evidence. *Health Policy, 91*(2), 121-134.

Leone, T. (2010). How can demography inform health policy? *Health Economics, Policy and Law, 5*(1), 1-11.

Lettieri, E., & Masella, C. (2009). Priority setting for technology adoption at a hospital level: Relevant issues from the literature. *Health Policy, 90*(1), 81-88.

Leutz, W. N. (1999). Five laws for integrating medical and social services: Lessons from the United States and the United Kingdom. *Milbank Quarterly, 77*(1), 77-110.

Leutz, W. (2005). Reflections on integrating medical and social care: Five laws revisited. *Journal of Integrated Care, 13*(5), 3-12.

Levin, L., Goeree, R., Levine, M., Krahn, M., Easty, T., Brown, A., et al. (2011). Coverage with evidence development: The Ontario experience. *International Journal of Technology Assessment in Health Care, 27*(2), 159-168.

Lewis, R., Smith, J., & Harrison, A. (2009). From quasi-market to market in the National Health Service in England: What does this mean for the purchasing of health services? *Journal of Health Services Research and Policy, 14*(1), 44-51.

Lewis, S. (2009). Pay for performance: The wrong time, the wrong place? *Healthcare Quarterly, 12*(3), 8-9.

Lewis, S. (2011). Securing a bright health infomation future: Context, culture and strategies. In C. M. Flood (Ed.), *Data data everywhere: Access and accountability?* Montreal: McGill-Queen's University Press.

Lewis, S., & Kouri, D. (2004). Regionalization: Making sense of the Canadian experience. *HealthcarePapers, 5*(1), 12-31.

Lexchin, J., Bero, L. A., Djulbergovic, B., & Clark, O. (2003). Pharmaceutical industry sponsorship and research outcome and quality: Systematic review. *BMJ, 326*(31 May), 1167-1177.

Leykum, L., Palmer, R., Lanham, H., Jordan, M., McDaniel, R., Noel, P., et al. (2011). Reciprocal learning and chronic care model implementation in primary care: Results from a new scale of learning in primary care settings. *BMC Health Services Research, 11*(44).

Liao, L., Chen, M., Rodrigues, J., Lai, X., & Vuong, S. (in press). A novel web-enabled healthcare solution on HealthVault System. *Journal of Medical Systems*, 1-11. Advance online publication.

Lindsay, N. (1918). *The magic pudding: Being the adventures of Bunyip Bluegum and his friends Bill Barnacle and Sam Sawnoff.* Sydney: Angus and Robertson.

Lipscombe, L. L., Austin, P. C., Manuel, D. G., Shah, B. R., Hux, J. E., & Booth, G. L. (2010). Income-related differences in mortality among people with diabetes mellitus. *Canadian Medical Association Journal, 182*(1), E1-E17.

Lockett, A., Currie, G., Waring, J., Finn, R., & Martin, G. (in press). The role of institutional entrepreneurs in reforming healthcare. *Social Science & Medicine.*

Lomas, J., & Brown, A. D. (2009). Research and advice giving: A functional view of evidence-informed policy advice in a Canadian ministry of health. *Milbank Quarterly, 87*(4), 903-926.

Lord, J., & Hutchison, P. (2003). Individualised support and funding: Building blocks for capacity building and inclusion. *Disability and Society, 18*(1), 71-86.

Lorenz, K. A., Lynn, J., Dy, S. M., Shugarman, L. R., Wilkinson, A., Mularski, R. A., et al. (2008). Evidence for improving palliative care at the end of life: A systematic review. *Annals of Internal Medicine, 148*(2), 147-159.

Lorig, K., Ritter, P., Laurent, D., & Plant, K. (2006). Internet-based chronic disease self-management: A randomized trial. *Medical Care, 44*(11), 964-971.

Lorig, K. R., Ritter, P., Stewart, A. L., Sobel, D. S., William Brown, B. J., Bandura, A., et al. (2001). Chronic disease self-management program: 2-year health status and health care utilization outcomes. *Medical Care, 39*(11), 1217-1223.

Lorig, K. R., Sobel, D. S., Stewart, A. L., Brown, B. W., Jr., Bandura, A., Ritter, P., et al. (1999). Evidence suggesting that a chronic disease self-management program can improve health status while reducing hospitalization: A randomized trial. *Medical Care, 37*(1), 5-14.

Low, L.-F., Yap, M., & Brodaty, H. (2011). A systematic review of different models of home and community care services for older persons. *BMC Health Services Research, 11*(93).

Lowthian, J. A., Curtis, A. J., Cameron, P. A., Comitti, B. L., Tomlinson, J., Stripp, A. M., et al. (2011). Streamlining elective surgery care in a public hospital: The Alfred experience. *Medical Journal of Australia, 194*(9), 448-451.

Ludwig, M., Van Merode, F., & Groot, W. (2010). Principal agent relationships and the efficiency of hospitals. *The European Journal of Health Economics, 11*(3), 291-304.

Lundsgaard, J. (2006). Choice and long-term care in OECD countries: Care outcomes, employment and fiscal sustainability. *European Societies, 8*(3), 361-383.

Luo, W., Morrison, H., de Groh, M., Waters, C., DesMeules, M., Jones-McLean, E., et al. (2007). The burden of adult obesity in Canada. *Chronic Diseases in Canada, 27*(4), 135-144.

Lurie, N. (2002). What the federal government can do about the nonmedical determinants of health. *Health Affairs, 21*(2), 94-106.

Lynch, T. (2011). Greening health care: How hard can that be? *Journal of Health Services Research & Policy, 16*(4), 247-248.

MacAdam, M. (2008). *Frameworks of integrated care for the elderly: A systematic review*. Ottawa: Canadian Policy Research Networks.

MacDonald, B.-J., Andrews, D., & Brown, R. L. (2010). The Canadian elder standard? Pricing the cost of basic needs for the Canadian elderly. *Canadian Journal on Aging, 29*[Special Issue 1], 39-56.

Macgregor, A. (2007). Chronic disease management—PLUS. In J. Dorland & M. A. McColl (Eds.), *Emerging approaches to chronic disease management in primary health care*. Montreal and Kingston: McGill-Queen's University Press.

Macinko, J. A., Shi, L., Starfield, B., & Wulu, J. T. (2003). Income inequality and health: A critical review of the literature. *Medical Care Research and Review, 60*(4), 407-452.

Macinko, J., Starfield, B., & Shi, L. (2003). The contribution of primary care systems to health outcomes within Organization for Economic Cooperation and Development (OECD) countries, 1970–1998. *Health Services Research, 38*(3), 831-865.

MacIntyre, C. R., Ruth, D., & Ansari, Z. (2002). Hospital in the home is cost saving for appropriately selected patients: A comparison with in-hospital care. *International Journal for Quality in Health Care, 14*(4), 285-293.

MacKay, C., Davis, A. M., Mahomed, N., & Badley, E. M. (2009). Expanding roles in orthopaedic care: A comparison of physiotherapist and orthopaedic surgeon recommendations for triage. *Journal of Evaluation in Clinical Practice, 15*(1), 178-183.

Mackenbach, J., & Bakker, M. (2002). *Reducing inequalities in health. A European perspective*. London: Routledge.

Mackenzie, H., & Rachlis, M. (2010). *The sustainability of Medicare*. Ottawa: Canadian Federation of Nurses Unions.

Mackey, H., & Nancarrow, S. (2005). Assistant practitioners: Issues of accountability, delegation and competence. *International Journal of Therapy & Rehabilitation, 12*(8), 331-338.

MacKinnon, J. C. (2004). The arithmetic of health care. *Canadian Medical Association Journal, 171*(6), 603.

Mackintosh, M. (2000). Flexible contracting? Economic cultures and implicit contracts in social care. *Journal of Social Policy, 29*(1), 1-19.

Maddison, A., Asada, Y., & Urquhart, R. (2011). Inequity in access to cancer care: A review of the Canadian literature. *Cancer Causes and Control, 22*(3), 359-366.

Madore, O. (2007). *The impact of economic instruments that promote healthy eating, encourage physical activity and combat obesity: Literature review*. Ottawa: Library of Parliament.

Mahon, R. (2008). Varieties of liberalism: Canadian social policy from the "golden age" to the present. *Social Policy and Administration, 42*(4), 342-361.

Maioni, A. (2010). Health care funding: Needs and reality. *Policy Options, 31*(5), 69-72.

Makarov, D. V., Yu, J. B., Desai, R. A., Penson, D. F., & Gross, C. P. (2011). The association between diffusion of the surgical robot and radical prostatectomy rates. *Medical Care, 49*(4), 333-339.

Mankins, J. C. (2009). Technology readiness and risk assessments: A new approach. *Acta Astronautica, 65*(9-10), 1208-1215.

Mannion, R. (2011). General practitioner-led commissioning in the NHS: Progress, prospects and pitfalls. *British Medical Bulletin, 97*(1), 7-15.

Manton, K. G. (2008). Recent declines in chronic disability in the elderly U.S. population: Risk factors and future dynamics. *Annual Review of Public Health, 29*(1), 91-113.

Manuel, D., Creatore, M., Rosella, L., & Henry, D. (2009). *What does it take to make a healthy province? A benchmark study of jurisdictions in Canada and around the world with the highest levels of health and the best health behaviours.* Toronto, ON: Institute for Clinical Evaluative Sciences.

Manzano-Santaella, A. (2010a). Disentangling the impact of multiple innovations to reduce delayed hospital discharges. *Journal of Health Services Research and Policy, 15*(1), 41-46.

Manzano-Santaella, A. (2010b). From bed-blocking to delayed discharges: Precursors and interpretations of a contested concept. *Health Services Management Research, 23*(3), 121-127.

Marchessault, G. (2011). The Manitoba Centre for Health Policy: A case study. *Healthcare Policy, 6*[Special Issue], 29-43.

Marchildon, G. P. (2005). The Chaoulli case: A two-tier Magna Carta? *Healthcare Quarterly, 8*(4), 49-52.

Marchildon, G. P., & Schrijvers, K. (2011). Physician resistance and the forging of public healthcare: A comparative analysis of the doctors' strikes in Canada and Belgium in the 1960s. *Medical History, 55*(2), 203-222.

Maric, B., Kaan, A., Ignaszewski, A., & Lear, S. A. (2009). A systematic review of telemonitoring technologies in heart failure. *European Journal of Heart Failure, 11*(5), 506-517.

Mark, B. A. (2006). Methodological issues in nurse staffing research. *Western Journal of Nursing Research, 28*(6), 694-709.

Mark, B. A., Harless, D. W., McCue, M., & Xu, Y. (2004). A longitudinal examination of hospital registered nurse staffing and quality of care. *Health Services Research, 39*(2), 279-300.

Mark, B. A., Jones, C. B., Lindley, L., & Ozcan, Y. A. (2009). An examination of technical efficiency, quality, and patient safety in acute care nursing units. *Policy, Politics, and Nursing Practice, 10*(3), 180-186.

Markel, H. (2010). Abraham Flexner and his remarkable report on medical education: A century later. *JAMA, 303*(9), 888-890.

Marklund, B., Ström, M., Månsson, J., Borgquist, L., Baigi, A., & Fridlund, B. (2007). Computer-supported telephone nurse triage: An evaluation of medical quality and costs. *Journal of Nursing Management, 15*(2), 180-187.

Marmor, T. R. (2007). *Fads, fallacies and foolishness in medical care management and policy.* Singapore: World Scientific Publishing.

Marmor, T., Freeman, R., & Okma, K. (2005). Comparative perspectives and policy learning in the world of health care. *Journal of Comparative Policy Analysis: Research and Practice, 7*(4), 331-348.

Marmor, T., Okma, K. G. H., & Latham, S. R. (2002). National values, institutions, and health policies: What do they imply for [Canadian] medicare reform? *Canadian-American Public Policy,* (November), 14-43.

Marmor, T. R., Okma, K. G. H., & Latham, S. R. (2010). National values, institutions and health policies: What do they imply for Medicare reform? *Journal of Comparative Policy Analysis: Research and Practice, 12*(1), 179-196.

Marriott, A., Reid, G., Jones, K., de Villiers, R., & Kennedy, C. (2005). Interdisciplinary working in intermediate care: Generic working or the key to a person centred approach? In B. H. Roe & R. Beech (Eds.), *Intermediate and continuing care: Policy and practice.* Oxford: Blackwell.

Marshall, M., & Øvretveit, J. (2011). Can we save money by improving quality? *BMJ Quality & Safety, 20*(4), 293-296.

Martin, G. P. (2008). "Ordinary people only": Knowledge, representativeness, and the publics of public participation in healthcare. *Sociology of Health and Illness, 30*(1), 35-54.

Martin, S., Kelly, G., George, K. W., McCreight, B., & Nugent, C. (2008). Smart home technologies for health and social care support. *Cochrane Database of Systematic Reviews* (4).

Masnick, K., & McDonnell, G. (2010). A model linking clinical workforce skill mix planning to health and health care dynamics. *Human Resources for Health, 8*(11).

Masuda, J. R., Poland, B., & Baxter, J. (2010). Reaching for environmental health justice: Canadian experiences for a comprehensive research, policy and advocacy agenda in health promotion. *Health Promotion International, 25*(4), 453-463.

Mattes, R. D., Shikany, J. M., Kaiser, K. A., & Allison, D. B. (2011). Nutritively sweetened beverage consumption and body weight: A systematic review and meta-analysis of randomized experiments. *Obesity Reviews, 12*(5), 346-365.

May, C., Finch, T., Cornford, J., Exley, C., Gately, C., Kirk, S., et al. (2011). Integrating telecare for chronic disease management in the community: What needs to be done? *BMC Health Services Research, 11*(131).

Mayer, T. (1999). Regaining control of your practice. Physician empowerment through active "followership." *Postgraduate Medicine, 106*(2), 15-16.

Mayes, D. C., & Mador, D. R. (2010). Evaluating the value and impact of an electronic health record in a complex health system. *ElectronicHealthcare, 8*(4), e3-e14.

Maynard, A., & Bloor, K. (2010). Patient reported outcome measurement: Learning to walk before we run. *Journal of the Royal Society of Medicine, 103*(4), 129-132.

Mays, G. P., & Smith, S. A. (2011). Evidence links increases in public health spending to declines in preventable deaths. *Health Affairs, 30*(8), 1585-1593.

McClellan, M. (2011). Reforming payments to healthcare providers: The key to slowing healthcare cost growth while improving quality? *Journal of Economic Perspectives, 25*(2), 69-92.

McColl, M. A., & Dorland, J. (2007). Conclusion and direction for the future. In J. Dorland & M. A. McColl (Eds.), *Emerging approaches to chronic disease management in primary health care.* Montreal and Kingston: McGill-Queen's University Press.

McDaniel, S. A. (2002). Intergenerational interlinkages: Public, family, and work. In D. Cheal (Ed.), *Aging and demographic change in Canadian context.* Toronto, ON: University of Toronto Press.

McDonagh, M. S., Smith, D. H., & Goddard, M. (2000). Measuring appropriate use of acute beds: A systematic review of methods and results. *Health Policy, 53*(3), 157-184.

McDonald, K. M., Romano, P. S., Geppert, J., Davies, S. M., Duncan, B. W., Shojania, K. G., et al. (2002). *Measures of patient safety based on hospital administrative data – the patient safety indicators*. Rockville, MD: U.S. Dept. of Health and Human Services, Public Health Service, Agency for Healthcare Research and Quality.

McDonald, R., White, J., & Marmor, T. R. (2009). Paying for performance in primary medical care: Learning about and learning from "success" and "failure" in England and California. *Journal of Health Politics Policy and Law, 34*(5), 747-776.

McGregor, M. J., Tate, R. B., McGrail, K. M., Ronald, L. A., Broemeling, A.-M., & Cohen, M. (2006). Care outcomes in long-term care facilities in British Columbia, Canada: Does ownership matter? *Medical Care, 44*(10), 929-935.

McIntosh, T. (2004). Intergovernmental relations, social policy and federal transfers after Romanow. *Canadian Public Administration, 47*(1), 27-51.

McKay, L. (2000). *Making the Lalonde Report*. Ottawa: Health Network, CPRN.

McKay, N. L., & Deily, M. E. (2005). Comparing high- and low-performing hospitals using risk-adjusted excess mortality and cost inefficiency. *Health Care Management Review, 30*(4), 347-360.

McKie, J., Richardson, J., Singer, P., & Kuhse, H. (1998). *The allocation of health care resources: An ethical evaluation of the "QALY" approach*. Aldershot: Ashgate/ Dartmouth.

McKillop, I. (2002). *Financial rules as a catalyst for change in the Canadian health care system*. Saskatoon, SK: Commission on the Future of Health Care in Canada.

McKillop, I. (2004). Financial rules as a catalyst for change in the canadian health care system. In P.-G. Forest, G. P. Marchildon, & T. McIntosh (Eds.), *Changing health care in Canada: The Romanow papers Vol. 2*. Toronto, ON: University of Toronto Press.

McLaren, L., McIntyre, L., & Kirkpatrick, S. (2010). Rose's population strategy of prevention need not increase social inequalities in health. *International Journal of Epidemiology, 39*(2), 372-377.

McManus, P., Donnelly, N., Henry, D., Hall, W., Primrose, J., & Lindner, J. (1996). Prescription drug utilization following patient co-payment changes in Australia. *Pharmacoepidemiology and Drug Safety, 5*, 385-392.

McNair, P. D., Luft, H. S., & Bindman, A. B. (2009). Medicare's policy not to pay for treating hospital-acquired conditions: The impact. *Health Affairs, 28*(5), 1485-1493.

McNutt, R., & Hasler, S. (2011). The hospital is not your home: Making safety safer (Swiss cheese is a culinary missed metaphor). *Quality Management in Health Care, 20*(3), 176-178.

Mechanic, R. E., & Altman, S. H. (2009). Payment reform options: Episode payment is a good place to start. *Health Affairs, 28*(2), w262-w271.

Megginson, W. L., & Netter, J. M. (2001). From state to market: A survey of empirical studies on privatization. *Journal of Economic Literature, 39*(2), 321-389.

Mendelsohn, M. (2002). *Canadians' thoughts on their health care system: Preserving the Canadian model through innovation*. Saskatoon, SK: Commission on the Future of Health Care in Canada.

Meng, H., Friedman, B., Dick, A. W., Wamsley, B. R., Eggert, G. M., & Mukamel, D. (2006). Effect of a voucher benefit on the demand for paid personal assistance. *The Gerontologist, 46*(2), 183-192.

Merani, S., Abdulla, S., Kwong, J. C., Rosella, L., Streiner, D. L., Johnson, I. L., et al. (2010). Increasing tuition fees in a country with two different models of medical education. *Medical Education, 44*(6), 577-586.

Messer, K., Pierce, J. P., Zhu, S.-H., Hartman, A. M., Al-Delaimy, W. K., Trinidad, D. R., et al. (2007). The California Tobacco Control Program's effect on adult smokers: (1) Smoking cessation. *Tobacco Control, 16*(2), 85-90.

Mhatre, S. L., & Deber, R. B. (1992). From equal access to health care to equitable access to health: A review of Canadian provincial health commissions and reports. *International Journal of Health Services, 22*(4), 645-668.

Michaud, P.-C., Goldman, D., Lakdawalla, D., Zheng, Y., & Gailey, A. (2009). Understanding the economic consequences of shifting trends in population health. *National Bureau of Economic Research Working Paper Series, No. 15231.*

Miller, C., Quester, P., Hill, D., & Hiller, J. (2011). Smokers' recall of Australian graphic cigarette packet warnings and awareness of associated health effects, 2005–2008. *BMC Public Health, 11*(238).

Miller, M. R., Elixhauser, A., Zhan, C., & Meyer, G. S. (2001). Patient safety indicators: Using administrative data to identify potential patient safety concerns. *Health Services Research, 36*(6), 110-132.

Miller, S. C., Miller, E. A., Jung, H.-Y., Sterns, S., Clark, M., & Mor, V. (2010). Nursing home organizational change: The "culture change" movement as viewed by long-term care specialists. *Medical Care Research and Review, 67*(Suppl. 4), 65S-81S.

Milligan, C., Roberts, C., & Mort, M. (2011). Telecare and older people: Who cares where? *Social Science & Medicine, 72*(3), 347-354.

Milstein, B., Homer, J., Briss, P., Burton, D., & Pechacek, T. (2011). Why behavioral and environmental interventions are needed to improve health at lower cost. *Health Affairs, 30*(5), 823-832.

Minister's Advisory Committee on Health. (2010). *A foundation for Alberta's health system.* Retrieved 16 August 2011 from http://www.health.alberta.ca/documents/MACH-Final-Report-2010-01-20.pdf

Mintzberg, H. (1979). *The structuring of organizations: A synthesis of the research.* Englewood Cliffs, NJ: Prentice-Hall.

Mir, H., Buchanan, D., Gilmore, A., McKee, M., Yusuf, S., & Chow, C. K. (2011). Cigarette pack labelling in 12 countries at different levels of economic development. *Journal of Public Health Policy, 32*(2), 146-164.

Mitton, C., Dionne, F., Peacock, S., & Sheps, S. (2006). Quality and cost in healthcare: A relationship worth examining. *Applied Health Economics and Health Policy, 5*(4), 201-208.

Mitton, C., Smith, N., Peacock, S., Evoy, B., & Abelson, J. (2009). Public participation in health care priority setting: A scoping review. *Health Policy, 91*(3), 219-228.

Moïse, P., & Jacobzone, S. (2003). Population ageing, health expenditure and treatment: An ARD perspective. In OECD (Ed.), *A disease-based comparison of health systems. What is best and at what cost?* (pp. 163-179). Paris: OECD.

Monk, A. H. B. (2008). The interplay between social welfare and competitiveness: The case of Canadian Medicare. *Geoforum, 39*(6), 2009-2018.

Montalto, M. (2010). The 500-bed hospital that isn't there: The Victorian Department of Health review of the Hospital in the Home program. *Medical Journal of Australia, 193*(10), 598-601.

Montalto, M., Lui, B., Mullins, A., & Woodmason, K. (2010). Medically-managed Hospital in the Home: 7 year study of mortality and unplanned interruption. *Australian Health Review, 34*(3), 269-275.

Mor, V., Miller, E. A., & Clark, M. (2010). The taste for regulation in long-term care. *Medical Care Research and Review, 67*(Suppl. 4), 38S-64S.

Moreno-Serra, R., & Wagstaff, A. (2010). System-wide impacts of hospital payment reforms: Evidence from Central and Eastern Europe and Central Asia. *Journal of Health Economics, 29*(4), 585-602.

Morgan, S. (2004). Drug spending in Canada: Recent trends and causes. *Medical Care, 42*(7), 635-642.

Morgan, S. (2008). Challenges and changes in Pharmacare: Could social insurance be the answer? In C. M. Flood, M. Stabile, & C. Tuohy (Eds.), *Exploring social insurance: Can a dose of Europe cure Canadian health care finance?* Montreal and Kingston: McGill-Queen's University Press.

Morgan, S., & Cunningham, C. (2011). Population aging and the determinants of healthcare expenditures: The case of hospital, medical and pharmaceutical care in British Columbia, 1996 to 2006. *Healthcare Policy, 7*(1), 68-79.

Morgan, S., McMahon, M., & Mitton, C. (2006). Centralising drug review to improve coverage decisions: Economic lessons from (and for) Canada. *Applied Health Economics and Health Policy, 5*(2), 67-73.

Morgan, S. G., & Willison, D. J. (2004). Post-Romanow Pharmacare: Last-dollar first … first-dollar lost? *HealthcarePapers, 4*(3), 10-20.

Morlacchi, P., & Nelson, R. R. (2011). How medical practice evolves: Learning to treat failing hearts with an implantable device. *Research Policy, 40*(4), 511-525.

Morra, D., Nicholson, S., Levinson, W., Gans, D. N., Hammons, T., & Casalino, L. P. (2011). US physician practices versus Canadians: Spending nearly four times as much money interacting with payers. *Health Affairs, 30*(8), 1443-1450.

Mortimer, D. (2010). Reorienting programme budgeting and marginal analysis (PBMA) towards disinvestment. *BMC Health Services Research, 10*(288).

Motiwala, S. S., Flood, C. M., Coyte, P. C., & Laporte, A. (2005). The First Ministers' Accord on Health Renewal and the Future of Home Care in Canada. *Longwoods Review, 2*(4), 2-10.

Moulton, B., & King, J. S. (2010). Aligning ethics with medical decision-making: The quest for informed patient choice. *Journal of Law, Medicine and Ethics, 38*(1), 85-97.

Moxey, A., Robertson, J., Newby, D., Hains, I., Williamson, M., & Pearson, S. A. (2010). Computerized clinical decision support for prescribing: Provision does not guarantee uptake. *Journal of the American Medical Informatics Association, 17*(1), 25-33.

Muenchberger, H., & Kendall, E. (2010). Predictors of preventable hospitalization in chronic disease: Priorities for change. *Journal of Public Health Policy, 31*(2), 150-163.

Mukamel, D. B., Ladd, H., Weimer, D. L., Spector, W. D., & Zinn, J. S. (2009). Is there evidence of cream skimming among nursing homes following the publication of the Nursing Home Compare Report Card? *The Gerontologist, 49*(6), 793-802.

Mukamel, D. B., Spector, W. D., Zinn, J. S., Huang, L., Weimer, D. L., & Dozier, A. (2007). Nursing homes' response to the Nursing Home Compare Report Card. *The Journals of Gerontology Series B: Psychological Sciences and Social Sciences, 62*, S218-S225.

Mukamel, D. B., Spector, W. D., Zinn, J., Weimer, D. L., & Ahn, R. (2010). Changes in clinical and hotel expenditures following publication of the Nursing Home Compare Report Card. *Medical Care, 48*(10), 869-874.

Mundinger, M. O., Kane, R. L., Lenz, E. R., Totten, A. M., Tsai, W.-Y., Cleary, P. D., et al. (2000). Primary care outcomes in patients treated by nurse practitioners or physicians: A randomized trial. *JAMA, 283*(1), 59-68.

Muntaner, C., & Chung, H. (2008). Macrosocial determinants, epidemiology, and health policy: Should politics and economics be banned from social determinants of health research? *Journal of Public Health Policy, 29*(3), 299-306.

Mustard, C. A., Bielecky, A., Etches, J., Wilkins, R., Tjepkema, M., Amick, B. C., et al. (2010). Avoidable mortality for causes amenable to medical care, by occupation in Canada, 1991–2001. *Canadian Journal of Public Health, 101*(6), 500-507.

Mutter, R. L., Rosko, M. D., & Wong, H. S. (2008). Measuring hospital inefficiency: The effects of controlling for quality and patient burden of illness. *Health Services Research, 43*(6), 1992-2013.

Naccarella, L., Southern, D., Furler, J., Scott, A., Prosser, L., Young, D., et al. (2008). Primary care funding and organisational policy options and implications: A narrative review of evidence from five comparator countries. *Medical Journal of Australia, 188*(Suppl. 8), S73-76.

Naiman, A., Glazier, R., & Moineddin, R. (2011). Is there an impact of public smoking bans on self-reported smoking status and exposure to secondhand smoke? Do smoking bans decrease exposure? *BMC Public Health, 11*(146).

Nasmith, L., Ballem, P., Baxter, R., Bergman, H., Colin-Thomé, D., Herbert, C., et al. (2010). *Transforming care for Canadians with chronic health conditions: Put people first, expect the best, manage for results.* Ottawa: Canadian Academy of Health Sciences.

National Forum on Health. (1997). Canada health action: Building on the legacy. Vol. 1. Retrieved 16 August 2011 from http://www.hc-sc.gc.ca/hcs-sss/pubs/renewal-renouv/1997-nfoh-fnss-v1/index-eng.php#message

National Nursing Research Unit King's College London, & NHS Institute for Innovation and Improvement. (2010). *Improving healthcare quality at scale and pace. Lessons from the productive ward: Releasing time to care programme.* Coventry: NHS Institute for Innovation and Improvement.

National Partnership for Action to End Health Disparities. (n.d.). *Toolkit for community action.* Washington: US Department of Health and Human Services. Retrieved 23 August 2011 from http://www.minorityhealth.hhs.gov/npa/files/Plans/Toolkit/NPA_Toolkit.pdf

Nauenberg, E., Flood, C., & Coyte, P. (2005). A complex taxonomy: Technology assessment in Canadian Medicare. In T. S. Jost (Ed.), *Health care coverage determinations: An international comparative study.* Maidenhead, Berkshire: Open University Press.

Naylor, C. D. (1986). *Private practice, public payment: Canadian medicine and the politics of health insurance, 1911–1966.* Kingston: McGill-Queen's University Press.

Naylor, C. D. (1999). Health care in Canada: Incrementalism under fiscal duress. *Health Affairs, 18*(3), 9-26.

Nelson, E. C., Batalden, P. B., & Godfrey, M. M. (2007). *Quality by design: A clinical microsystems approach.* San Francisco: Jossey-Bass/Wiley.

Nembhard, I. M., Alexander, J. A., Hoff, T. J., & Ramanujam, R. (2009). Why does the quality of health care continue to lag? Insights from management research. *Academy of Management Perspectives, 23*(1), 24-42.

Neumann, P. J. (2005). *Using cost-effectiveness analysis to improve health care: Opportunities and barriers.* Oxford: Oxford University Press.

Neumann, P. J., Sandberg, E. A., Bell, C. M., Stone, P. W., & Chapman, R. H. (2000). Are pharmaceuticals cost-effective? A review of the evidence. *Health Affairs, 19,* 92-109.

Newhouse, J. P. (1977). Medical-care expenditure: A cross-national survey. *The Journal of Human Resources, 12*(1), 115-125.

Newhouse, J. P., & the Health Insurance Experiment Group. (1993). *Free for all? Lessons from the RAND health insurance experiment.* Cambridge, MA: Harvard University Press.

NHS Modernisation Agency. (2003). *Changing workforce programme pilot sites progress report - Spring 2003.* NHS Modernisation Agency.

Nicholson, S., Pauly, M. V., Wu, A. Y. J., Murray, J. F., Teutsch, S. M., & Berger, M. L. (2008). Getting real performance out of pay-for-performance. *Milbank Quarterly, 86*(3), 435-457.

Niemeijer, G. C., Trip, A., Does, R. J. M. M., De Mast, J., & Van Den Heuvel, J. (2011). Generic project definitions for improvement of health care delivery: A case-based approach. *Quality Management in Health Care, 20*(2), 152-164.

Nienaber, J., & Wildavsky, A. (1973). *The budgeting and evaluation of federal recreation programs or money doesn't grow on trees.* New York: Basic Books.

Noble, D. J., Panesar, S. S., & Pronovost, P. J. (2011). A public health approach to patient safety reporting systems is urgently needed. *Journal of Patient Safety, 7*(2), 109-112.

Nolte, E., & McKee, M. (2008). Measuring the health of nations: Updating an earlier analysis. *Health Affairs, 27*(1), 58-71.

Nordström, J., & Thunström, L. (2009). The impact of tax reforms designed to encourage healthier grain consumption. *Journal of Health Economics, 28*(3), 622-634.

Normand, S.-L. T. (2010). Large data streams and the power of numbers. In L. Olsen & J. M. McGinnis (Eds.), *Redesigning the clinical effectiveness research paradigm: Innovation and practice-based approaches* [Workshop summary]. Washington, DC: National Academies Press.

Noro, A., Poss, J., Hirdes, J., Finne-Soveri, H., Ljunggren, G., Bjornsson, J., et al. (2011). Method for assigning priority levels in acute care (MAPLe-AC) predicts outcomes of acute hospital care of older persons: A cross-national validation. *BMC Medical Informatics and Decision Making, 11*(39).

Norquay, G. (2010). The gathering storm in federal-provincial relations. *Policy Options, 31*(5), 16-22.

Nutting, P. A., Crabtree, B. F., Miller, W. L., Stange, K. C., Stewart, E., & Jaén, C. (2011). Transforming physician practices to patient-centered medical homes: Lessons from the National Demonstration Project. *Health Affairs, 30*(3), 439-445.

Oberlander, J., & White, J. (2009). Public attitudes toward health care spending aren't the problem; prices are. *Health Affairs, 28*(5), 1285-1293.

O'Brien-Pallas, L., Alksnis, C., Wang, S., Birch, S., Tomblin Murphy, G., Roy, F. A., et al. (2003). Early retirement among RNs: Estimating the size of the problem in Canada. *Healthcare Quarterly, 7*(1), 2-9.

O'Connor, A., Bennett, C., Stacey, D., Barry, M., Col, N., Eden, K., et al. (2009). Decision aids for people facing health treatment or screening decisions. *Cochrane Database of Systematic Reviews, 3,* CD001431.

O'Connor, A. M., Wennberg, J. E., Legare, F., Llewellyn-Thomas, H. A., Moulton, B. W., Sepucha, K. R., et al. (2007). Toward the "tipping point": Decision aids and informed patient choice. *Health Affairs, 26*(3), 716-725.

OECD. (2010a). *Economic survey of Canada 2010*(14). Retrieved from http://www. oecd.org/document/56/0,3746,en_2649_34569_45925432_1_1_1_1,00.html

OECD. (2010b). Health data 2010. Retrieved 15 August 2011 from http://www. oecd.org/document/16/0,3746,en_2649_37407_2085200_1_1_1_37407, 00.html

OECD. (2010c). *Improving health sector efficiency: The role of information and communication technologies.* Paris: OECD.

OECD. (2010d). *Improving value in health care: Measuring quality.* Paris: OECD.

OECD. (2010e). *Value for money in health spending.* Paris: OECD.

Oelke, N., Cunning, L., Andrews, K., Martin, D., MacKay, A., Kuschminder, K., et al. (2009). Organizing care across the continuum: Primary care, specialty services, acute and long-term care. *Healthcare Quarterly, 13*[Special issue], 75-79.

Office of the Auditor General of Canada. (2002). Health Canada – Federal support for health care delivery. In *2002 September status report of the Auditor General of Canada.* Retrieved from http://www.oag-bvg.gc.ca/internet/English/ parl_oag_200209_03_e_12388.html#ch3hd4b

Office of the Auditor General of Canada. (2008). Reporting on health indicators – Health Canada. In *2008 report of the Auditor General of Canada* (Chapter 8). Retrieved 26 August 2011 from http://www.oag-bvg.gc.ca/internet/English/ parl_oag_200812_08_e_31832.html

Office of the Auditor General of Canada. (2010). *Electronic health records in Canada: An overview of federal and provincial audit reports.* Ottawa: Author.

Oldmeadow, L., Bedi, H., Burch, H., Smith, J., Leahy, E., & Goldwasser, M. (2007). Experienced physiotherapists as gatekeepers to hospital orthopaedic outpatient care. *Medical Journal of Australia, 186*(12), 625-628.

Olsen, L., & McGinnis, J. M. (Eds.). (2010). *Redesigning the clinical effectiveness research paradigm: Innovation and practice-based approaches* [Workshop summary]. Washington, DC: National Academies Press.

Olshansky, S. J. (1988). On forecasting mortality. *Milbank Quarterly, 66*(3), 482-530.

Olshansky, S. J., Goldman, D. P., Zheng, Y., & Rowe, J. W. (2009). Aging in America in the twenty-first century: Demographic forecasts from the Macarthur Foundation Research Network on an aging society. *Milbank Quarterly, 87*(4), 842-862.

Olshansky, S. J., Passaro, D. J., Hershow, R. C., Layden, J., Carnes, B. A., Brody, J., et al. (2005). A potential decline in life expectancy in the United States in the 21st century. *New England Journal of Medicine, 352*(11), 1138-1145.

Omachonu, V. K., & Einspruch, N. G. (2010). Innovation in healthcare delivery systems: A conceptual framework. *Innovation Journal, 15*(1), 1-20.

Ombudsman Ontario. (2007). *Annual report 2006–07.* Toronto, ON: Author.

Ombudsman Saskatchewan. (2010). *Recommendations 2010: Third quarter update.* Regina, SK: Author.

Ong, M.-S., & Coiera, E. (2011). A systematic review of failures in handoff communication during intrahospital transfers. *Joint Commission Journal on Quality and Patient Safety, 37*(6), 274-284.

Or, Z., Cases, C., Lisac, M., Vrangbæk, K., Winblad, U., & Bevan, G. (2010). Are health problems systemic? Politics of access and choice under Beveridge and Bismarck systems. *Health Economics, Policy and Law, 5*(3), 269-293.

Ottmann, G., Allen, J., & Feldman, P. (2009). *Self-directed community aged care for people with complex needs: A literature review.* Melbourne: Uniting Care Community Option/Deakin University.

Oxley, H. (2009). Improving health care system performance through better co-ordination of care. In OECD (Ed.), *Achieving better value for money in health care.* Paris: OECD Publishing.

Oxman, A. D., Bjorndal, A., Becerra-Posada, F., Gibson, M., Block, M. A., Haines, A., et al. (2010). A framework for mandatory impact evaluation to ensure well informed public policy decisions. *Lancet, 375*(9712), 427-431.

Oxman, A. D., Sackett, D. L., Chalmers, I., & Prescott, T. E. (2005). A surrealistic mega-analysis of redisorganization theories. *Journal of the Royal Society of Medicine, 98*(12), 563-568.

Palangkaraya, A., & Yong, J. (2009). Population ageing and its implications on aggregate health care demand: Empirical evidence from 22 OECD countries. *International Journal of Health Care Finance and Economics, 9*(4), 391-402.

Palley, H. A., Pomey, M.-P., & Forest, P.-G. (2011). Examining private and public provision in Canada's provincial health care systems: Comparing Ontario and Quebec. *International Political Science Review, 32*(1), 79-94.

Paré, G., Jaana, M., & Sicotte, C. (2007). Systematic review of home telemonitoring for chronic diseases: The evidence base. *Journal of the American Medical Informatics Association, 14*(3), 269-277.

Paré, G., Moqadem, K., Pineau, G., & St-Hilaire, C. (2010). Clinical effects of home telemonitoring in the context of diabetes, asthma, heart failure and hypertension: A systematic review. *Journal of Medical Internet Research, 12*, e21.

Parkin, D., McGuire, A., & Yule, B. (1987). Aggregate health care expenditures and national income: Is health care a luxury good? *Journal of Health Economics, 6*(2), 109-127.

Parmelli, E., Flodgren, G., Beyer, F., Baillie, N., Schaafsma, M., & Eccles, M. (2011). The effectiveness of strategies to change organisational culture to improve health-care performance: A systematic review. *Implementation Science, 6*(33).

Patented Medicine Prices Review Board. (2011a.) *Annual report 2010.* Ottawa: Author.

Patented Medicine Prices Review Board. (2011b.) *Generic drugs in Canada: International price comparisons and potential cost savings.* Ottawa: Author.

Patra, J., Popova, S., Rehm, J., Bondy, S., Flint, R., & Giesbrecht, N. (2007). *Economic cost of chronic disease in Canada 1995–2003.* Ottawa: Ontario Chronic Disease Prevention Alliance and the Ontario Public Health Association.

Patry, R. A., & Eiland, L. S. (2007). Addressing the shortage of pharmacy faculty and clinicians: The impact of demographic changes. *American Journal of Health-System Pharmacy, 64*(7), 773-775.

Paulus, R. A., Davis, K., & Steele, G. D. (2008). Continuous innovation in health care: Implications of the Geisinger experience. *Health Affairs, 27*(5), 1235-1245.

Payne, G., Laporte, A., Deber, R., & Coyte, P. C. (2007). Counting backward to health care's future: Using time-to-death modeling to identify changes in end-of-life morbidity and the impact of aging on health care expenditures. *Milbank Quarterly, 85*(2), 213-257.

Perneger, T. (2005). The Swiss cheese model of safety incidents: Are there holes in the metaphor? *BMC Health Services Research, 5*(1), 71.

Perrier, L., Mrklas, K., Lavis, J., & Straus, S. (2011). Interventions encouraging the use of systematic reviews by health policymakers and managers: A systematic review. *Implementation Science, 6*(43).

Perrow, C. (1999). *Normal accidents: Living with high-risk technologies.* Princeton: Princeton University Press.

Perry, S. J., Wears, R. L., & Cook, R. I. (2005). The role of automation in complex system failures. *Journal of Patient Safety, 1*(1), 56-61.

Peters, L., & Sellick, K. (2006). Quality of life of cancer patients receiving inpatient and home-based palliative care. *Journal of Advanced Nursing, 53*(5), 524-533.

Petersen, L. A., Woodard, L. D., Urech, T., Daw, C., & Sookanan, S. (2006). Does pay-for-performance improve the quality of health care? *Annals of Internal Medicine, 145*(4), 265-272.

Petrie, D., Tang, K. K., & Rao, D. S. P. (2009). *Measuring avoidable health inequality with realization of conditional potential life years (RCPLY).* Dundee: Department of Economic Studies, University of Dundee.

Petrou, S., & Gray, A. (2011). Economic evaluation using decision analytical modelling: Design, conduct, analysis, and reporting. *BMJ, 342*(7808), 1195-1198.

Petticrew, M. (2007). "More research needed": Plugging gaps in the evidence base on health inequalities. *European Journal of Public Health, 17*(5), 411-413.

Petticrew, M., Whitehead, M., Macintyre, S. J., Graham, H., & Egan, M. (2004). Evidence for public health policy on inequalities: 1: The reality according to policymakers. *Journal of Epidemiology and Community Health, 58*(10), 811-816.

Phillips, C. J., Fordham, R., Marsh, K., Bertranou, E., Davies, S., Hale, J., et al. (2011). Exploring the role of economics in prioritization in public health: What do stakeholders think? *European Journal of Public Health, 21*(5), 578-584.

Pink, D. H. (2006). *A whole new mind: Why right-brainers will rule the future.* New York: Riverhead Books.

Ploeg, A. J., Lange, C. P. E., Lardenoye, J.-W., & Breslau, P. J. (2008). The incidence of unplanned returns to the operating room after peripheral arterial bypass surgery and its value as indicator of quality of care. *Vascular and Endovascular Surgery, 42*(1), 19-24.

Poder, T. G., Bellemare, C., Bédard, S. K., He, J., & Lemieux, R. (2010). New design of care: Assessment of an interdisciplinary orthopaedic clinic with a pivot nurse in the province of Quebec. *Orthopaedic Nursing, 29*(6), 381-389.

Poksinska, B. (2010). The current state of Lean implementation in health care: Literature review. *Quality Management in Health Care, 19*(4), 319-329.

Poland, B., Frohlich, K., Haines, R. J., Mykhalovskiy, E., Rock, M., & Sparks, R. (2006). The social context of smoking: The next frontier in tobacco control? *Tobacco Control, 15*(1), 59-63.

Polisena, J., Coyle, D., Coyle, K., & McGill, S. (2009). Home telehealth for chronic disease management: A systematic review and an analysis of economic evaluations. *International Journal of Technology Assessment in Health Care, 25*(3), 339-349.

Polisena, J., Tran, K., Cimon, K., Hutton, B., McGill, S., Palmer, K., et al. (2010). Home telemonitoring for congestive heart failure: A systematic review and meta-analysis. *Journal of Telemedicine and Telecare, 16*(2), 68-76.

Pollitt, C. (1993). The struggle for quality: The case of the National Health Service. *Policy and Politics, 21*(3), 161-170.

Pollock, A. M., & Kirkwood, G. (2009). Independent sector treatment centres: The first independent evaluation, a Scottish case study. *Journal of the Royal Society of Medicine, 102*(7), 278-286.

Pollock, A. M., & Price, D. (2011). How the secretary of state for health proposes to abolish the NHS in England. *BMJ, 342.*

Polyzos, N. P., Valachis, A., Mauri, D., & Ioannidis, J. P. A. (2011). Industry involvement and baseline assumptions of cost-effectiveness analyses: Diagnostic accuracy of the Papanicolaou test. *Canadian Medical Association Journal, 183*(6), E337-E343.

Pomey, M.-P., Forest, P.-G., Sanmartin, C., De Coster, C., & Drew, M. (2010). Wait time management strategies for scheduled care: What makes them succeed? *Healthcare Policy, 5*(3), 66-81.

Poss, J. W., Hirdes, J. P., Fries, B. E., McKillop, I., & Chase, M. (2008). Validation of Resource Utilization Groups Version III for Home Care (RUG-III/HC): Evidence from a Canadian home care jurisdiction. *Medical Care, 46*(4), 380-387.

Potrafke, N. (2010). The growth of public health expenditures in OECD countries: Do government ideology and electoral motives matter? *Journal of Health Economics, 29*(6), 797-810.

Powell Davies, G., Harris, M., Perkins, D., Roland, M., Williams, A., Larsen, K., et al. (2006). *Coordination of care within primary health care and with other sectors: A systematic review.* Kensington: Research Centre for Primary Health Care and Equity, School of Public Health and Community Medicine, UNSW.

Praxia Information Intelligence & Gartner, Inc. (2011). *Telehealth benefits and adoption: Connecting people and providers across Canada.* A study commissioned by Canada Health Infoway. Retrieved from https://www2.infoway-inforoute.ca/Documents/telehealth_report_summary_2010_en.pdf

Predy, G., Edwards, J., Fraser-Lee, N., Ladd, B., Moore, K., Lightfoot, P., & Spinola, C. (2008). *Poverty and health in Edmonton.* Edmonton: Alberta Health Services.

Preker, A. S., & Harding, A. (Eds.). (2003). *Innovations in health service delivery. The corporatization of public hospitals.* Washington, DC: World Bank.

Prémont, M. C. (2007). Wait-time guarantees for health services: An analysis of Quebec's reaction to the Chaoulli Supreme Court decision. *Health Law Journal, 15*, 43-86.

Pressman, J., & Wildavsky, A. (1973). *Implementation: How great expectations in Washington are dashed in Oakland or, why it's amazing that federal programs work at all, this being a saga of the Economic Development Administration as told by two sympathetic observers who seek to build morals on a foundation of ruined hopes.* Berkeley: California University Press.

Price, R. A., Frank, R. G., Cleary, P. D., & Goldie, S. J. (2011). Effects of direct-to-consumer advertising and clinical guidelines on appropriate use of human papillomavirus DNA tests. *Medical Care, 49*(2), 132-138.

Prime Minister's Strategy Unit. (2006). *The UK government's approach to public service reform.* London: Cabinet Office.

Pritchard, C., & Wallace, M. S. (2011). Comparing the USA, UK and 17 Western countries' efficiency and effectiveness in reducing mortality. *Journal of the Royal Society of Medicine* [*Short Reports*], *2*(7).

Pronovost, P. J., & Lilford, R. (2011). A road map for improving the performance of performance measures. *Health Affairs, 30*(4), 569-573.

Pronovost, P. J., Marsteller, J. A., & Goeschel, C. A. (2011). Preventing bloodstream infections: A measurable national success story in quality improvement. *Health Affairs, 30*(4), 628-634.

Pronovost, P., Weast, B., Rosenstein, B., Sexton, J. B., Holzmueller, C. G., Paine, L., et al. (2005). Implementing and validating a comprehensive unit-based safety program. *Journal of Patient Safety, 1*(1), 33-40.

Propper, C. (2003). Expenditure on healthcare in the UK: A review of the issues. In D. Miles, G. Myles, & I. Preston (Eds.), *The economics of public spending* (pp. 89-119). Oxford: Oxford University Press.

Propper, C., Sutton, M., Whitnall, C., & Windmeijer, F. (2008). Did "targets and terror" reduce waiting times in England for hospital care? *The B.E. Journal of Economic Analysis & Policy, 8*(2).

Propper, C., Sutton, M., Whitnall, C., & Windmeijer, F. (2010). Incentives and targets in hospital care: Evidence from a natural experiment. *Journal of Public Economics, 94*(3-4), 318-335.

Provost, S., Pineault, R., Levesque, J.-F., Groulx, S., Baron, G., Roberge, D., et al. (2010). Does receiving clinical preventive services vary across different types of primary healthcare organizations? Evidence from a population-based survey. *Healthcare Policy, 6*(2), 67-83.

Public Health Agency of Canada. (2009). *Report from the National Diabetes Surveillance System: Diabetes in Canada, 2009.* Ottawa: Author.

Public Health Agency of Canada & Canadian Institute for Health Information. (2011). *Obesity in Canada: A joint report from the Public Health Agency of Canada and the Canadian Institute for Health Information.* Ottawa: Authors.

Purc-Stephenson, R. J., & Thrasher, C. (2010). Nurses' experiences with telephone triage and advice: A meta-ethnography. *Journal of Advanced Nursing, 66*(3), 482-494.

Puska, P., & Ståhl, T. (2010). Health in all policies – the Finnish initiative: Background, principles, and current issues. *Annual Review of Public Health, 31*(1), 315-328.

Putnam, S., & Galea, S. (2008). Epidemiology and the macrosocial determinants of health. *Journal of Public Health Policy, 29*(3), 275-289.

Raleigh, V. S., & Foot, C. (2010). *Getting the measure of quality: Opportunities and challenges.* London: King's Fund.

Raphael, D. (Ed.). (2009). *Social determinants of health: Canadian perspectives* (2nd ed.). Toronto: Canadian Scholars' Publishing.

Rasanathan, K., Montesinos, E. V., Matheson, D., Etienne, C., & Evans, T. (2011). Primary health care and the social determinants of health: Essential and complementary approaches for reducing inequities in health. *Journal of Epidemiology and Community Health, 65*(8), 656-660.

Rashman, L., Withers, E., & Hartley, J. (2009). Organizational learning and knowledge in public service organizations: A systematic review of the literature. *International Journal of Management Reviews, 11*(4), 463-494.

Reason, J. (1990). *Human error.* Cambridge: Cambridge University Press.

Reason, J. (2000). Human error: Models and management. *BMJ, 320*(7237), 768-770.

Reason, J. T. (1997). *Managing the risks of organizational accidents.* Aldershot, England: Ashgate.

Reay, T., Berta, W., & Kohn, M. K. (2009). What's the evidence on evidence-based management? *Academy of Management Perspectives, 23*(4), 5-18.

Reda, A. A., Kaper, J., Fikrelter, H., Severens, J. L., & van Schayck, C. P. (2009). Healthcare financing systems for increasing the use of tobacco dependence treatment. *Cochrane Database of Systematic Reviews, 15*(2), CD004305.

Regan, S., Thorne, S., & Mildon, B. (2009). Uncovering blind spots in education and practice leadership: Towards a collaborative response to the nurse shortage. *Nursing Leadership, 22*(2), 30-40.

Reid, J. L., & Hammond, D. (2011). *Tobacco use in Canada: Patterns and trends.* Waterloo, ON: Propel Centre for Population Health Impact, University of Waterloo.

Reinhardt, U. E. (2003). Does the aging of the population really drive the demand for health care? *Health Affairs, 22*(6), 27-39.

Reither, E. N., Olshansky, S. J., & Yang, Y. (2011). New forecasting methodology indicates more disease and earlier mortality ahead for today's younger Americans. *Health Affairs, 30*(8), 1562-1568.

Reitsma-van Rooijen, M., de Jong, J., & Rijken, M. (2011). Regulated competition in health care: Switching and barriers to switching in the Dutch health insurance system. *BMC Health Services Research, 11*(95).

Resar, R. K., Griffin, F. A., Kabcenell, A., & Bones, C. (2011). *Hospital inpatient waste identification tool.* IHI Innovation Series white paper. Cambridge, MA: Institute for Healthcare Improvement. Retrieved 15 August 2011 from http://www.ihi.org/IHI/Results/WhitePapers/HospitalInpatientWasteIDToolWhitePaper.htm

Reshef, Y., & Lam, H. (1999). Union responses to quality improvement initiatives: Factors shaping support and resistance. *Journal of Labor Research, 20*(1), 111-131.

Reti, S. R., Feldman, H. J., Ross, S. E., & Safran, C. (2010). Improving personal health records for patient-centered care. *Journal of the American Medical Informatics Association, 17*(2), 192-195.

Rice, T. (2002). Addressing cost pressures in health care systems. In Productivity Commission and Melbourne Institute of Applied Economic and Social Research (Ed.), *Health policy roundtable* (pp. 67-119). Melbourne: Productivity Commission and Melbourne Institute of Applied Economic and Social Research.

Richard, L., Gauvin, L., & Raine, K. (2011). Ecological models revisited: Their uses and evolution in health promotion over two decades. *Annual Review of Public Health, 32*(1), 307-326.

Ricketts, T. C. (2011). The health care workforce: Will it be ready as the boomers age? A review of how we can know (or not know) the answer. *Annual Review of Public Health, 32*(1), 417-430.

Rijckmans, M. J. N., Bongers, I. M. B., Garretsen, H. F. L., & Van de Goor, I. A. M. (2007). A clients' perspective on demand-oriented and demand-driven health care. *International Journal of Social Psychiatry, 53*(1), 48-62.

Riley, G. F., & Lubitz, J. D. (2010). Long-term trends in Medicare payments in the last year of life. *Health Services Research, 45*(2), 565-576.

Ring, I., & O'Brien, J. (2007). Our hearts and minds – What would it take for Australia to become the healthiest country in the world? *Medical Journal of Australia, 187*(8), 447-451.

Rittel, H. W. J., & Webber, M. M. (1973). Dilemmas in a general theory of planning. *Policy Sciences, 4*(2), 155-169.

Rittenhouse, D. R., Casalino, L. P., Shortell, S. M., McClellan, S. R., Gillies, R. R., Alexander, J. A., et al. (2011). Small and medium-size physician practices use few patient-centered medical home processes. *Health Affairs, 30*(8), 1575-1584.

Rivard, P. E., Luther, S. L., Christiansen, C. L., Zhao, S., Loveland, S., Elixhauser, A., et al. (2008). Using patient safety indicators to estimate the impact of potential adverse events on outcomes. *Medical Care Research and Review, 65*(1), 67-87.

Robinson, J. (2001). Theory and practice in the design of physician payment incentives. *Milbank Quarterly, 79*(2), 149.

Robinson, J. C., Shortell, S. M., Li, R., Casalino, L. P., & Rundall, T. (2004). The alignment and blending of payment incentives within physician organizations. *Health Services Research, 39*(5), 1589-1606.

Roblin, D. W., Howard, D. H., Becker, E. R., Adams, E. K., & Roberts, M. H. (2004). Use of midlevel practitioners to achieve labor cost savings in the primary care practice of an MCO. *Health Services Research, 39*(3), 607-625.

Rochester, P., Townsend, J., Given, L., Krebill, H., Balderrama, S., & Vinson, C. (2010). Comprehensive cancer control: Progress and accomplishments. *Cancer Causes and Control, 21*(12), 1967-1977.

Rodin, J., & Langer, E. J. (1977). Long-term effects of a control-relevant intervention with the institutionalized aged. *Journal of Personality and Social Psychology, 35*(12), 897-902.

Roebuck, M. C., Liberman, J. N., Gemmill-Toyama, M., & Brennan, T. A. (2011). Medication adherence leads to lower health care use and costs despite increased drug spending. *Health Affairs, 30*(1), 91-99.

Roehrig, C. S., & Rousseau, D. M. (2011). The growth in cost per case explains far more of US health spending increases than rising disease prevalence. *Health Affairs, 30*(9), 1657-1663.

Roemer, M. (1961). Bed supply and hospital utilization: A natural experiment. *Hospitals: Journal of the American Hospitals Association, 35*, 36-42.

Rokholm, B., Baker, J. L., & Sørensen, T. I. A. (2010). The levelling off of the obesity epidemic since the year 1999 – A review of evidence and perspectives. *Obesity Reviews, 11*(12), 835-846.

Roland, M., & Rosen, R. (2011). English NHS embarks on controversial and risky market-style reforms in health care. *New England Journal of Medicine, 364*(14), 1360-1366.

Romano, M. J., & Stafford, R. S. (2011). Electronic health records and clinical decision support systems: Impact on national ambulatory care quality. *Archives of Internal Medicine, 171*(10), 897-903.

Roos, L. L., Menec, V., & Currie, R. J. (2004). Policy analysis in an information-rich environment. *Social Science & Medicine, 58*, 2231-2241.

Roos, N. P., & Roos, L. L. (2011). Administrative data and the Manitoba Centre for Health Policy: Some reflections. *Healthcare Policy, 6*[Special issue], 16-28.

Rose, G. (1985). Sick individuals and sick populations. *International Journal of Epidemiology, 14*(1), 32-38.

Rose, G. (2001). Sick individuals and sick populations. *International Journal of Epidemiology, 30*(3), 427-432.

Rosenbaum, S., Frankford, D. M., & Moore, B. (1999). Who should determine when health care is medically necessary? *New England Journal of Medicine, 340*(3), 229-232.

Rosenthal, M. (2007). P4P: Rumors of its demise may be exaggerated. *American Journal of Managed Care,* (7 May), 238-239.

Rosenthal, M. B. (2008). Beyond pay for performance – Emerging models of provider-payment reform. *New England Journal of Medicine, 359*(12), 1197-1200.

Rosenthal, M., & Frank, R. (2006). What is the empirical basis for paying for quality in health care? *Medical Care Research and Review, 63*(2), 135-157.

Rosko, M. D., & Mutter, R. L. (2008). Stochastic frontier analysis of hospital inefficiency: A review of empirical issues and an assessment of robustness. *Medical Care Research and Review, 65*(2), 131-166.

Rothemich, S. F., Woolf, S. H., Johnson, R. E., Devers, K. J., Flores, S. K., Villars, P., et al. (2010). Promoting primary care smoking-cessation support with quitlines: The quitlink randomized controlled trial. *American Journal of Preventive Medicine, 38*(4), 367-374.

Rothstein, J., & Rouse, C. E. (2011). Constrained after college: Student loans and early-career occupational choices. *Journal of Public Economics, 95*(1-2), 149-163.

Rotter, T., Kinsman, L., James, E., Machotta, A., Gothe, H., Willis, J., et al. (2010). Clinical pathways: Effects on professional practice, patient outcomes, length of stay and hospital costs. *Cochrane Database of Systematic Reviews* (3).

Rouppe van der Voort, M. M. B. V., van Merode, F. G. G., & Berden, B. H. J. J. M. (2010). Making sense of delays in outpatient specialty care: A system perspective. *Health Policy, 97*(1), 44-52.

Rowbottom, R. (1973). *Hospital organization: A progress report on the Brunel Health Services Organization Project.* London: Heinemann Educational Books.

Rozenblum, R., Jang, Y., Zimlichman, E., Salzberg, C., Tamblyn, M., Buckeridge, D., et al. (2011). A qualitative study of Canada's experience with the implementation of electronic health information technology. *Canadian Medical Association Journal, 183*(5), E281-E288.

Runciman, W., Hibbert, P., Thomson, R., Van Der Schaaf, T., Sherman, H., & Lewalle, P. (2009). Towards an international classification for patient safety: Key concepts and terms. *International Journal for Quality in Health Care, 21*(1), 18-26.

Runnels, V., Labonte, R., & Packer, C. (2011). Reflections on the ethics of recruiting foreign-trained human resources for health. *Human Resources for Health, 9*(1), 2.

Rush, B., Shiell, A., & Hawe, P. (2004). A census of economic evaluations in health promotion. *Health Education Research, 19*(6), 707-719.

Russell, G. M., Hogg, W., & Lemelin, J. (2010). Integrated primary care organizations. *Canadian Family Physician, 56*(3), 216-218.

Russell, J., Greenhalgh, T., Burnett, A., & Montgomery, J. (2011). "No decisions about us without us"? Individual healthcare rationing in a fiscal ice age. *BMJ, 342.*

Russell, L. B. (1986). *Is prevention better than cure?* Washington, DC: Brookings Institution.

Russell, L. B. (1989). *Medicare's new hospital payment system: Is it working?* Washington, DC: Brookings Institution.

Russell, L. B. (2009). Preventing chronic disease: An important investment, but don't count on cost savings. *Health Affairs, 28*(1), 42-45.

Ryan, R., Davoren, J., Grant, H., & Delbridge, L. (2004). A 23-hour care centre model for the management of surgical patients. *ANZ Journal of Surgery, 74*(9), 754-759.

Sabik, L., & Lie, R. (2008). Priority setting in health care: Lessons from the experiences of eight countries. *International Journal for Equity in Health, 7*(4).

Safaei, J. (2006). Is democracy good for health? *International Journal of Health Services, 36*(4), 767-786.

Saito, A., Landrum, M. B., Neville, B., Ayanian, J., & Earle, C. (2011). The effect on survival of continuing chemotherapy to near death. *BMC Palliative Care, 10*(14).

Saltman, R. B., Busse, R., & Mossialos, E. (Eds.). (2002). *Regulating entrepreneurial behaviour in European health care systems.* Buckingham, UK: Open University Press.

Saltman, R. B., & Ferroussier-Davis, O. (2000). The concept of stewardship in health policy. *Bulletin of the World Health Organization, 78*(6), 732-739.

Saltman, R. B., & von Otter, C. (Eds.). (1995). *Implementing planned markets in health care: Balancing social and economic responsibility.* London, UK: Open University Press.

Saltman, R. B., & Young, D. W. (1981). The hospital power equilibrium: An alternative view of the cost containment dilemma. *Journal of Health Politics, Policy and Law, 6*(3), 391-418.

Samoocha, D., Bruinvels, D. J., Elbers, N. A., Anema, J. R., & van der Beek, A. J. (2010). Effectiveness of web-based interventions on patient empowerment: A systematic review and meta-analysis. *Journal of Medical Internet Research, 12*(2), e23.

Sanchez, M., Vellanky, S., Herring, J., Liang, J., & Jia, H. (2008). Variations in Canadian rates of hospitalization for ambulatory care sensitive conditions. *Healthcare Quarterly, 11*(4), 20-22.

Sanders, D., Baum, F. E., Benos, A., & Legge, D. (2011). Revitalising primary health-care requires an equitable global economic system – now more than ever. *Journal of Epidemiology and Community Health, 65*(8), 661-665.

Sanmartin, C. A., & the Steering Committee of the Western Canada Waiting List Project. (2003). Toward standard definitions for waiting times. *Healthcare Management Forum, 16*(2), 49-53.

Sanmartin, C., Khan, S., & LHAD Research Team. (2011). *Hospitalizations for Ambulatory Care Sensitive Conditions (ACSC): The factors that matter.* Ottawa: Statistics Canada.

Sarma, S., Devlin, R. A., Belhadji, B., & Thind, A. (2010). Does the way physicians are paid influence the way they practice? The case of Canadian family physicians' work activity. *Health Policy, 98*(2-3), 203-217.

Sarma, S., Devlin, R. A., & Hogg, W. (2010). Physician's production of primary care in Ontario, Canada. *Health Economics, 19*(1), 14-30.

Sax, S. (1984). *A strife of interests: Politics and policies in Australian health services.* North Sydney: Allen & Unwin.

Scanlon, D., Swaminathan, S., Lee, W., & Chernew, M. (2008). Does competition improve health care quality? *Health Services Research, 43*(6), 1931-1951.

Schneeweiss, S., & Avorn, J. (2005). A review of uses of health care utilization databases for epidemiologic research on therapeutics. *Journal of Clinical Epidemiology, 58*, 232-337.

Schneider, E. C., Hussey, P. S., & Schnyer, C. (2011). *Payment reform: Analysis of models and performance measurement implications.* Santa Monica, CA: Rand Corporation.

Schneider, J., Waterbury, A., Feldstein, A., Donovan, J., Vollmer, W. M., Dubanoski, J., et al. (2011). Maximizing acceptability and usefulness of an automated telephone intervention. *Health Informatics Journal, 17*(1), 72-88.

Schoder, J., & Zweifel, P. (2011). Flat-of-the-curve medicine: A new perspective on the production of health. *Health Economics Review, 1*(2).

Schoen, C., Osborn, R., Doty, M. M., Bishop, M., Peugh, J., & Murukutla, N. (2007). Toward higher-performance health systems: Adults' health care experiences in seven countries, 2007. *Health Affairs, 26*(6), w717-w734.

Schoen, C., Osborn, R., Squires, D., Doty, M. M., Pierson, R., & Applebaum, S. (2010). How health insurance design affects access to care and costs, by income, in eleven countries. *Health Affairs, 29*(12), 2323-2334.

Schoeni, R. F., Freedman, V. A., & Martin, L. G. (2008). Why is late-life disability declining? *Milbank Quarterly, 86*(1), 47-89.

Schouten, L. M., Hulscher, M. E., van Everdingen, J. J., Huijsman, R., & Grol, R. P. (2008). Evidence for the impact of quality improvement collaboratives: Systematic review. *BMJ (Clinical research ed.), 336*(7659), 1491-1494.

Schulz, J. A. (1998). The economics and financing of long-term care. *The Australasian Journal on Ageing, 17*(Suppl. 1), 82-84.

Scitovsky, A. A. (2005). "The high cost of dying": What do the data show? *Milbank Quarterly, 83*(4), 825-841.

Scott, A., Schurer, S., Jensen, P. H., & Sivey, P. (2009). The effects of an incentive program on quality of care in diabetes management. *Health Economics, 18*(9), 1091-1108.

Scott, C., & Hofmeyer, A. (2007). Networks and social capital: A relational approach to primary healthcare reform. *Health Research Policy and Systems, 5*(9).

Scott, I. A. (2010). Public hospital bed crisis: Too few or too misused? *Australian Health Review, 34*(3), 317-324.

Scott, I. A., Wills, R.-A., Coory, M., Watson, M. J., Butler, F., Waters, M., et al. (2011). Impact of hospital-wide process redesign on clinical outcomes: A comparative study of internally versus externally led intervention. *BMJ Quality & Safety, 20*(6), 539-548.

Sears, R. V. (2010). The next federal-provincial battles: This time it's different. *Policy Options, 31*(5), 23-30.

Self, P. (1975). *Econocrats and the policy process: The politics and philosophy of cost-benefit analysis.* London: Macmillan.

Sen, A., Entezarkheir, M., & Wilson, A. (2010). Obesity, smoking, and cigarette taxes: Evidence from the Canadian Community Health Surveys. *Health Policy, 97*(2-3), 180-186.

Senate. Standing Committee on Social Affairs, Science and Technology (Chair: Senator Michael Kirby). (2002a). *The health of Canadians: The federal role. Final report on the state of the health care system in Canada.* Ottawa: Senate of Canada.

Senate. Standing Committee on Social Affairs, Science and Technology (Chair: Senator Michael Kirby). (2002b). *The health of Canadians: The federal role. Vol. 5: Principles and recommendations for reform.* Ottawa: Senate of Canada.

Senate. Standing Committee on Social Affairs, Science and Technology (Chair: Senator Michael Kirby). (2006). *Out of the shadows at last: Transforming mental health, mental illness and addiction services in Canada.* Final report. Ottawa: Senate of Canada.

Senate. Subcommittee on Population Health (Chair: Senator Wilbert Keon). (2009). *A healthy, productive Canada: A determinant of health approach.* Final report. Ottawa: Senate of Canada.

Seshamani, M., & Gray, A. M. (2004). A longitudinal study of the effects of age and time to death on hospital costs. *Journal of Health Economics, 23*, 217-235.

Seto, E. (2008). Cost comparison between telemonitoring and usual care of heart failure: A systematic review. *Telemedicine and e-Health, 14*(7), 679-686.

Shahian, D. M., Wolf, R. E., Iezzoni, L. I., Kirle, L., & Normand, S.-L. T. (2010). Variability in the measurement of hospital-wide mortality rates. *New England Journal of Medicine, 363*(26), 2530-2539.

Shapiro, E., & Tate, R. B. (1995). Monitoring the outcomes of quality of care in nursing homes using administrative data. *Canadian Journal on Aging, 14*(4), 755-768.

Sharpe, A., Messinger, H., & Bradley, C. (2007). *The measurement of output and productivity in the health care sector in Canada: An overview.* Ottawa: Centre for the Study of Living Standards.

Shechter, S. M. (2011). Treatment evolution and new standards of care: Implications for cost-effectiveness analysis. *Medical Decision Making, 31*(1), 35-42.

Shekelle, P., Morton, S., & Keeler, E. (2006). *Costs and benefits of health information technology.* Rockville, MD: Agency for Healthcare Research and Quality.

Shepperd, S., Doll, H., Angus, R. M., Clarke, M. J., Iliffe, S., Kalra, L., et al. (2008). Admission avoidance hospital at home. *Cochrane Database of Systematic Reviews* (4).

Shiell, A., Hawe, P., Perry, R., & Matthias, S. (2009). How health managers think about risk and the implications for portfolio theory in health systems. *Health, Risk & Society, 11*(1), 71-85.

Shiell, A., & McIntosh, K. (2006). Some economics of health promotion: What we know, don't know and need to know before spending to promote public health. *Harvard Health Policy Review, 7*(2), 21-31.

Shonkoff, J. P. (2010). Building a new biodevelopmental framework to guide the future of early childhood policy. *Child Development, 81*(1), 357-367.

Shonkoff, J. P., & Phillips, D. A. (2000). *From neurons to neighborhoods: The science of early child development.* Washington, DC: National Academies Press.

Shortt, S. E. D. (1998). *The doctor dilemma: Public policy and the changing role of physicians under Ontario Medicare.* Montreal: McGill-Queen's University Press.

Shukla, R. K., Pestian, J., & Clement, J. (1997). A comparative analysis of revenue and cost-management strategies of not-for-profit and for-profit hospitals. *Hospital and Health Services Adminstration, 42*(1), 117-134.

Shwartz, M., Cohen, A. B., Restuccia, J. D., Ren, Z. J., Labonte, A., Theokary, C., et al. (2011). How well can we identify the high-performing hospital? *Medical Care Research and Review, 68*(3), 290-310.

Siciliani, L., & Hurst, J. (2005). Tackling excessive waiting times for elective surgery: A comparative analysis of policies in 12 OECD countries. *Health Policy, 72,* 201-215.

Sigerist, H. E. (1941). *Medicine and human welfare.* New Haven, CT: Yale University Press.

Simborg, D. W. (1981). DRG creep: A new hospital-acquired disease. *New England Journal of Medicine, 304*(26), 1602-1604.

Simmons, A. B. (2011). Population growth: From fast growth to possible decline. In B. Edmonston & E. Fong (Eds.), *The changing Canadian population.* Montreal and Kingston: McGill-Queen's University Press.

Simoens, S., & Giuffrida, A. (2004). The impact of physician payment methods on raising the efficiency of the healthcare system: An international comparison. *Applied Health Economics & Health Policy, 3*(1), 39-46.

Simoens, S., Villeneuve, M., & Hurst, J. (2005). *Tackling nurse shortages in OECD countries* (No. 19). Paris: OECD.

Simons, P. (2010, 13 November). Our health-care system is failing us miserably. *Edmonton Journal*. Retrieved 23 August 2011 from http://www2.canada.com/edmontonjour-nal/news/cityplus/story.html?id=847f5d81-19bf-40b9-a486-d2d7f2ed427c&p=1

Simpson, J. (2005). Sorting our priorities: The funding gap between health care and higher education. *Policy Options, 26*(5), 47-52.

Sinclair, D. G., Rochon, M., & Leatt, P. (2005). *Riding the third rail: The story of Ontario's Health Services Restructuring Commission, 1996–2000.* Montreal: Institute for Research on Public Policy.

Singer, S. J., Burgers, J., Friedberg, M., Rosenthal, M. B., Leape, L., & Schneider, E. (2011). Defining and measuring integrated patient care: Promoting the next frontier in health care delivery. *Medical Care Research and Review, 68*(1), 112-127.

Singer, S., Lin, S., Falwell, A., Gaba, D., & Baker, L. (2009). Relationship of safety climate and safety performance in hospitals. *Health Services Research, 44*(2 Pt. 1), 399-421.

Singla, A. K., Kitch, B. T., Weissman, J. S., & Campbell, E. G. (2006). Assessing patient safety culture: A review and synthesis of the measurement tools. *Journal of Patient Safety, 2*(3), 105-115.

Sinha, A. (2000). An overview of telemedicine: The virtual gaze of health care in the next century. *Medical Anthropology Quarterly, 14*, 291-309.

Sinha, S. K. (2011). Why the elderly could bankrupt Canada and how demographic imperatives will force the redesign of acute care service delivery. *Healthcare-Papers, 11*(1), 46-51.

Sistrom, C. L., Dang, P. A., Dreyer, K. J., Rosenthal, D. I., Thrall, J. H., & Weilburg, J. B. (2009). Effect of computerized order entry with integrated decision support on the growth of outpatient procedure volumes: Seven-year time series analysis. *Radiology, 251*(1), 147-155.

Skinner, B. J., & Rovere, M. (2009). *Paying more, getting less: Measuring the sustainability of government health spending in Canada. 2009 Report.* Vancouver, BC: Fraser Institute.

Skinner, B. J., & Rovere, M. (2011). *Canada's Medicare bubble: Is government health spending sustainable without user-based funding?* Vancouver, BC: Fraser Institute.

Slaughter, S., & Leslie, L. L. (1997). *Academic capitalism. Politics, policies, and the entrepreneurial university.* Baltimore, MA: Johns Hopkins University Press.

Smith, C. M. (2005). Origin and uses of primum non nocere – Above all, do no harm! *The Journal of Clinical Pharmacology, 45*(4), 371-377.

Smith, G. C. S., & Pell, J. P. (2003). Parachute use to prevent death and major trauma related to gravitational challenge: Systematic review of randomised controlled trials. *BMJ, 327*(7429), 1459-1461.

Smith, P., Mossialos, E., Papanicolas, I., & Leatherman, S. (Eds.). (2009). *Performance measurement for health system improvement: Experiences, challenges, and prospects.* Cambridge: Cambridge University Press.

Smith, P. C., & Street, A. (2007). The measurement of non-market output in education and health. *Economic and Labour Market Review, 1*(6), 46-52.

Smith, S., Newhouse, J. P., & Freeland, M. S. (2009). Income, insurance, and technology: Why does health spending outpace economic growth? *Health Affairs, 28*(5), 1276-1284.

Smylie, J. (2009). The health of Aboriginal peoples. In D. Raphael (Ed.), *Social determinants of health: Canadian perspectives* (2nd ed.). Toronto, ON: Canadian Scholars' Publishing.

Snowdon, W., Potter, J.-L., Swinburn, B., Schultz, J., & Lawrence, M. (2010). Prioritizing policy interventions to improve diets? Will it work, can it happen, will it do harm? *Health Promotion International, 25*(1), 123-133.

Solberg, L. I., Hroscikoski, M. C., Sperl-Hillen, J. M., O'Connor, P. J., & Crabtree, B. F. (2004). Key issues in transforming health care organizations for quality: The case of advanced access. *Joint Commission Journal on Quality and Patient Safety, 30*(1), 15-24.

Sood, N., Huckfeldt, P. J., Escarce, J. J., Grabowski, D. C., & Newhouse, J. P. (2011). Medicare's bundled payment pilot for acute and postacute care: Analysis and recommendations on where to begin. *Health Affairs, 30*(9), 1708-1717.

Soroka, S. N. (2007). *Canadian perceptions of the health care system: A report to the Health Council of Canada.* Toronto, ON: Health Council of Canada.

Spalding, K. L., Williams, A. P., & Watkins, J. R. (2006). *Self-managed care programs in Canada: A report to Health Canada* (No. 9780662463511 066246351X). Ottawa: Health Care Policy Directorate, Health Canada.

Spanier, P. A., Marshall, S. J., & Faulkner, G. E. (2006). Tackling the obesity pandemic: A call for sedentary behaviour research. *Canadian Journal of Public Health, 97*(3), 255-257.

Stabile, M. (2008). Private financing outside the publicly funded system. In M. Lu & E. Jonsson (Eds.), *Financing health care: New ideas for a changing society.* Weinheim: Wiley-VCH.

Stabile, M., & Ward, C. (2005). The effects of delisting publicly funded health-care services. In C. M. Beach, R. P. Chaykowski, S. Shortt, F. St-Hilaire, & A. Sweetman (Eds.), *Health services restructuring in Canada: New evidence and new directions.* Kingston, ON: John Deutsch Institute for the Study of Economic Policy, Queen's University.

Stacey, R. D. (2007). *Strategic management and organisational dynamics: The challenge of complexity to ways of thinking about organizations* (5th ed.). Harlow, England: Financial Times Prentice Hall.

Stacey, R. D. (2010). *Strategic management and organisational dynamics: The challenge of complexity (to ways of thinking about organizations).* Gardners Books.

Stainkey, L. A., Seidl, I. A., Johnson, A. J., Tulloch, G. E., & Pain, T. (2010). The challenge of long waiting lists: How we implemented a GP referral system for non-urgent specialist appointments at an Australian public hospital. *BMC Health Services Research, 10*(303).

Stanley, K. (2007). Evaluation of randomized controlled trials. *Circulation, 115*(13), 1819-1822.

Starfield, B. (1992). *Primary care: Concept, evaluation and policy.* New York: Oxford University Press.

Starfield, B., Hyde, J., Gervas, J., & Heath, I. (2008). The concept of prevention: A good idea gone astray? *Journal of Epidemiology and Community Health, 62,* 580-583.

Starfield, B., Shi, L., & Macinko, J. (2005). Contribution of primary care to health systems and health. *Milbank Quarterly, 83*(3), 457-502.

Starky, S. (2005). The obesity epidemic in Canada. Library of Parliament, Parliamentary Information and Research Service, Ottawa.

Statistics Canada. (2010). *Population projections for Canada, provinces and territories.* Ottawa: Author.

Statistics Canada. (2011). *Residential care facilities 2008/2009* (Catalogue no. 83-237-X). Ottawa: Author.

Stausberg, J., Halim, A., & Faerber, R. (2011). Concordance and robustness of quality indicator sets for hospitals: An analysis of routine data. *BMC Health Services Research, 11*(106).

Stavins, R. N., Wagner, A. F., & Wagner, G. (2003). Interpreting sustainability in economic terms: Dynamic efficiency plus intergenerational equity. *Economics Letters, 79*(3), 339-343.

Steele, G. D., Haynes, J. A., Davis, D. E., Tomcavage, J., Stewart, W. F., Graf, T. R., et al. (2010). How Geisinger's advanced medical home model argues the case for rapid-cycle innovation. *Health Affairs, 29*(11), 2047-2053.

Steffen, M. (2005). Comparing complex policies: Lessons from a public health case. *Journal of Comparative Policy Analysis: Research and Practice, 7*(4), 267-290.

Steinbrook, R. (2008). Personally controlled online health data: The next big thing in medical care? *New England Journal of Medicine, 358*(16), 1653-1656.

Stevens, A. J., Jensen, J. J., Wyller, K., Kilgore, P. C., Chatterjee, S., & Rohrbaugh, M. L. (2011). The role of public-sector research in the discovery of drugs and vaccines. *New England Journal of Medicine, 364*(6), 535-541.

Stevenson, H. M., Williams, A. P., & Vayda, E. (1988). Medical politics and Canadian Medicare: Professional response to the *Canada Health Act. Milbank Quarterly, 66*(1), 65-104.

Stoddart, G. L., Barer, M. L., & Evans, R. G. (1993). *User charges, snares and delusions: Another look at the literature.* Vancouver, BC: Health Policy Research Unit, University of British Columbia.

Stone, D. (2004). Shopping for long-term care. *Health Affairs, 23*(4), 191-196.

Stone, R. I. (2004). The direct care worker: The third rail of home care policy. *Annual Review of Public Health, 25*(1), 521-537.

Stone, R., & Wiener, J. M. (2001). *Who will care for us? Addressing the long-term care workforce crisis.* Washington, DC: Urban Institute.

Strating, M. M. H., Nieboer, A. P., Zuiderent-Jerak, T., & Bal, R. A. (2011). Creating effective quality-improvement collaboratives: A multiple case study. *BMJ Quality and Safety, 20*(4), 344-350.

Street, A., & Duckett, S. (1996). Are waiting lists inevitable? *Health Policy, 36*, 1-15.

Street, A., & Maynard, A. (2007a). Activity based financing in England: The need for continual refinement of payment by results. *Health Economics, Policy and Law, 2*(4), 419-427.

Street, A., & Maynard, A. (2007b). Payment by results: Qualified ambition? *Health Economics, Policy and Law, 2*(4), 445-448.

Stuart, B., Davidoff, A., Lopert, R., Shaffer, T., Samantha Shoemaker, J., & Lloyd, J. (2011). Does medication adherence lower medicare spending among beneficiaries with diabetes? *Health Services Research, 46*(4), 1180-1199.

Stuart, T. E., Ozdemir, S. Z., & Ding, W. W. (2007). Vertical alliance networks: The case of university-biotechnology-pharmaceutical alliance chains. *Research Policy, 36*, 477-498.

Subramanian, S. V., & Kawachi, I. (2004). Income inequality and health: What have we learned so far? *Epidemiologic Reviews, 26*, 78-91.

Sullivan, T., & Baranek, P. M. (2002). *First do no harm: Making sense of Canadian health reform.* Vancouver: University of British Columbia Press.

Suryawanshi, S., Zhang, L., Pfister, M., & Meibohm, B. (2010). The current role of model-based drug development. *Expert Opinion on Drug Discovery, 5*(4), 311-321.

Susser, M., & Susser, E. (1996). Choosing a future for epidemiology: 1. Eras and paradigms. *American Journal of Public Health, 86*(5), 668-673.

Sutcliffe, K. M., Lewton, E., & Rosenthal, M. M. (2004). Communication failures: An insidious contributor to medical mishaps. *Academic Medicine, 79*(2), 186-194.

Sutherland, J. (2011). *Hospital payment mechanisms: An overview and options for Canada.* Ottawa: Canadian Health Services Research Foundation.

Sutherland, J. M., Barer, M. L., Evans, R. G., & Crump, R. T. (2011). Will paying the piper change the tune? *Healthcare Policy, 6*(4), 14-21.

Swan, M. (2009). Emerging patient-driven health care models: An examination of health social networks, consumer personalized medicine and quantified self-tracking. *International Journal of Environmental Research and Public Health, 6*(2), 492-525.

Swaminathan, S., Chernew, M., & Scanlon, D. P. (2008). Persistence of HMO performance measures. *Health Services Research, 43*(6), 2033-2049.

Swensen, S. J., Meyer, G. S., Nelson, E. C., Hunt, G. C., Pryor, D. B., Weissberg, J. I., et al. (2010). Cottage industry to postindustrial care – The revolution in health care delivery. *New England Journal of Medicine, 362*(5).

Swerissen, H., & Crisp, B. R. (2004). The sustainability of health promotion interventions for different levels of social organization. *Health Promotion International, 19*(1), 123-130.

Swift, R. (2011). The relationship between health and GDP in OECD countries in the very long run. *Health Economics, 20*(3), 306-322.

Swinburn, B. A., Sacks, G., Hall, K. D., McPherson, K., Finegood, D. T., Moodie, M. L., & Gortmaker, S.L. (2011). The global obesity pandemic: Shaped by global drivers and local environments. *The Lancet, 378*(9793), 804-814.

Syrett, K. (2003). A technocratic fix to the "legitimacy problem"? The Blair government and health care rationing in the United Kingdom. *Journal of Health Politics, Policy and Law, 28*(4), 715-746.

Tamblyn, R., Laprise, R., Hanley, J. A., Abrahamowicz, M., Scott, S., Mayo, N., et al. (2001). Adverse events associated with prescription drug cost-sharing among poor and elderly persons. *JAMA, 285*(4), 421-429.

Tanenbaum, S. J. (2009). Pay for performance in Medicare: Evidentiary irony and the politics of value. *Journal of Health Politics, Policy and Law, 34*(5), 717-746.

Tang, P. C., Ash, J. S., Bates, D. W., Overhage, J. M., & Sands, D. Z. (2006). Personal health records: Definitions, benefits, and strategies for overcoming barriers to adoption. *Journal of the American Medical Informatics Association, 13*(2), 121-126.

Tannahill, A. (2008). Beyond evidence – to ethics: A decision-making framework for health promotion, public health and health improvement. *Health Promotion International, 23*(4), 380-390.

Taplin, S., Galvin, M. S., Payne, T., Coole, D., & Wagner, E. (1998). Putting population-based care into practice: Real option or rhetoric? *Journal of the American Board of Family Practice, 11*(2), 116-126.

Tarrant, C., Dixon-Woods, M., Colman, A. M., & Stokes, T. (2010). Continuity and trust in primary care: A qualitative study informed by game theory. *Annals of Family Medicine, 8*(5), 440-446.

Tarride, J. E., McCarron, C. E., Lim, M., Bowen, J. M., Blackhouse, G., Hopkins, R., et al. (2008). Economic evaluations conducted by Canadian health technology assessment agencies: Where do we stand? *International Journal of Technology Assessment in Health Care, 24*(4), 437-444.

Taylor, M. G. (1978). *Health insurance and Canadian public policy: The seven decisions that created the Canadian health insurance system.* Montreal: Institute of Public Administration of Canada and McGill Queen's University Press.

Telford, H. (2003). The federal spending power in Canada: Nation-building or nation-destroying? *Publius: The Journal of Federalism, 33*(1), 23-44.

Tenbensel, T. (2010). Public participation in health policy in high income countries – A review of why, who, what, which, and where? *Social Science & Medicine, 71*(9), 1537-1540.

Teno, J. M., Gruneir, A., Schwartz, Z., Nanda, A., & Wetle, T. (2007). Association between advance directives and quality of end-of-life care: A national study. *Journal of the American Geriatrics Society, 55*(2), 189-194.

Terris, M. (1984). Newer perspectives on the health of Canadians: Beyond the Lalonde report. The Rosenstadt lecture. *Journal of Public Health Policy, 5*(3), 327-337.

Thomas, E. J. (2011). Improving teamwork in healthcare: Current approaches and the path forward. *BMJ Quality & Safety, 20*(8), 647-650.

Thompson, C. R., & McKee, M. (2011). An analysis of hospital capital planning and financing in three European countries: Using the principal-agent approach to identify the potential for economic problems. *Health Policy, 99*(2), 158-166.

Thomson, S., Foubister, T., Figueras, J., Kutzin, J., Permanand, G., & Bryndová, L. (2009). *Addressing financial sustainability in health systems.* Copenhagen: World Health Organization.

Thornley, C. (2003). What future for health care assistants: High road or low road. In C. Davies (Ed.), *The future health workforce.* Basingstoke: Palgrave Macmillan.

Thorpe, K. E. (2005). The rise in health care spending and what to do about it. *Health Affairs, 24*(6), 1436-1445.

Thorpe, K. E., Florence, C. S., Howard, D. H., & Joski, P. (2005). The rising prevalence of treated disease: Effects on private health insurance spending. *Health Affairs (Web exclusive)*, w5, 317-325.

Thorpe, K. E., Florence, C. S., & Joski, P. (2004). Which medical conditions account for the rise in health care spending? *Health Affairs (Millwood), 23*(Web Suppl. 2), w4, 437-445.

Tieman, J., Mitchell, G., Shelby-James, T., Currow, D., Fazekas, B., O Doherty, L., et al. (2006). *Integration, coordination and multidisciplinary approaches in primary care: A systematic investigation of the literature.* Canberra: Australian Primary Health Care Research Institute and Flinders University Department of Palliative and Supportive Services.

Timonen, V., Convery, J., & Cahill, S. (2006). Care revolutions in the making? A comparison of cash-for-care programmes in four European countries. *Ageing & Society, 26*(3), 455-474.

Tinghög, G., Carlsson, P., & Lyttkens, C. H. (2010). Individual responsibility for what? A conceptual framework for exploring the suitability of private financing in a publicly funded health-care system. *Health Economics, Policy and Law, 5*(2), 201-223.

Tomblin Murphy, G., Kephart, G., Lethbridge, L., O'Brien-Pallas, L., & Birch, S. (2009). Planning for what? Challenging the assumptions of health human resources planning. *Health Policy, 92*(2), 225-233.

Torjesen, I. (2011). Pressure grows for government to "grasp the nettle" and close hospitals. *BMJ, 342,* 1381.

Toth, F. (2010). Healthcare policies over the last 20 years: Reforms and counter-reforms. *Health Policy, 95*(1), 82-89.

Toussaint, J. (2009). Writing the new playbook for U.S. health care: Lessons from Wisconsin. *Health Affairs, 28*(5), 1343-1350.

Town, R., Kane, R., Johnson, P., & Butler, M. (2005). Economic incentives and physicians' delivery of preventive care: A systematic review. *American Journal of Preventive Medicine, 28*(2), 234-240.

Tracey, J., & Zelmer, J. (2005). Volumes and outcomes for surgical services in Canada. *Healthcare Quarterly, 8*(4), 28-30.

Trogdon, J. G., Nonnemaker, J., & Pais, J. (2008). Peer effects in adolescent over-weight. *Journal of Health Economics, 27*(5), 1388-1399.

Trottier, H., Martel, L., Houle, C., Berthelot, J. M., & Légaré, J. (2000). Living at home or in an institution: What makes the difference for seniors? *Health Reports 11*(4), 49-61.

Trovato, F. (2011). Canada's age and sex composition. In B. Edmonston & E. Fong (Eds.), *The changing Canadian population.* Montreal and Kingston: McGill-Queen's University Press.

Tsai, A., Morton, S., Mangione, C., & Keeler, E. (2005). A meta-analysis of interventions to improve care for chronic illnesses. *American Journal of Managed Care, 11*(8), 478-488.

Tsasis, P., & Bains, J. (2009). Chronic disease: Shifting the focus of healthcare in Canada. *Healthcare Quarterly, 12*(2), e1-e11.

Tu, K., Cauch-Dudek, K., & Chen, Z. (2009). Comparison of primary care physician payment models in the management of hypertension. *Canadian Family Physician, 55*(7), 719-727.

Tuohy, C. H. (1999). *Accidental logics: The dynamics of change in the health care arena in the United States, Britain, and Canada.* New York: Oxford University Press.

Tuohy, C. H. (2009). Single payers, multiple systems: The scope and limits of sub-national variation under a federal health policy framework. *Journal of Health Politics, Policy and Law, 34*(4), 453-496.

Tuohy, C. H., Flood, C. M., & Stabile, M. (2004). How does private finance affect public health care systems? Marshaling the evidence from OECD nations. *Journal of Health Politics, Policy and Law, 29*(3), 359-396.

Tuohy, C. J. (1988). Medicine and the state in Canada: The extra-billing issue in perspective. *Canadian Journal of Political Science, 21*(2), 267-296.

Urbach, D., Stukel, T., Croxford, R., & MacCallum, N. L. (2005). *Analysis of current research related to the impact of low-volume procedures/surgery and care on outcomes of care.* Toronto, ON: Institute for Clinical Evaluative Science and Canadian Institute for Health Information.

Vabø, M. (2006). Caring for people or caring for proxy consumers? *European Societies, 8*(3), 403-422.

van Baal, P. H. M., Polder, J. J., de Wit, G. A., Hoogenveen, R. T., Feenstra, T. L., Boshuizen, H. C., et al. (2008). Lifetime medical costs of obesity: Prevention no cure for increasing health expenditure. *PLoS Medicine, 5*(2), e29.

Van De Belt, T. H., Engelen, L. J., Berben, S. A., & Schoonhoven, L. (2010). Definition of Health 2.0 and Medicine 2.0: A systematic review. *Journal of Medical Internet Research, 12*, e18.

Van de Ven, W. P. M. M. (2011). Risk adjustment and risk equalization: What needs to be done? *Health Economics, Policy and Law, 6*(1), 147-156.

van der Zee, J., & Kroneman, M. (2007). Bismarck or Beveridge: A beauty contest between dinosaurs. *BMC Health Services Research, 7*, 94.

van Dishoeck, A.-M., Lingsma, H. F., Mackenbach, J. P., & Steyerberg, E. W. (2011). Random variation and rankability of hospitals using outcome indicators. *BMJ Quality and Safety, 20*(10), 869-874.

van Dishoeck, A. M., Looman, C. W. N., van der Wilden-van Lier, E. C. M., Mackenbach, J. P., & Steyerberg, E. W. (2011). Displaying random variation in comparing hospital performance. *BMJ Quality and Safety, 20*(8), 651-657.

van Gils, P. F., Tariq, L., Verschuuren, M., & van den Berg, M. (2011). Cost-effectiveness research on preventive interventions: A survey of the publications in 2008. *European Journal of Public Health, 21*(2), 260-264.

Van Herck, P., De Smedt, D., Annemans, L., Remmen, R., Rosenthal, M., & Sermeus, W. (2010). Systematic review: Effects, design choices, and context of pay-for-performance in health care. *BMC Health Services Research, 10*(247).

van Rijnsoever, F. J., van Lente, H., & van Trijp, H. C. M. (2011). Systemic policies towards a healthier and more responsible food system. *Journal of Epidemiology and Community Health, 65*(9), 737-739.

van Walraven, C., Bennett, C., Jennings, A., Austin, P. C., & Forster, A. J. (2011). Proportion of hospital readmissions deemed avoidable: A systematic review. *Canadian Medical Association Journal, 183*(7), E391-402.

van Walraven, C., Dhalla, I. A., Bell, C., Etchells, E., Stiell, I. G., Zarnke, K., et al. (2010). Derivation and validation of an index to predict early death or unplanned readmission after discharge from hospital to the community. *Canadian Medical Association Journal, 182*(6), 551-557.

Vandergrift, M., & Kanavos, P. (1997). Health policy versus industrial policy in the pharmaceutical sector: The case of Canada. *Health Policy, 41*, 241-260.

Vanhaecht, K., Panella, M., Van Zelm, R., & Sermeus, W. (2009). Is there a future for pathways? Five pieces of the puzzle. *Journal of Integrated Care Pathways, 13*(2), 82-86.

Vemer, P., & Rutten-van Mölken, M. (2011). Largely ignored: The impact of the threshold value for a QALY on the importance of a transferability factor. *European Journal of Health Economics, 12*(5), 397-404.

Verma, S., Paterson, M., & Medves, J. (2006). Core competencies for health care professionals: What medicine, nursing, occupational therapy, and physiotherapy share. *Journal of Allied Health, 35*, 109-115.

Vest, J. R., Bolin, J. N., Miller, T. R., Gamm, L. D., Siegrist, T. E., & Martinez, L. E. (2010). Medical homes: "Where you stand on definitions depends on where you sit." *Medical Care Research and Review, 67*(4), 393-411.

Visscher, T. L., & Seidell, J. C. (2001). The public health impact of obesity. *Annual Review of Public Health, 22*(1), 355-375.

Vladeck, B. C., & Rice, T. (2009). Market failure and the failure of discourse: Facing up to the power of sellers. *Health Affairs, 28*(5), 1305-1315.

von Tigerstrom, B., Larre, T., & Sauder, J. (2011). Using the tax system to promote physical activity: Critical analysis of Canadian initiatives. *American Journal of Public Health, 101*(8), e10-16.

Vos, L., Wagner, C., Duckers, M. L. A., & van Merode, G. G. (2010). Does case-mix based reimbursement stimulate the development of process-oriented care delivery? *Health Policy, 98*(1), 74-80.

Vos, T., Carter, R., Barendregt, J., Mihalopoulos, C., Veerman, L., Magnus, A., et al. (2010). *Assessing cost-effectiveness in prevention (ACE–Prevention): Final report.* Brisbane and Melbourne: University of Queensland and Deakin University.

Vujicic, M., & Evans, R. G. (2005). The impact of deficit reduction on the nursing labour market in Canada: Unintended consequences of fiscal reform. *Applied Health Economics and Health Policy, 4*(2), 99-110.

Vujicic, M., Onate, K., Laporte, A., & Deber, R. (2011). Hospital expenditure as a major driver of nurse labour force participation: Evidence from a 10-year period in Canada. *Healthcare Policy, 6*(4), 62-71.

Wachter, R. M., & Pronovost, P. J. (2009). Balancing "no blame" with accountability in patient safety. *New England Journal of Medicine, 361*(14), 1401-1406.

Wagner, E. H., Davis, C., Schaefer, J., Von Korff, M., & Austin, B. (1999). A survey of leading chronic disease management programs: Are they consistent with the literature? *Managed Care Quarterly, 7*(3), 56-66.

Wagner, E. H., Glasgow, R. E., Davis, C., Bonomi, A. E., Provost, L., McCulloch, D., et al. (2001). Quality improvement in chronic illness care: A collaborative approach. *Joint Commission Journal on Quality Improvement, 27*(2), 63-80.

Wagstaff, A. (2010). Social health insurance reexamined. *Health Economics, 19*(5), 503-517.

Wait Time Alliance. (2010). *No time for complacency: Report card on wait times in Canada.* Ottawa: Author.

Wakefield, M., & Chaloupka, F. (2000). Effectiveness of comprehensive tobacco control programmes in reducing teenage smoking in the USA. *Tobacco Control, 9*(2), 177-186.

Walker, A., & Maynard, A. (2003). Managing medical workforces: From relative stability to disequilibrium in the UK NHS. *Applied Health Economics and Health Policy, 2*(1), 25-36.

Walker, J. D., Teare, G. F., Hogan, D. B., Lewis, S., & Maxwell, C. J. (2009). Identifying potentially avoidable hospital admissions from Canadian long-term care facilities. *Medical Care, 47*(2), 250-254.

Wallerstein, N. (2006). *What is the evidence on effectiveness of empowerment to improve health?* Copenhagen, Denmark: World Health Organization, Regional Office for Europe.

Walshe, K. (2009). Pseudoinnovation: The development and spread of healthcare quality improvement methodologies. *International Journal for Quality in Health Care, 21*(3), 153-159.

Walshe, K., & Ham, C. (2011). Can the government's proposals for NHS reform be made to work? *BMJ, 342*, d2038.

Wansink, B. (2002). Changing eating habits on the home front: Lost lessons from World War II research. *Journal of Public Policy and Marketing, 21*(1), 90-99.

Watson, D. (2003). *Death sentence: The decay of public language.* Milsons Point, New South Wales: Vintage Australia.

Watson, D. (2004). *Watson's dictionary of weasel words, contemporary clichés, cant and management jargon.* Milsons Point, New South Wales: Vintage Australia.

Watson, D. E., Barer, M. L., Matkovich, H. M., & Gagnon, M. L. (2007). Wait time benchmarks, research evidence and the knowledge translation process. *Healthcare Policy, 2*(3), 56-61.

Weale, A., & Clark, S. (2010). Co-payments in the NHS: An analysis of the normative arguments. *Health Economics, Policy and Law, 5*(2), 225-246.

Weber, V., & Joshi, M. S. (2000). Effecting and leading change in health care organizations. *Joint Commission Journal on Quality and Patient Safety, 26*(7), 388-399.

Weiner, B. J., Alexander, J. A., Baker, L. C., Shortell, S. M., & Becker, M. (2006). Quality improvement implementation and hospital performance on patient safety indicators. *Medical Care Research and Review, 63*(1), 29-57.

Weiner, B. J., Alexander, J., Shortell, S., Baker, L., Becker, M., & Geppert, J. (2006). Qualtiy improvement implementation and hospital performance on quality indicators. *Health Services Research, 41*(2), 307-334.

Weiner, B. J., Hobgood, C., & Lewis, M. A. (2008). The meaning of justice in safety incident reporting. *Social Science & Medicine, 66*(2), 403-413.

Weinstein, M. C., & Skinner, J. A. (2010). comparative effectiveness and health care spending: Implications for reform. *New England Journal of Medicine, 362*(5), 460-465.

Weissert, W., Chernew, M., & Hirth, R. (2003). Titrating versus targeting home care services to frail elderly clients: An application of agency theory and cost-benefit analysis to home care policy. *Journal of Aging and Health, 15*(1), 99-123.

Wendt, C., & Kohl, J. (2010). Translating monetary inputs into health care provision: A comparative analysis of the impact of different modes of public policy. *Journal of Comparative Policy Analysis: Research and Practice, 12*(1), 11-31.

Wennberg, D. E., Marr, A., Lang, L., O'Malley, S., & Bennett, G. (2010). A randomized trial of a telephone care-management strategy. *New England Journal of Medicine, 363*(13), 1245-1255.

Wennberg, J. E. (2010). *Tracking medicine a researcher's quest to understand health care.* New York: Oxford University Press.

Wensing, M., Wollersheim, H., & Grol, R. (2006). Organizational interventions to implement improvements in patient care: A structured review of reviews. *Implementation Science, 1*(2).

Whicher, D. M., Chalkidou, K., Dhalla, I. A., Levin, L., & Tunis, S. (2009). Comparative effectiveness research in Ontario, Canada: Producing relevant and timely information for health care decision makers. *Milbank Quarterly, 87*(3), 585-606.

White, D., Oelke, N. D., Besner, J., Doran, D., McGillis Hall, L., & Giovannetti, P. (2008). Nursing scope of practice: Descriptions and challenges. *Nursing Leadership, 21*(1), 44-57.

White, J. (1999). Targets and systems of health care cost control. *Journal of Health Politics, Policy and Law, 24*(4), 1-44.

White, J. (2001). *False alarm: Why the greatest threat to social security and Medicare is the campaign to save them.* Baltimore: Johns Hopkins University Press.

White, J. (2011). Prices, volume, and the perverse effects of the variations crusade. *Journal of Health Politics, Policy and Law, 36*(4), 775-790.

Whitehead, M. (2007). A typology of actions to tackle social inequalities in health. *Journal of Epidemiology and Community Health, 61*(6), 473-478.

Whitehead, M., Petticrew, M., Graham, H., Macintyre, S. J., Bambra, C., & Egan, M. (2004). Evidence for public health policy on inequalities: 2. Assembling the evidence jigsaw. *Journal of Epidemiology and Community Health, 58*(10), 817-821.

Whiteside, H. (2009). Canada's health care "crisis": Accumulation by dispossession and the neoliberal fix. *Studies in Political Economy, 84,* 79-100.

WHO Europe. (2011a). *Governance for health in the 21st century: A study conducted for the WHO Regional Office for Europe.* Copenhagen: WHO Regional Office for Europe.

WHO Europe. (2011b). *Impact of economic crises on mental health.* Copenhagen: WHO Regional Office for Europe.

WHO Europe. Health Evidence Network. (2006). *What is known about the effectiveness of economic instruments to reduce consumption of foods high in saturated fats and other energy-dense foods for preventing and treating obesity?* Copenhagen: WHO Regional Office for Europe.

Wildavsky, A. B. (1988). *The new politics of the budgetary process.* Glenview, IL: Scott, Foresman.

Wilkins, K. (2006). Government-subsidized home care. *Health Reports, 17,* 39-42.

Wilkinson, R. G., & Pickett, K. (2010). *The spirit level: Why equality is better for everyone.* London: Penguin.

Williamson, D. L., Milligan, C. D., Kwan, B., Frankish, C. J., & Ratner, P. A. (2003). Implementation of provincial/territorial health goals in Canada. *Health Policy 64*(2), 173-191.

Williamson, O. E. (1975). *Markets and hierarchies: Analysis and antitrust implications.* New York: Free Press.

Williamson, O. E. (1986). *Economic organization: Firms, markets and policy control.* Hemel Hempstead, England: Wheatsheaf Books.

Williamson, O. E. (2002). The theory of the firm as governance structure: From choice to contract. *Journal of Economic Perspectives, 16*(3), 171-195.

Wister, A. V., & Wanless, D. (2007). A health profile of community-living nonagenarians in Canada. *Canadian Journal on Aging, 26*(1), 1-18.

Withrow, D., & Alter, D. A. (2011). The economic burden of obesity worldwide: A systematic review of the direct costs of obesity. *Obesity Reviews, 12*(2), 131-141.

Wolff, A. C., Regan, S., Pesut, B., & Black, J. (2010). Ready for what? An exploration of the meaning of new graduate nurses' readiness for practice. *International Journal of Nursing Education Scholarship, 7*(1).

Wolfson, M. C. (2007). Population ageing and health – Empirical needs for effective foresight. In A. Gupta & A. Harding (Eds.), *Modelling our future: Population ageing, health and aged care.* Amsterdam: Elsevier.

Womack, J. P., & Jones, D. T. (2003). *Lean thinking: Banish waste and create wealth in your corporation.* New York: Free Press.

Wong, E., & Stewart, M. (2010). Predicting the scope of practice of family physicians. *Canadian Family Physician, 56*(6), e219-e225.

Wong, G., Pawson, R., & Owen, L. (2011). Policy guidance on threats to legislative interventions in public health: A realist synthesis. *BMC Public Health, 11*(222).

Woodcock, J. (2007). The prospects for "personalized medicine" in drug development and drug therapy. *Clinical Pharmacology and Therapeutics, 81*(2), 164-169.

Woodcock, J., & Woosley, R. (2008). The FDA critical path initiative and its influence on new drug development. *Annual Review of Medicine, 59*(1), 1-12.

Woodward, H. I., Mytton, O. T., Lemer, C., Yardley, I. E., Ellis, B. M., Rutter, P. D., et al. (2010). What have we learned about interventions to reduce medical errors? *Annual Review of Public Health, 31*(1), 479-497.

Woolhandler, S., Campbell, T., & Himmelstein, D. U. (2003). Costs of health care administration in the United States and Canada. *New England Journal of Medicine, 349*(8), 768-775.

World Alliance for Patient Safety Drafting Group, Sherman, H., Castro, G., Fletcher, M., Hatlie, M., Hibbert, P., et al. (2009). Towards an international classification for patient safety: The conceptual framework. *International Journal for Quality in Health Care, 21*(1), 2-8.

Worthington, A. C. (2004). Frontier efficiency measurement in health care: A review of empirical techniques and selected applications. *Medical Care Research and Review, 61*(2), 135-170.

Wranik, D. W., & Durier-Copp, M. (2009). Physician remuneration methods for family physicians in Canada: Expected outcomes and lessons learned. *Health Care Analysis, 18*(1), 35-59.

Wright, D. B., & Ricketts, T. C. (2011). The road to efficiency? Re-examining the impact of the primary care physician workforce on health care utilization rates. *Social Science & Medicine, 70*(12), 2006-2010.

Wright, J. G., Hawker, G. A., Bombardier, C., Croxford, R., Dittus, R. S., Freund, D. A., et al. (1999). Physician enthusiasm as an explanation for area variation in the utilization of knee replacement surgery. *Medical Care, 37*(9), 946-956.

Wyatt, G., & Black, K. M. (2011). Reimbursing a drug "off-label": It's what you don't know. *Policy Options, 32*(2), 69-74.

Xi, G., McDowell, I., Nair, R., & Spasoff, R. (2005). Income inequality and health in Ontario: A multilevel analysis. *Canadian Journal of Public Health, 96*(3), 206-211.

Yeo, M., Emery, J. C. H., & Kary, D. (2009). *The private insurance debate in Canadian health policy: Making the values explicit.* Calgary, AB: School of Public Policy, University of Calgary.

You, J. J., Alter, D. A., Iron, K., Slaughter, P. M., Kopp, A., Przbysz, R., et al. (2007). *Diagnostic services in Ontario: Descriptive analysis and jurisdictional review.* Toronto, ON: Institute for Clinical Evaluative Sciences.

Young, D. W., & Saltman, R. B. (1985). *The hospital power equilibrium: Physician behaviour and cost control.* Baltimore: Johns Hopkins University Press.

Zeithaml, V. A., Parasuraman, A., & Berry, L. L. (1990). *Delivering quality service: Balancing customer perceptions and expectations.* New York: Free Press.

Zimmerman, D. R. (2003). Improving nursing home quality of care through outcomes data: The MDS quality indicators. *International Journal of Geriatric Psychiatry, 18*(3), 250-257.

Zinn, J., & Flood, A. B. (2009). Slack resources in health care organizations – Fat to be trimmed or muscle to be exercised? *Health Services Research, 44*(3), 812-820.

Zinn, J. S., Weimer, D. L., Spector, W., & Mukamel, D. B. (2010). Factors influencing nursing home response to quality measure publication: A resource dependence perspective. *Health Care Management Review, 35*, 256-265.

Zulman, D., Vijan, S., Omenn, G., & Hayward, R. (2008). The relative merits of population-based and targeted prevention strategies. *Milbank Quarterly, 86*(4), 557-580.

Zurn, P., Dal Poz, M., Stilwell, B., & Adams, O. (2004). Imbalance in the health workforce. *Human Resources for Health, 2*(13).

Zweifel, P., Steinmann, L., & Eugster, P. (2005). The Sisyphus syndrome in health revisited. *International Journal of Health Care Finance and Economics, 5*(2), 127-145.

# INDEX

# ABOUT THE AUTHOR

Stephen Duckett, an economist, is a professor in the School of Public Health at the University of Alberta. In 2009 he was appointed inaugural president and chief executive officer of Alberta Health Services, Canada's largest provider of health care, a position he held until November 2010. He oversaw the integration of the previous 12 regions and provincewide boards, which were merged to form the new organization, and fostered innovative responses to address health needs in a fiscally constrained environment.

Formerly, he was secretary (deputy minister) of the Australian health department from 1994 to 1996 and has held leadership positions in the Queensland and Victorian health departments.

Stephen also has a distinguished academic career, publishing extensively on health policy and financing, and on the Australian health care system. He was elected a Fellow of the Academy of the Social Sciences in Australia in 2004, and was awarded the Sidney Sax Medal of the Australian Healthcare Association in the same year and an Australian Centenary Medal in 2003. Stephen has a reputation as a policy innovator in areas as diverse as hospital funding (he was responsible for the introduction of activity-based funding for hospitals in Australia) and quality (developing new systems to measure safety of hospital care and associated accountability mechanisms to address safety issues).

# Queen's Policy Studies
## Recent Publications

The Queen's Policy Studies Series is dedicated to the exploration of major public policy issues that confront governments and society in Canada and other nations. **Manuscript submission.** We are pleased to consider new book proposals and manuscripts. Preliminary enquiries are welcome. A subvention is normally required for the publication of an academic book. Please direct questions or proposals to the Publications Unit by email at spspress@queensu.ca, or visit our website at: www.queensu.ca/sps/books, or contact us by phone at (613) 533-2192.

Our books are available from good bookstores everywhere, including the Queen's University bookstore (http://www.campusbookstore.com/). McGill-Queen's University Press is the exclusive world representative and distributor of books in the series. A full catalogue and ordering information may be found on their web site (http://mqup.mcgill.ca/).

## School of Policy Studies

*International Migration in Uncertain Times,* John Nieuwenhuysen, Howard Duncan, and Stine Neerup (eds.) 2012. ISBN 978-1-55339-308-5

*Life After Forty: Official Languages Policy in Canada/Après quarante ans, les politiques de langue officielle au Canada,* Jack Jedwab and Rodrigue Landry (eds.) 2011. ISBN 978-1-55339-279-8

*From Innovation to Transformation: Moving up the Curve in Ontario Healthcare,* Hon. Elinor Caplan, Dr. Tom Bigda-Peyton, Maia MacNiven, and Sandy Sheahan 2011. ISBN 978-1-55339-315-3

*Academic Reform: Policy Options for Improving the Quality and Cost-Effectiveness of Undergraduate Education in Ontario,* Ian D. Clark, David Trick, and Richard Van Loon 2011. ISBN 978-1-55339-310-8

*Integration and Inclusion of Newcomers and Minorities across Canada,* John Biles, Meyer Burstein, James Frideres, Erin Tolley, and Robert Vineberg (eds.) 2011. ISBN 978-1-55339-290-3

*A New Synthesis of Public Administration: Serving in the 21st Century,* Jocelyne Bourgon, 2011. Paper ISBN 978-1-55339-312-2 Cloth ISBN 978-1-55339-313-9

*Recreating Canada: Essays in Honour of Paul Weiler,* Randall Morck (ed.), 2011. ISBN 978-1-55339-273-6

*Data Data Everywhere: Access and Accountability?* Colleen M. Flood (ed.), 2011. ISBN 978-1-55339-236-1

*Making the Case: Using Case Studies for Teaching and Knowledge Management in Public Administration,* Andrew Graham, 2011. ISBN 978-1-55339-302-3

*Canada's Isotope Crisis: What Next?* Jatin Nathwani and Donald Wallace (eds.), 2010. Paper ISBN 978-1-55339-283-5 Cloth ISBN 978-1-55339-284-2

*Pursuing Higher Education in Canada: Economic, Social, and Policy Dimensions,* Ross Finnie, Marc Frenette, Richard E. Mueller, and Arthur Sweetman (eds.), 2010. Paper ISBN 978-1-55339-277-4 Cloth ISBN 978-1-55339-278-1

*Canadian Immigration: Economic Evidence for a Dynamic Policy Environment,* Ted McDonald, Elizabeth Ruddick, Arthur Sweetman, and Christopher Worswick (eds.), 2010. Paper ISBN 978-1-55339-281-1 Cloth ISBN 978-1-55339-282-8

*Taking Stock: Research on Teaching and Learning in Higher Education*, Julia Christensen Hughes and Joy Mighty (eds.), 2010. Paper ISBN 978-1-55339-271-2 Cloth ISBN 978-1-55339-272-9

## Centre for the Study of Democracy

*Jimmy and Rosalynn Carter: A Canadian Tribute*, Arthur Milnes (ed.), 2011. Paper ISBN 978-1-55339-300-9 Cloth ISBN 978-1-55339-301-6

*Unrevised and Unrepented II: Debating Speeches and Others By the Right Honourable Arthur Meighen*, Arthur Milnes (ed.), 2011. Paper ISBN 978-1-55339-296-5 Cloth ISBN 978-1-55339-297-2

## Centre for International and Defence Policy

*Security Operations in the 21st Century: Canadian Perspectives on the Comprehensive Approach*, Michael Rostek and Peter Gizewski (eds.), 2011. ISBN 978-1-55339-351-1

*Europe Without Soldiers? Recruitment and Retention across the Armed Forces of Europe*, Tibor Szvircsev Tresch and Christian Leuprecht (eds.), 2010. Paper ISBN 978-1-55339-246-0 Cloth ISBN 978-1-55339-247-7

*Mission Critical: Smaller Democracies' Role in Global Stability Operations*, Christian Leuprecht, Jodok Troy, and David Last (eds.), 2010. ISBN 978-1-55339-244-6

## John Deutsch Institute for the Study of Economic Policy

*The 2009 Federal Budget: Challenge, Response and Retrospect*, Charles M. Beach, Bev Dahlby and Paul A.R. Hobson (eds.), 2010. Paper ISBN 978-1-55339-165-4 Cloth ISBN 978-1-55339-166-1

*Discount Rates for the Evaluation of Public Private Partnerships*, David F. Burgess and Glenn P. Jenkins (eds.), 2010. Paper ISBN 978-1-55339-163-0 Cloth ISBN 978-1-55339-164-7

## Institute of Intergovernmental Relations

*The Evolving Canadian Crown*, Jennifer Smith and D. Michael Jackson (eds.), 2011. ISBN 978-1-55339-202-6

*The Federal Idea: Essays in Honour of Ronald L. Watts*, Thomas J. Courchene, John R. Allan, Christian Leuprecht, and Nadia Verrelli (eds.), 2011. Paper ISBN 978-1-55339-198-2 Cloth ISBN 978-1-55339-199-9

*Canada: The State of the Federation 2009*, vol. 22, *Carbon Pricing and Environmental Federalism*, Thomas J. Courchene and John R. Allan (eds.), 2010. Paper ISBN 978-1-55339-196-8 Cloth ISBN 978-1-55339-197-5

---

Our publications may be purchased at leading bookstores, including the Queen's University Bookstore (http://www.campusbookstore.com/) or can be ordered online from: McGill-Queen's University Press, at **http://mqup.mcgill.ca/ordering.php**

For more information about new and backlist titles from Queen's Policy Studies, visit http://www.queensu.ca/sps/books or visit the McGill-Queen's University Press web site at: **http://mqup.mcgill.ca/**